2012
YEAR BOOK OF
ENDOCRINOLOGY®

The 2012 Year Book Series

Year Book of Anesthesiology and Pain Management™: Drs Chestnut, Abram, Black, Gravlee, Lien, Mathru, and Roizen

Year Book of Cardiology®: Drs Gersh, Cheitlin, Elliott, Gold, Graham, and Thourani

Year Book of Critical Care Medicine®: Drs Dries, Zanotti-Cavazzoni, Latenser, Martinez, Rincon, and Zwank

Year Book of Dermatology and Dermatologic Surgery™: Dr Del Rosso

Year Book of Diagnostic Radiology®: Drs Elster, Abbara, Oestreich, Offiah, Rosado de Christenson, Stephens, and Strickland

Year Book of Emergency Medicine®: Drs Hamilton, Bruno, Handly, Minczak, Mullin, Quintana, and Ramoska

Year Book of Endocrinology®: Drs Schott, Apovian, Clarke, Eugster, Meikle, Oetgen, Ovalle, Schteingart, and Toth

Year Book of Hand and Upper Limb Surgery®: Drs Yao, Adams, Isaacs, Lee, and Rizzo

Year Book of Medicine®: Drs Barker, Garrick, Gersh, Khardori, LeRoith, Panush, Talley, and Thigpen

Year Book of Neonatal and Perinatal Medicine®: Drs Fanaroff, Benitz, Donn, Neu, Papile, Polin, and Van Marter

Year Book of Neurology and Neurosurgery®: Drs Klimo, Minagar, Gandhi, House, Kevill, Liu, Mazia, Panagariya, Ragel, Riesenburger, Robottom, Schwendimann, Shafazand, Uhm, and Yang

Year Book of Obstetrics, Gynecology, and Women's Health®: Drs Dungan and Shulman

Year Book of Oncology®: Drs Arceci, Bauer, Chiorean, Gordon, Lawton, Murphy, Thigpen, and Tsao

Year Book of Ophthalmology®: Drs Rapuano, Cohen, Flanders, Hammersmith, Milman, Myers, Nagra, Nelson, Penne, Pyfer, Sergott, Shields, Talekar, and Vander

Year Book of Orthopedics®: Drs Morrey, Huddleston, Rose, Swiontkowski, and Trigg

Year Book of Otolaryngology-Head and Neck Surgery®: Drs Sindwani, Balough, Franco, Gapany, and Mitchell

Year Book of Pathology and Laboratory Medicine®: Drs Raab and Bissell

Year Book of Pediatrics®: Dr Stockman

Year Book of Plastic and Aesthetic Surgery™: Drs Miller, Gosman, Gurtner, Gutowski, Ruberg, Salisbury, and Smith

Year Book of Psychiatry and Applied Mental Health®: Drs Talbott, Ballenger, Buckley, Frances, Krupnick, and Mack

Year Book of Pulmonary Disease®: Drs Barker, Jones, Maurer, Spradley, Tanoue, and Willsie

Year Book of Sports Medicine®: Drs Shephard, Cantu, Feldman, Galea, Jankowski, Janssen, Lebrun, and Nieman

Year Book of Surgery®: Drs Copeland, Behrns, Daly, Eberlein, Fahey, Huber, Klodell, Mozingo, and Pruett

Year Book of Urology®: Drs Andriole and Coplen

Year Book of Vascular Surgery®: Drs Moneta, Gillespie, Starnes, and Watkins

2012

The Year Book of ENDOCRINOLOGY®

Editor-in-Chief
Matthias Schott, MD, PhD
Associate Professor, Deputy Director of the Department of Endocrinology, Diabetology and Rheumatology, University Hospital of Düsseldorf, Düsseldorf, Germany

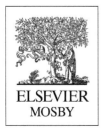

ELSEVIER
MOSBY

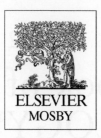

ELSEVIER
MOSBY

Vice President, Continuity: Kimberly Murphy
Developmental Editor: Patrick Manley
Production Supervisor, Electronic Year Books: Donna M. Skelton
Electronic Article Manager: Mike Sheets
Senior Illustrations and Permissions Coordinator: Dawn Vohsen

2012 EDITION

Printed and bound by CPI Group (UK) Ltd, Croydon, CR0 4YY

Transferred to Digital Print 2012

Composition by TNQ Books and Journals Pvt Ltd, India

Editorial Office:
Elsevier
Suite 1800
1600 John F. Kennedy Blvd
Philadelphia, PA 19103-2899

International Standard Serial Number: 0084-3741
International Standard Book Number: 978-0-323-08879-4

Associate Editors

Caroline M. Apovian, MD, FACP, FACN
Associate Professor of Medicine and Pediatrics, Boston University School of Medicine; Director, Center for Nutrition and Weight Management, Boston Medical Center, Boston, Massachusetts

Bart L. Clarke, MD
Associate Professor of Medicine, Mayo Clinic College of Medicine; Consultant, St. Mary's Hospital; Consultant, Rochester Methodist Hospital, Rochester, Minnesota

Erica Eugster, MD
Professor of Pediatrics, Director, Section of Pediatric Endocrinology/ Diabetology, Riley Hospital for Children, Indiana University School of Medicine, Indianapolis, Indiana

A. Wayne Meikle, MD
Professor of Medicine and Pathology, University of Utah School of Medicine; Director of Endocrine Testing, ARUP Laboratories, The University of Utah Hospitals, Salt Lake City, Utah

Elke Oetjen
Professor Institute for Clinical Pharmacology and Toxicology University Medical Center Hamburg-Eppendorf

David E. Schteingart, MD
Professor, Department of Internal Medicine, Division of Metabolism, Endocrinology and Diabetes, University of Michigan Health System, Ann Arbor, Michigan

Peter P. Toth, MD, PhD, FAAFP, FICA, FAHA, FCCP, FACC
Director of Preventive Cardiology, Sterling Rock Falls Clinic, Ltd; Clinical Professor, University of Illinois College of Medicine, Peoria, Illinois

Contributing Editors

Thomas Baehring, PhD
University Hospital of Düsseldorf, Düsseldorf, Germany

Rosane Ness-Abramof, MD
Meir Hospital, Kfar Saba, Israel, and Sackler School of Medicine, Tel Aviv, Israel

Amanda G. Powell, MD
Instructor of Medicine, Boston University School of Medicine, Boston, MA

Pornpoj (Piam) Pramyothin, MD
Endocrine Fellow at Boston Medical Center, Boston, MA

Megan Ruth, PhD
Post-doctoral Fellow, Endocrinology, Diabetes and Nutrition, Boston University School of Medicine, Boston, Massachusetts

Dr. Annette Thiel, MD
University Hospital of Düsseldorf, Düsseldorf, Germany

Table of Contents

Journals Represented

Journals represented in this YEAR BOOK are listed below.

Acta Paediatrica
American Heart Journal
American Journal of Clinical Nutrition
American Journal of Hypertension
American Journal of Medicine
Annals of Internal Medicine
Annals of Thoracic Surgery
Archives of Internal Medicine
BioMedical Central Pediatrics
British Medical Journal
Cancer
Cancer Genetics
Cancer Research
Cardiovascular Diabetology
Circulation
Clinical Endocrinology
Current Opinion in Pediatrics
Diabetes
Diabetes Care
Endocrinology
Fertility and Sterility
Gut
Heart
Human Reproduction
International Journal of Cardiology
International Journal of Obesity
International Journal of Radiation Oncology Biology Physics
Journal of Bone Mineral Research
Journal of Clinical Endocrinology & Metabolism
Journal of Clinical Investigation
Journal of Clinical Oncology
Journal of Diabetic Complications
Journal of Immunology
Journal of Pediatrics
Journal of the American College of Cardiology
Journal of the American Medical Association
Journal of Ultrasound in Medicine
Lancet
Metabolism
Metabolism Clinical and Experimental
Modern Pathology
Nature
New England Journal of Medicine
Osteoporosis International
Pediatric Blood & Cancer
Pediatrics
Proceedings of the National Academy of Sciences of the United States of America

Public Library of Science One
Radiology
Stroke
Surgery
Thyroid
Urology

STANDARD ABBREVIATIONS

The following terms are abbreviated in this edition: adrenocorticotropin hormone (ACTH); acquired immunodeficiency syndrome (AIDS); cardiopulmonary resuscitation (CPR); central nervous system (CNS); cerebrospinal fluid (CSF); computed tomography (CT); corticotropin-releasing hormone (CRH); deoxyribonucleic acid (DNA); electrocardiography (ECG); follicle-stimulating hormone (FSH); gonadotropin-releasing hormone (GnRH); growth hormone (GH); health maintenance organization (HMO); high-density lipoprotein (HDL); human immunodeficiency virus (HIV); insulin-dependent diabetes mellitus (IDDM); insulin-like growth factor I (IGF-I); intensive care unit (ICU); intermediate-density lipoprotein (IDL); intramuscular (IM); intravenous (IV); low-density lipoprotein (LDL); luteinizing hormone (LH); magnetic resonance (MR) imaging (MRI); multiple endocrine neoplasia (MEN); non-insulin-dependent diabetes mellitus (NIDDM); parathyroid hormone (PTH); prolactin (PRL); releasing hormone (RH); ribonucleic acid (RNA); thyrotropin-releasing hormone (TRH); thyroid-stimulating hormone or thyrotropin (TSH); thyroxine (T_4); triiodothyronine (T_3); ultrasound (US); and very-low-density lipoprotein (VLDL).

NOTE

The YEAR BOOK OF ENDOCRINOLOGY is a literature survey service providing abstracts of articles published in the professional literature. Every effort is made to assure the accuracy of the information presented in these pages. Neither the editor nor the publisher of the YEAR BOOK OF ENDOCRINOLOGY can be responsible for errors in the original materials. The editors' comments are their own opinions. Mention of specific products within this publication does not constitute endorsement.

To facilitate the use of the YEAR BOOK OF ENDOCRINOLOGY as a reference tool, all illustrations and tables included in this publication are now identified as they appear in the original article. This change is meant to help the reader recognize that any illustration or table appearing in the YEAR BOOK OF ENDOCRINOLOGY may be only one of many in the original article. For this reason, figure and table numbers appear to be out of sequence within the YEAR BOOK OF ENDOCRINOLOGY.

Introduction

The number of scientific articles is largely increasing every year. Before I started to write this introduction, I performed a PubMed search for the keyword "hyperthyroidism." The search yielded about 788 articles. When entering the keyword "diabetes mellitus," the results are even more impressive, with 16 813 articles showing up on the computer screen. Because of that, the editorial board has no chance to review all articles in order to select the best ones. Nonetheless, we all tried to do our best to select the articles that have the highest impact from the clinical and the basic research point of view.

Out of the selected articles, this year's Editor's Choice is the article by Samual Wells and coworkers, which investigated the role of vandetanib for the treatment of metastasized medullary thyroid cancer (MTC).[1] Vandetanib is an oral agent that selectively targets different tyrosine kinases, including RET, VEGFR, and EGFR signaling. The aim of this study was to investigate the effectiveness of vandetanib in an international, randomized, placebo-controlled, double-blind, phase III trial (ZETA) in patients with locally advanced or metastatic MTC. More than 330 patients were randomly assigned to receive vandetanib or placebo. The study met its primary objective of PFS prolongation with vandetanib versus placebo. Statistically significant advantages for vandetanib were also seen for objective response rate, disease control rate, and biochemical response. The benefit that was demonstrated in PFS for patients receiving vandetanib compared with placebo was observed in patients with the hereditary or the sporadic form of MTC. These data are highly promising for physicians treating patients with metastasized MTC. Up to now there is absolutely no effective treatment available for the treatment of these patients. Therefore, vandetanib is the first drug with the potential of reaching clinical effectiveness in a broad number of patients with advanced (and growing) MTC.

The editors hope that all selected articles and their accompanying editorial comments provide our readers fresh insight into endocrine problems encountered in everyday practice. In the name of all editors ...

Matthias Schott, MD, PhD

Reference

1. Wells SA Jr, Robinson BG, Gagel RF, et al. Vandetanib in patients with locally advanced or metastatic medullary thyroid cancer: a randomized, double-blind phase III trial. *J Clin Oncol.* 2012;30:134-141.

1 Diabetes

Complications

Long-Term Effects of Intensive Glucose Lowering on Cardiovascular Outcomes

The Accord Study Group (McMaster Univ and Hamilton Health Sciences, Ontario, Canada; Wake Forest Univ School of Medicine, Winston-Salem, NC; Case Western Reserve Univ, Cleveland, OH)
N Engl J Med 364:818-828, 2011

Background.—Intensive glucose lowering has previously been shown to increase mortality among persons with advanced type 2 diabetes and a high risk of cardiovascular disease. This report describes the 5-year outcomes of a mean of 3.7 years of intensive glucose lowering on mortality and key cardiovascular events.

Methods.—We randomly assigned participants with type 2 diabetes and cardiovascular disease or additional cardiovascular risk factors to receive intensive therapy (targeting a glycated hemoglobin level below 6.0%) or standard therapy (targeting a level of 7 to 7.9%). After termination of the intensive therapy, due to higher mortality in the intensive-therapy group, the target glycated hemoglobin level was 7 to 7.9% for all participants, who were followed until the planned end of the trial.

Results.—Before the intensive therapy was terminated, the intensive-therapy group did not differ significantly from the standard-therapy group in the rate of the primary outcome (a composite of nonfatal myocardial infarction, nonfatal stroke, or death from cardiovascular causes) ($P=0.13$) but had more deaths from any cause (primarily cardiovascular) (hazard ratio, 1.21; 95% confidence interval [CI], 1.02 to 1.44) and fewer nonfatal myocardial infarctions (hazard ratio, 0.79; 95% CI, 0.66 to 0.95). These trends persisted during the entire follow-up period (hazard ratio for death, 1.19; 95% CI, 1.03 to 1.38; and hazard ratio for nonfatal myocardial infarction, 0.82; 95% CI, 0.70 to 0.96). After the intensive intervention was terminated, the median glycated hemoglobin level in the intensive-therapy group rose from 6.4% to 7.2%, and the use of glucose-lowering medications and rates of severe hypoglycemia and other adverse events were similar in the two groups.

Conclusions.—As compared with standard therapy, the use of intensive therapy for 3.7 years to target a glycated hemoglobin level below 6%

reduced 5-year nonfatal myocardial infarctions but increased 5-year mortality. Such a strategy cannot be recommended for high-risk patients with advanced type 2 diabetes. (Funded by the National Heart, Lung and Blood Institute; ClinicalTrials.gov number, NCT00000620.)

▶ Cardiovascular diseases are the main cause of death in people suffering from diabetes. It is, therefore, tempting to assume that an intensive glucose-lowering treatment might prevent cardiovascular events in diabetics. The aim of the Action to Control Cardiovascular Risk in Diabetes (ACCORD) trial was to investigate whether lowering glycated hemoglobin (HbA1c) level below 6.0% (corresponding to the normal range) would reduce cardiovascular events. Persons suffering from diabetes for a median of 10 years with HbA1c of 7.5% or higher and who had a high risk of cardiovascular diseases were enrolled. In this high-risk cohort, an intensive glucose-lowering treatment cannot be recommended because increased 5-year mortality was observed in the intensive-treatment group. The outcome of this trial suggests that starting an intensive glucose-lowering therapy after approximately 10 years of diabetes is too late. However, intensive therapy directly after diagnosing diabetes might still be beneficial.

E. Oetjen, MD

Acute Hypoglycemia Decreases Myocardial Blood Flow Reserve in Patients With Type 1 Diabetes Mellitus and in Healthy Humans
Rana O, Byrne CD, Kerr D, et al (Poole Hosp and Bournemouth Univ, UK; Univ of Southampton and Southampton Univ Hosp Trust, UK; Bournemouth Univ, Dorset, UK; et al)
Circulation 124:1548-1556, 2011

Background.—Hypoglycemia is associated with increased cardiovascular mortality, but the reason for this association is poorly understood. We tested the hypothesis that the myocardial blood flow reserve (MBFR) is decreased during hypoglycemia using myocardial contrast echocardiography in patients with type 1 diabetes mellitus (DM) and in healthy control subjects.

Methods and Results.—Twenty-eight volunteers with DM and 19 control subjects underwent hyperinsulinemic clamps with maintained sequential hyperinsulinemic euglycemia (plasma glucose, 90 mg/dL [5.0 mmol/L]) followed by hyperinsulinemic hypoglycemia (plasma glucose, 50 mg/dL [2.8 mmol/L]) for 60 minutes each. Low-power real-time myocardial contrast echocardiography was performed with flash impulse imaging using low-dose dipyridamole stress at baseline and during hyperinsulinemic euglycemia and hyperinsulinemic hypoglycemia. In control subjects, MBFR increased during hyperinsulinemic euglycemia by 0.57 U (22%) above baseline (B coefficient, 0.57; 95% confidence interval, 0.38 to 0.75; $P<0.0001$) and decreased during hyperinsulinemic hypoglycemia by 0.36 U (14%) below baseline values (B coefficient, -0.36; 95% confidence interval, -0.50 to -0.23; $P<0.0001$). Although MBFR was lower in patients with DM at baseline by 0.37 U (14%; B coefficient, -0.37; 95% confidence interval, −0.55 to −0.19; $P = 0.0002$) compared with control subjects at baseline, the subsequent changes in MBFR during hyperinsulinemic euglycemia and hyperinsulinemic hypoglycemia in DM patients were similar to that observed in control subjects. Finally, the presence of microvascular complications in the patients with DM was associated with a reduction in MBFR of 0.52 U (24%; B coefficient, −0.52; 95% confidence interval, −0.70 to −0.34; $P<0.0001$).

Conclusions.—Hypoglycemia decreases MBFR in both healthy humans and patients with DM. This finding may explain the association between hypoglycemia and increased cardiovascular mortality in susceptible individuals.

▶ Ever since the first publication of the ACCORD study in 2008 demonstrating that intensive glucose-lowering therapy in people suffering from type 2 diabetes increased mortality, attempts have been undertaken to explain how hypoglycemia might result in increased mortality risk. In the study of Rana et al, the myocardial blood flow reserve was investigated in type 1 diabetic patients and in healthy volunteers. Although this study is rather small, it provides a first link to how hypoglycemia affects the myocardial blood flow reserve and results in increased cardiovascular risk. It should be noted that other changes within the myocardium might occur as well.

E. Oetjen, MD

Intensive glycemic control has no impact on the risk of heart failure in type 2 diabetic patients: Evidence from a 37,229 patient meta-analysis
Castagno D, Baird-Gunning J, Jhund PS, et al (Univ of Turin, Italy; Univ of Glasgow, UK; et al)
Am Heart J 162:938-948.e2, 2011

Background.—More intensive glycemic control reduces the risk of microvascular disease in patients with diabetes mellitus but has not been proven to reduce the risk of macrovascular events such as myocardial infarction and stroke. Poorer glycemic control, as indicated by glycated hemoglobin level concentration, is associated with an increased risk of heart failure (HF), but it is not known whether improved glycemic control reduces this risk. We conducted a meta-analysis of randomized controlled trials comparing strategies of more versus less intensive glucose-lowering that reported HF events.

Methods.—Two investigators independently searched PubMed, the Cochrane CENTRAL register of controlled trials, metaRegister, pre-MEDLINE, and CINAHL from January 1970 to October 2010 for prospective controlled randomized trials comparing a more intensive glucose-lowering regimen to a standard regimen. The outcome of interest was HF-related events (both fatal and nonfatal). Odds ratios (ORs) were calculated from published data from relevant trials and pooled with a random-effects meta-analysis.

Results.—A total of 37,229 patients from 8 randomized trials were included in the analysis. Follow-up ranged from 2.3 to 10.1 years, and the overall number of HF-related events was 1469 (55% in the intensive treatment arm). The mean difference in glycated hemoglobin level between patients given standard treatment and those allocated to a more intensive regimen was 0.9%. Overall, the risk of HF-related events did not differ significantly between intensive glycemic control and standard treatment (OR 1.20, 95% CI 0.96-1.48), but the effect estimate was highly heterogeneous ($I^2 = 69\%$). At subgroup analysis, intensive glycemic control achieved with high thiazolidinediones use significantly increased HF risk (OR 1.33, 95% CI 1.02-1.72).

Conclusions.—More intensive glycemic control in patients with type 2 diabetes mellitus did not reduce the occurrence of HF events. Furthermore, intensive glycemic control with thiazolidinediones increased the risk of HF. These findings question a direct mechanistic link between hyperglycemia and HF.

▶ Diabetes mellitus is a major risk factor for cardiovascular disease, and poor glycemic control is associated with a higher rate of heart failure. It is tempting to speculate that intensive glucose-lowering therapies result in a reduced risk of heart failure. That this is not the case is demonstrated by the meta-analysis of Castagno et al. It should be noted that different studies with very different anti-diabetic treatments were included in this analysis, including those studies using pioglitazone and rosiglitazone, known to impair heart function. In addition, the impact of the duration of diabetes was not considered. It will remain difficult to elucidate whether hyperglycemia per se is a risk factor for the development of heart failure or whether heart failure-associated comorbidities like obesity and hypertension are the "real" risk factors. The answer to this question might have impact on the therapy of newly diagnosed diabetic patients.

E. Oetjen, MD

The duration of diabetes affects the response to intensive glucose control in type 2 subjects: the VA Diabetes Trial

Duckworth WC, for the Investigators of the VADT (Phoenix VA Health Care Ctr, AZ; et al)
J Diabetes Complications 25:355-361, 2011

Background.—The goal of the VA Diabetes Trial (VADT) was to determine the effect of intensive glucose control on macrovascular events in subjects with difficult-to-control diabetes. No significant benefit was found. This report examines predictors of the effect of intensive therapy on the primary outcome in this population.

Methods.—This trial included 1791 subjects. Baseline cardiovascular risk factors were collected by interview and the VA record. The analyses were done by intention to treat.

Findings.—Univariate analysis at baseline of predictors of a primary cardiovascular (CV) event included a prior CV event, age, insulin use at baseline, and duration of diagnosed diabetes (all $P<.0001$). Multivariable modeling revealed a U-shaped relationship between duration of diabetes and treatment. Modeled estimates for the hazard ratios (HRs) for treatment show that subjects with a short duration (3 years or less) of diagnosed diabetes have a nonsignificant increase in risk (HR >1.0) after which the HR is below 1.0. From 7 to 15 years' duration at entry, subjects have HRs favoring intensive treatment. Thereafter the HR approaches 1.0 and over-21-years' duration approaches 2.0. Duration over 21 years resulted in a HR of 1.977 (CI 1.77–3.320, $P<.01$). Baseline c-peptide levels progressively declined up to 15 years and were stable subsequently.

Interpretation.—In difficult-to-control older subjects with type 2 DM, duration of diabetes altered the response to intensive glucose control. Intensive therapy may reduce CV events in subjects with a duration of 15 years or less and may increase risks in those with longer duration.

▶ The findings of the Action to Control Cardiovascular Risk in Diabetes (ACCORD) Study Group were corroborated in the Veteran's Affairs Diabetes Trial (VADT), stating that an intensive glucose-lowering treatment failed to reduce major cardiovascular events significantly. In this post hoc analysis, the influence of the duration of diabetes on the response to intensive glucose-lowering treatment was analyzed in a difficult-to-control cohort. It should be noted that in this study, people were enrolled with mean glycated hemoglobin (HbA1c) levels of 9.4%. The mean HbA1c level in the standard treated group was 8.4%, that in the intensive treatment group was 6.9%. Both values are considerably higher than in the ACCORD study. However, the results of both studies are the same. Thus, an early intensive glucose-lowering therapy might be beneficial to prevent major cardiovascular events.

E. Oetjen, MD

Epidemiology

New-onset diabetes and cardiovascular events in essential hypertensives: A 6-year follow-up study
Tsiachris D, Tsioufis C, Thomopoulos C, et al (Univ of Athens Med School, Greece; et al)
Int J Cardiol 153:154-158, 2011

Background.—Controversy still exists regarding the impact of new-onset diabetes (NOD) on CV outcomes among patients with hypertension. Our aim was to determine the incidence of NOD in essential hypertensives and to evaluate its association with major cardiovascular (CV) events.

Methods.—We followed-up for a mean period of 6 years 1572 essential hypertensives (mean age 54.3 years, 696 males) for the incidence of NOD, as well as of fatal and non-fatal coronary artery disease and stroke. Based on the development of NOD, the cohort was divided into patients with pre-existing diabetes (10%), patients with NOD (10%) and those who remained free from diabetes.

Results.—During the follow-up period, new or recurrent cases of coronary artery disease and stroke events occurred at a rate of 5.6% (n = 88) and 4.65% (n = 73). The independent predictors for NOD were age (OR = 1.026, $p = 0.041$), waist circumference (OR = 1.044, $p<0.001$), family history of diabetes (OR = 2.173, $p = 0.003$) and systolic BP at follow-up (OR 1.022, $p = 0.044$). The presence of NOD was independently associated with greater incidence of stroke (HR 2.404, $p = 0.046$), along with age (HR 1.078, $p<0.001$), duration of hypertension (HR 1.039, $p = 0.017$) and office systolic blood pressure at follow-up (HR 1.022, $p = 0.026$), whereas development of NOD had no relationship with the incidence of coronary artery disease.

Conclusions.—Our findings indicate the high incidence of NOD and its close association with stroke in essential hypertension. Poorer control of hypertension appears to be a common denominator of both NOD and stroke in this setting.

▶ Uncontrolled hypertension is associated with an increased risk of new-onset diabetes (NOD), and the treatment of hypertension, especially with a combination of thiazide diuretics and β-blockers, impairs glucose tolerance and increases the risk of NOD as well. The study of Tsiachris et al aimed to evaluate the incidence of NOD in essentially hypertensive patients and its association with major cardiovascular events like stroke and fatal or nonfatal coronary artery disease. Given the distinct effects of antihypertensive drugs on glucose homeostasis (β-blockers and thiazide as opposed to the angiotensin-converting-enzyme inhibitors and AT1-receptor blockers), it is unfortunate that the cohort was not distinguished for drug treatment. Nonetheless, it is to be hoped that the result of this study will enliven studies on the association of diabetes, hypertension, and cerebrovascular diseases.

E. Oetjen, MD

Utility of Hemoglobin A$_{1c}$ for Diagnosing Prediabetes and Diabetes in Obese Children and Adolescents
Nowicka P, Santoro N, Liu H, et al (Yale Univ School of Medicine, New Haven, CT; Yale Ctr for Clinical Investigation of Yale Univ School of Medicine, New Haven, CT)
Diabetes Care 34:1306-1311, 2011

Objective.—Hemoglobin A$_{1c}$ (A1C) has emerged as a recommended diagnostic tool for identifying diabetes and subjects at risk for the disease. This recommendation is based on data in adults showing the relationship between A1C with future development of diabetes and microvascular complications. However, studies in the pediatric population are lacking.

Research Design and Methods.—We studied a multiethnic cohort of 1,156 obese children and adolescents without a diagnosis of diabetes (male, 40%/female, 60%). All subjects underwent an oral glucose tolerance test (OGTT) and A1C measurement. These tests were repeated after a follow-up time of ~2 years in 218 subjects.

Results.—At baseline, subjects were stratified according to A1C categories: 77% with normal glucose tolerance (A1C <5.7%), 21% at risk for diabetes (A1C 5.7—6.4%), and 1% with diabetes (A1C >6.5%). In the at risk for diabetes category, 47% were classified with prediabetes or diabetes, and in the diabetes category, 62% were classified with type 2 diabetes by the OGTT. The area under the curve receiver operating characteristic for A1C was 0.81 (95% CI 0.70—0.92). The threshold for identifying type 2 diabetes was 5.8%, with 78% specificity and 68% sensitivity. In the subgroup with repeated measures, a multivariate analysis showed that the strongest predictors of 2-h glucose at follow-up were baseline A1C and 2-h glucose, independently of age, ethnicity, sex, fasting glucose, and follow-up time.

Conclusions.—The American Diabetes Association suggested that an A1C of 6.5% underestimates the prevalence of prediabetes and diabetes in obese children and adolescents. Given the low sensitivity and specificity, the use of A1C by itself represents a poor diagnostic tool for prediabetes and type 2 diabetes in obese children and adolescents.

▶ Given that a prediabetic metabolic condition and diabetes do not hurt and that an early therapeutic intervention will retard the pathogenesis of diabetes-associated diseases, the identification of people suffering ignorantly from diabetes or being at risk for diabetes is important. This is especially true in obese children and adolescents. Because HbA1c usually reflects the glucose homeostasis of the previous 3 to 4 months, does not require fasting for accurate measurements, and has low intraindividual variability, its determination is considered a reliable marker and is recommended by the American Diabetes Association. However, this recommendation is based on studies in adults. In a multiethnic cohort of obese children and adolescents with a 2-year follow-up, the reliability of HbA1c to identify diabetics or persons at risk for diabetes was compared with that of an oral glucose tolerance test.

E. Oetjen, MD

Glycemic Control

Antidiabetic actions of a non—agonist PPARγ ligand blocking Cdk5—mediated phosphorylation
Choi JH, Banks AS, Kamenecka TM, et al (Harvard Med School, Boston, MA; The Scripps Res Inst, Jupiter, FL; et al)
Nature 477:477-481, 2011

PPARγ is the functioning receptor for the thiazolidinedione (TZD) class of antidiabetes drugs including rosiglitazone and pioglitazone. These drugs are full classical agonists for this nuclear receptor, but recent data have shown that many PPARγ-based drugs have a separate biochemical activity, blocking the obesity-linked phosphorylation of PPARγ by Cdk5 (ref. 2). Here we describe novel synthetic compounds that have a unique mode of binding to PPARγ, completely lack classical transcriptional agonism and block the Cdk5-mediated phosphorylation in cultured adipocytes and in insulin-resistant mice. Moreover, one such compound, SR1664, has potent antidiabetic activity while not causing the fluid retention and weight gain that are serious side effects of many of the PPARγ drugs. Unlike TZDs, SR1664 also does not interfere with bone formation in culture. These data illustrate that new classes of antidiabetes drugs can be developed by specifically targeting the Cdk5-mediated phosphorylation of PPARγ.

▶ Thiazolidindiones like pioglitazone and rosiglitazone functioning as agonists of the peroxisome proliferator activated receptor (PPAR) γ are potent antidiabetic drugs, but their widespread use is hampered by several undesired effects, among them fluid retention with increased cardiac failure and osteoporosis. Like the desired antidiabetic effects, these undesired effects are due to the activation of PPAR-γ in diverse tissues. A selective PPAR-γ modulator, activating this nuclear receptor only in specific tissues and preventing the obesity-induced phosphorylation of PPAR-γ, might exert only the antidiabetic actions but none of the undesired actions. Such an agonist is described by Choi et al. Thus, the concept first described for the selective estrogen receptor modulators is now applied to PPAR-γ agonists, making it possible to envision new antidiabetic drugs targeting PPAR-γ but minimizing the undesired effects of the thiazolidindiones.

E. Oetjen, MD

Donor Islet Endothelial Cells in Pancreatic Islet Revascularization
Nyqvist D, Speier S, Rodriguez-Diaz R, et al (Karolinska Institutet, Stockholm, Sweden; Univ of Miami, FL; et al)
Diabetes 60:2571-2577, 2011

Objective.—Freshly isolated pancreatic islets contain, in contrast to cultured islets, intraislet endothelial cells (ECs), which can contribute to the formation of functional blood vessels after transplantation. We have characterized how donor islet endothelial cells (DIECs) may contribute to the revascularization rate, vascular density, and endocrine graft function after transplantation of freshly isolated and cultured islets.

Research Design and Methods.—Freshly isolated and cultured islets were transplanted under the kidney capsule and into the anterior chamber of the eye. Intravital laser scanning microscopy was used to monitor the revascularization process and DIECs in intact grafts. The grafts' metabolic function was examined by reversal of diabetes, and the ultrastructural morphology by transmission electron microscopy.

Results.—DIECs significantly contributed to the vasculature of fresh islet grafts, assessed up to 5 months after transplantation, but were hardly detected in cultured islet grafts. Early participation of DIECs in the revascularization process correlated with a higher revascularization rate of freshly isolated islets compared with cultured islets. However, after complete revascularization, the vascular density was similar in the two groups, and host ECs gained morphological features resembling the endogenous islet vasculature. Surprisingly, grafts originating from cultured islets reversed diabetes more rapidly than those originating from fresh islets.

Conclusions.—In summary, DIECs contributed to the revascularization of fresh, but not cultured, islets by participating in early processes of vessel formation and persisting in the vasculature over long periods of time. However, the DIECs did not increase the vascular density or improve the endocrine function of the grafts.

▶ Islet transplantation offers the possibility to restore glucose homeostasis in patients suffering from type 1 diabetes. After transplantation, islets are revascularized by blood vessels from the host organ via angiogenesis. However, during the first avascular engraftment period, loss of insulin content and a high rate of cell death are observed, impeding the restoration of glucose homeostasis. Nyqvist et al show that donor islet endothelial cells, which are more abundant in freshly isolated than in cultured islets, do not improve endocrine function of the grafts. Thus, islet transplantation is far from being the ultimate therapy for type 1 diabetes, and crucial factors determining what factors lead to successful islet transplantation need to be identified.

E. Oetjen, MD

Pathogenesis

Dual elimination of the glucagon and GLP-1 receptors in mice reveals plasticity in the incretin axis

Ali S, Lamont BJ, Charron MJ, et al (Univ of Toronto, Ontario, Canada; Albert Einstein College of Medicine, NY)
J Clin Invest 121:1917-1929, 2011

Disordered glucagon secretion contributes to the symptoms of diabetes, and reduced glucagon action is known to improve glucose homeostasis. In mice, genetic deletion of the glucagon receptor (*Gcgr*) results in increased levels of the insulinotropic hormone glucagon-like peptide 1 (GLP-1), which may contribute to the alterations in glucose homeostasis observed in $Gcgr^{-/-}$ mice. Here, we assessed the contribution of GLP-1 receptor (GLP-1R) signaling to the phenotype of $Gcgr^{-/-}$ mice by generating $Gcgr^{-/-}Glp1r^{-/-}$ mice. Although insulin sensitivity was similar in all genotypes, fasting glucose was increased in $Gcgr^{-/-}Glp1r^{-/-}$ mice. Elimination of the *Glp1r* normalized gastric emptying and impaired intraperitoneal glucose tolerance in $Gcgr^{-/-}$ mice. Unexpectedly, deletion of *Glp1r* in $Gcgr^{-/-}$ mice did not alter the improved oral glucose tolerance and increased insulin secretion characteristic of that genotype. Although $Gcgr^{-/-}Glp1r^{-/-}$ islets exhibited increased sensitivity to the incretin glucose-dependent insulinotropic polypeptide (GIP), mice lacking both $Glp1r$ and the GIP receptor ($Gipr$) maintained preservation of the enteroinsular axis following reduction of $Gcgr$ signaling. Moreover, $Gcgr^{-/-}Glp1r^{-/-}$ islets expressed increased levels of the cholecystokinin A receptor ($Cckar$) and G protein—coupled receptor 119 ($Gpr119$) mRNA transcripts, and $Gcgr^{-/-}Glp1r^{-/-}$ mice exhibited increased sensitivity to exogenous CCK and the GPR119 agonist AR231453. Our data reveal extensive functional plasticity in the enteroinsular axis via induction of compensatory mechanisms that control nutrient-dependent regulation of insulin secretion.

▶ Using different genetic mouse models and diverse receptor agonists and antagonists, the authors show that various compensatory mechanisms within the entero—insular axis exist to maintain nutrient-dependent regulation on insulin secretion. This article carefully differentiates between the various metabolic effects because of glucagon receptor knockout and highlights the importance of as yet not fully appreciated incretin receptors such as cholecystokinin-A receptor and the G-protein—coupled receptor 119. It thereby reveals a capacity of β-cell adaptation to loss of insulinotropic receptor signaling and might help to identify new targets to preserve β-cell function.

E. Oetjen, MD

A genetically engineered human pancreatic β cell line exhibiting glucose-inducible insulin secretion

Ravassard P, Hazhouz Y, Pechberty S, et al (Université Pierre et Marie Curie-Paris 6, France; CNRS, UMR 7225, Paris, France; Endocells, Paris, France; et al)
J Clin Invest 121:3589-3597, 2011

Despite intense efforts over the past 30 years, human pancreatic β cell lines have not been available. Here, we describe a robust technology for producing a functional human β cell line using targeted oncogenesis in human fetal tissue. Human fetal pancreatic buds were transduced with a lentiviral vector that expressed SV40LT under the control of the insulin promoter. The transduced buds were then grafted into SCID mice so that they could develop into mature pancreatic tissue. Upon differentiation, the newly formed SV40LT-expressing β cells proliferated and formed insulinomas. The resulting β cells were then transduced with human telomerase reverse transcriptase (hTERT), grafted into other SCID mice, and finally expanded in vitro to generate cell lines. One of these cell lines, EndoC-βH1, expressed many β cell—specific markers without any substantial expression of markers of other pancreatic cell types. The cells secreted insulin when stimulated by glucose or other insulin secretagogues, and cell transplantation reversed chemically induced diabetes in mice. These cells represent a unique tool for large-scale drug discovery and provide a preclinical model for cell replacement therapy in diabetes. This technology could be generalized to generate other human cell lines when the cell type—specific promoter is available.

▶ Although primary cells are considered the gold standard to investigate physiological and pathophysiological mechanisms within cells, it is often difficult to obtain them in an adequate amount and under standardized conditions. This holds especially true for rodent and even more so for human beta cells. Although many rodent beta-cell lines already exist, mimicking more or less faithfully primary beta-cell features, to date few human beta-cell lines have been described, and these are capable of producing insulin for only a few passages. Given the differences between rodent and human beta cells, a human beta-cell line has long been awaited. Ravassard et al describe the generation of a promising new human beta-cell line showing most of the characteristics of primary beta cells. Thus, this cell line might be an important tool to elucidate the regulation of human beta cells.

E. Oetjen, MD

MicroRNAs in β-Cell Biology, Insulin Resistance, Diabetes and Its Complications
Fernandez-Valverde SL, Taft RJ, Mattick JS (Univ of Queensland, St Lucia, Australia)
Diabetes 60:1825-1831, 2011

Background.—MicroRNAs (miRNAs) are small nucleotide RNA molecules that regulate protein expression in eukaryotic cells and strongly influence differentiation and developmental processes. The known and proposed roles and effects of miRNAs in type 1 (T1D) and type 2 (T2D) diabetes were assessed, focusing specifically on β-cell biology, altered expression related to obesity, and dysfunction in organs and tissues in later stages of diabetes.

β-Cell Biology.—Pancreatic β-cells release insulin in response to glucose levels in the bloodstream, then the insulin triggers glucose uptake in target tissues. However, β-cells can be missing or malfunctioning. T1D is characterized by a lack of insulin-producing cells, whereas T2D demonstrates an inability to increase insulin levels sufficiently to stimulate glucose uptake in the presence of insulin resistance. MiRNAs are implicated in pancreatic development and may produce aberrant β-cells. Changes in miRNA expression in regulatory T cells of patients with T1D may lead to the autoimmune destruction of β-cells. In T2D, low levels of some miRNAs may induce insulin secretion by de-repressing targets, or the overexpression of other miRNAs can attenuate proliferation and insulin gene transcription while reducing glucose-induced insulin secretion. MiR-375 targets genes that negatively regulate cellular growth and proliferation. Aberrant loss of miR-375 reduces β-cell mass, causing low insulin levels, hyperglycemia, and diabetes. MiR-9, miR-96, and miR-124a are also critical in the insulin exocytosis of β-cells. MiR-7 and miR-375 are expressed in brain as well as β-cell islets, possibly producing neurologic effects related to the diabetic state.

Obesity.—The onset of T2D is strongly related to the presence of obesity, hyperlipidemia, and insulin resistance. Obesity-induced molecular changes and environmental signals have a strong dysregulatory effect on miRNAs in adipose tissue. MiRNAs such as those in the miR-29 family, miR-320, and miR-27b target conserved core cell-regulatory pathways that are locally and systematically altered by obesity and diabetes. Obesity also triggers macrophage infiltration and cytokine release in adipose tissue, altering miRNA expression and affecting both lipid levels and adipogenesis. Many cytokines interfere with insulin signaling and inhibit adipogenesis, which affects the induction of several miRNAs. The connection between miRNA expression and cytokine exposure may suggest treatment options for the morbidly obese.

Diabetic Complications.—Diabetes adversely affects cardiac and skeletal muscle, the liver, the kidney, and the endothelium; MiRNA expression is also altered in these tissues in diabetes. Normally insulin activates the transcription of sterol regulatory element-n-binding protein 1, which represses miR-1 and miR-133 transcription. This repression is impaired in T2D patients, contributing to poor muscle function. The links between miR-133 and miR-1 and cardiomyocyte responses to insulin and glucose are complex, but their study may provide insight into how muscle cells respond to physiologic stimuli.

MiRNA expression profiles related to liver and kidney function can also be abnormal in the late stages of diabetes. In the diabetic kidney, transforming growth factor-β and miR-129 induce the expression of miR-216a and miR-217, leading to Akt activation by targeting phosphatase and tensin homolog (PTEN). MiR-126 levels and the onset of diabetic vascular complications show a strong negative correlation. MiR-126 may be both a biomarker for early detection of vascular complications of diabetes and a possible RNA-based therapeutic element for diabetes-induced atherosclerosis.

Conclusions.—MiRNAs carry out important regulatory functions. Understanding their roles may expand current knowledge regarding the effects of diabetes and other systemic diseases on tissues in the heart, brain, and other organs. Studies of miRNA must be integrated into existing resources to facilitate the development of such insights.

▶ Since the discovery of a pancreatic-specific microRNA-regulating insulin secretion by Poy et al in 2004, the number of microRNAs is increasing. It is now generally accepted that microRNAs are important regulators of diverse cellular functions, often in a tissue-specific manner, and might pose a drug target. This article provides an excellent overview for most of the microRNAs implicated in diabetes and its complications. It is therefore indispensible for everyone working in this field.

E. Oetjen, MD

Genome-Wide Association Identifies Nine Common Variants Associated With Fasting Proinsulin Levels and Provides New Insights Into the Pathophysiology of Type 2 Diabetes
Strawbridge RJ, Dupuis J, Prokopenko I, et al (Karolinska Univ Hosp Solna, Stockholm, Sweden; Boston Univ School of Public Health, MA; Univ of Oxford, UK; et al)
Diabetes 60:2624-2634, 2011

Objective.—Proinsulin is a precursor of mature insulin and C-peptide. Higher circulating proinsulin levels are associated with impaired β-cell function, raised glucose levels, insulin resistance, and type 2 diabetes (T2D). Studies of the insulin processing pathway could provide new insights about T2D pathophysiology.

Research Design and Methods.—We have conducted a meta-analysis of genome-wide association tests of ~2.5 million genotyped or imputed single nucleotide polymorphisms (SNPs) and fasting proinsulin levels in 10,701 nondiabetic adults of European ancestry, with follow-up of 23 loci in up to 16,378 individuals, using additive genetic models adjusted for age, sex, fasting insulin, and study-specific covariates.

Results.—Nine SNPs at eight loci were associated with proinsulin levels ($P < 5 \times 10^{-8}$). Two loci (*LARP6* and *SGSM2*) have not been previously related to metabolic traits, one (*MADD*) has been associated with fasting glucose, one (PCSK1) has been implicated in obesity, and four (*TCF7L2, SLC30A8, VPS13C/C2CD4A/B*, and *ARAP1*, formerly *CENTD2*) increase T2D risk. The proinsulin-raising allele of *ARAP1* was associated with a lower fasting glucose ($P = 1.7 \times 10^{-4}$), improved β-cell function ($P = 1.1 \times 10^{-5}$), and lower risk of T2D (odds ratio 0.88; $P = 7.8 \times 10^{-6}$). Notably, PCSK1 encodes the protein prohormone convertase 1/3, the first enzyme in the insulin processing pathway. A genotype score composed of the nine proinsulin-raising alleles was not associated with coronary disease in two large case-control datasets.

Conclusions.—We have identified nine genetic variants associated with fasting proinsulin. Our findings illuminate the biology underlying glucose homeostasis and T2D development in humans and argue against a direct role of proinsulin in coronary artery disease pathogenesis.

► Increased levels of proinsulin in relation to circulating levels of mature insulin are suggestive of beta-cell stress due to insulin resistance, impaired beta-cell function, or abnormal insulin processing and secretion. Evidence suggests that increases in proinsulin levels predict the development of diabetes mellitus type 2 (T2DM) or coronary artery disease (CAD). In an elaborate 2-stage analysis, 9 loci associated with fasting proinsulin levels were identified, both proinsulin-increasing and proinsulin-decreasing alleles. Several but not all of these loci are well known to increase the risk of T2DM. No association was found with CAD. This analysis tempts a more detailed study of the dysregulation of insulin secretion resulting in enhanced proinsulin levels.

E. Oetjen, MD

Hepatic Glucagon Action Is Essential for Exercise-Induced Reversal of Mouse Fatty Liver

Berglund ED, Lustig DG, Baheza RA, et al (Vanderbilt Univ School of Medicine, Nashville, TN; et al)
Diabetes 60:2720-2729, 2011

Objective.—Exercise is an effective intervention to treat fatty liver. However, the mechanism(s) that underlie exercise-induced reductions in fatty liver are unclear. Here we tested the hypothesis that exercise requires hepatic glucagon action to reduce fatty liver.

Research Design and Methods.—C57BL/6 mice were fed high-fat diet (HFD) and assessed using magnetic resonance, biochemical, and histological techniques to establish a timeline for fatty liver development over 20 weeks. Glucagon receptor null ($gcgr^{-/-}$) and wild-type ($gcgr^{+/+}$) littermate mice were subsequently fed HFD to provoke moderate fatty liver and then performed either 10 or 6 weeks of running wheel or treadmill exercise, respectively.

Results.—Exercise reverses progression of HFD-induced fatty liver in $gcgr^{+/+}$ mice. Remarkably, such changes are absent in $gcgr^{-/-}$ mice, thus confirming the hypothesis that exercise-stimulated hepatic glucagon receptor activation is critical to reduce HFD-induced fatty liver.

Conclusions.—These findings suggest that therapies that use antagonism of hepatic glucagon action to reduce blood glucose may interfere with the ability of exercise and perhaps other interventions to positively affect fatty liver.

► Nonalcoholic fatty liver (fatty liver) is associated with obesity, insulin resistance, and diabetes mellitus type 2 and might progress into more severe dysfunctions. Evidence in rodents and humans suggested that exercise positively affects fatty liver. Berglund et al confirm in mice that indeed exercise reduced fat content in the liver in part independent of a reduction in body weight. Glucagon is secreted in the fasting state and primarily acts on the liver to induce hepatic glucose release, and it participates in reducing fatty liver (this study). Thus, despite a better metabolic profile in mice lacking the glucagon receptor, exercise was not able to prevent fatty liver induced by high-fat diet in these mice. This study suggests that inhibition of glucagon action as a new target in antidiabetic should be considered carefully.

E. Oetjen, MD

A small molecule differentiation inducer increases insulin production by pancreatic β cells
Dioum EM, Osborne JK, Goetsch S, et al (Univ of Texas Southwestern Med Ctr, Dallas)
Proc Natl Acad Sci U S A 108:20713-20718, 2011

New drugs for preserving and restoring pancreatic β-cell function are critically needed for the worldwide epidemic of type 2 diabetes and the cure for type 1 diabetes. We previously identified a family of neurogenic 3,5-disubstituted isoxazoles (Isx) that increased expression of neurogenic differentiation 1 (NeuroD1, also known as BETA2); this transcription factor functions in neuronal and pancreatic β-cell differentiation and is essential for insulin gene transcription. Here, we probed effects of Isx on human cadaveric islets and MIN6 pancreatic β cells. Isx increased the expression and secretion of insulin in islets that made little insulin after prolonged ex vivo culture and increased expression of neurogenic differentiation 1 and other regulators of islet differentiation and insulin gene transcription. Within the first few hours of exposure, Isx caused biphasic activation of ERK1/2 and increased bulk histone acetylation. Although there was little effect on histone deacetylase activity, Isx increased histone acetyl transferase activity in nuclear extracts. Reconstitution assays indicated that Isx increased the activity of the histone acetyl transferase p300 through an ERK1/2-dependent mechanism. In summary, we have identified a small molecule with antidiabetic activity, providing a tool for exploring islet function and a possible lead for therapeutic intervention in diabetes.

▶ The maintenance of beta-cell function for insulin secretion as well as insulin production is an important aim in the therapy of diabetes. However, most actual antidiabetic therapy does not target the beta-cell to preserve its function and mass. In the study of Dioum et al, a small molecule is described that is dependent on either calcium influx or activation of ERK and activates beta-cell transcription factors and the histone acetyltransferase activity of p300. Given that it is the combination of transcription factors that determines tissue-specific expression of genes and that p300 is an important transcriptional coactivator of many transcription factors, it would be interesting to know how beta-cell-specific this small molecule acts.

E. Oetjen, MD

Prevention and Reversal of Diabetes

Management of type 2 diabetes: new and future developments in treatment

Tahrani AA, Bailey CJ, Del Prato S, et al (Univ of Birmingham, UK; Aston Univ, Birmingham, UK; Univ of Pisa, Italy)
Lancet 378:182-197, 2011

The increasing prevalence, variable pathogenesis, progressive natural history, and complications of type 2 diabetes emphasise the urgent need for new treatment strategies. Long acting (eg, once weekly) agonists of the glucagon-like-peptide-1 receptor are advanced in development, and they improve prandial insulin secretion, reduce excess glucagon production, and promote satiety. Trials of inhibitors of dipeptidyl peptidase 4, which enhance the effect of endogenous incretin hormones, are also nearing completion. Novel approaches to glycaemic regulation include use of inhibitors of the sodium–glucose cotransporter 2, which increase renal glucose elimination, and inhibitors of 11β-hydroxysteroid dehydrogenase 1, which reduce the glucocorticoid effects in liver and fat. Insulin-releasing glucokinase activators and pancreatic-G-protein-coupled fatty-acid-receptor agonists, glucagon-receptor antagonists, and metabolic inhibitors of hepatic glucose output are being assessed. Early proof of principle has been shown for compounds that enhance and partly mimic insulin action and replicate some effects of bariatric surgery.

▶ Considering the increase in diabetes mellitus type 2 worldwide and its severe complications, the need for new treatment strategies is obvious. Tahrani et al describe in detail obvious and not-so-obvious drug targets for the treatment of diabetes type 2. By this description, pathophysiological features of diabetes, clinical studies, and a summary of available drugs are depicted, giving a thorough picture of the future of diabetes treatment, including possible adverse effects.

E. Oetjen, MD

Insulin Receptor Substrate 1 Gene Variation Modifies Insulin Resistance Response to Weight-Loss Diets in a 2-Year Randomized Trial: The Preventing Overweight Using Novel Dietary Strategies (POUNDS LOST) Trial

Qi Q, Bray GA, Smith SR, et al (Brigham and Women's Hosp and Harvard Med School, Boston, MA; Pennington Biomedical Res Ctr of the Louisiana State Univ System, Baton Rouge; Translational Res Inst for Metabolism and Diabetes, Winter Park, FL)
Circulation 124:563-571, 2011

Background.—Common genetic variants in the insulin receptor substrate 1 (*IRS1*) gene have been recently associated with insulin resistance and hyperinsulinemia. We examined whether the best-associated variant modifies the long-term changes in insulin resistance and body weight in response to weight-loss diets in Preventing Overweight Using Novel Dietary Strategies (POUNDS LOST) trial.

Methods and Results.—We genotyped *IRS1* rs2943641 in 738 overweight adults (61% were women) who were randomly assigned to 1 of 4 diets varying in macronutrient contents for 2 years. We assessed the progress in fasting insulin, homeostasis model assessment of insulin resistance (HOMA-IR) and weight loss by genotypes. At 6 months, participants with the risk-conferring CC genotype had greater decreases in insulin ($P=0.009$), HOMA-IR ($P=0.015$), and weight loss ($P=0.018$) than those without this genotype in the highest-carbohydrate diet group whereas an opposite genotype effect on changes in insulin and HOMA-IR ($P\leq0.05$) was observed in participants assigned to the lowest-carbohydrate diet group. No significant differences were observed across genotypes in the other 2 diet groups. The tests for genotype by intervention interactions were all significant ($P<0.05$). At 2 years, the genotype effect on changes in insulin and HOMA-IR remained significant in the highest-carbohydrate diet group ($P<0.05$). The highest carbohydrate diet led to a greater improvement of insulin and HOMA-IR (P for genotype—time interaction ≤0.009) in participants with the CC genotype than those without this genotype across 2-year intervention.

Conclusions.—Individuals with the *IRS1* rs2943641 CC genotype might obtain more benefits in weight loss and improvement of insulin resistance than those without this genotype by choosing a high-carbohydrate and low-fat diet.

▶ In their study, Qi et al show that the genotype and the composition of nutrition contribute to the success of weight loss and the improvement of metabolic parameters. Thus, depending on the genotype, the same nutrient composition of a diet might exert different effects on weight loss and insulin resistance. It would be interesting to know whether and how genotypes in other genes implicated in metabolism contribute to a nutritional effect and whether these genotypes influence the preference for certain foods. In the future, maybe genotyping will be necessary prior to a weight reduction to determine the most effective composition of a diet.

E. Oetjen, MD

Valsartan Improves β-Cell Function and Insulin Sensitivity in Subjects With Impaired Glucose Metabolism: A randomized controlled trial
van der Zijl NJ, Moors CCM, Goossens GH, et al (Vrije Univ Med Ctr, Amsterdam, The Netherlands; Maastricht Univ Med Ctr, The Netherlands)
Diabetes Care 34:845-851, 2011

Objective.—Recently, the Nateglinide and Valsartan in Impaired Glucose Tolerance Outcomes Research Trial demonstrated that treatment with the angiotensin receptor blocker (ARB) valsartan for 5 years resulted in a relative reduction of 14% in the incidence of type 2 diabetes in subjects with impaired glucose metabolism (IGM). We investigated whether improvements in β-cell function and/or insulin sensitivity underlie these preventive effects of the ARB valsartan in the onset of type 2 diabetes.

Research Design and Methods.—In this randomized controlled, double-blind, two-center study, the effects of 26 weeks of valsartan (320 mg daily; $n = 40$) or placebo ($n = 39$) on β-cell function and insulin sensitivity were assessed in subjects with impaired fasting glucose and/or impaired glucose tolerance, using a combined hyperinsulinemic-euglycemic and hyperglycemic clamp with subsequent arginine stimulation and a 2-h 75-g oral glucose tolerance test (OGTT). Treatment effects were analyzed using ANCOVA, adjusting for center, glucometabolic status, and sex.

Results.—Valsartan increased first-phase ($P = 0.028$) and second-phase ($P = 0.002$) glucose-stimulated insulin secretion compared with placebo, whereas the enhanced arginine-stimulated insulin secretion was comparable between groups ($P = 0.25$). In addition, valsartan increased the OGTT-derived insulinogenic index (representing first-phase insulin secretion after an oral glucose load; $P = 0.027$). Clamp-derived insulin sensitivity was significantly increased with valsartan compared with placebo ($P = 0.049$). Valsartan treatment significantly decreased systolic and diastolic blood pressure compared with placebo ($P < 0.001$). BMI remained unchanged in both treatment groups ($P = 0.89$).

Conclusions.—Twenty-six weeks of valsartan treatment increased glucose-stimulated insulin release and insulin sensitivity in normotensive subjects with IGM. These findings may partly explain the beneficial effects of valsartan in the reduced incidence of type 2 diabetes.

▶ Drugs interfering with the renin-angiotensin system, such as the inhibitors of the angiotensin-converting enzyme and the antagonists of the angiotensin 2 subtype 1 receptor (ARB), have been suggested to improve glucose homeostasis in patients with hypertensive diabetes. Furthermore, the Nateglinide and Valsartan in Impaired Glucose Tolerance Outcomes Research Trial demonstrated that treatment with the ARB valsartan for 5 years significantly reduced the incidence of diabetes type 2 in people with impaired glucose metabolism. The aim of the present study was to elucidate preventive effects of valsartan on glucose homeostasis. The study points to an improvement in insulin secretion and insulin sensitivity due to valsartan therapy. It remains to be investigated whether this is a compound or a class effect. Taken together, the present study strongly suggests that hypertensive patients with impaired glucose metabolism benefit from the treatment with ARB respective to their metabolic condition.

E. Oetjen, MD

Body Weight, Not Insulin Sensitivity or Secretion, May Predict Spontaneous Weight Changes in Nondiabetic and Prediabetic Subjects: The RISC Study

Rebelos E, Muscelli E, Natali A, et al (Univ of Pisa, Italy; et al)
Diabetes 60:1938-1945, 2011

Objective.—Previous studies have found that high insulin sensitivity predicts weight gain; this association has not been confirmed. Our aim was to systematically analyze metabolic predictors of spontaneous weight changes.

Research Design and Methods.—In 561 women and 467 men from the Relationship Between Insulin Sensitivity and Cardiovascular Disease (RISC) cohort (mean age 44 years, BMI range 19—44 kg/m^2, 9% impaired glucose tolerance) followed up for 3 years, we measured insulin sensitivity (by a euglycemic clamp) and β-cell function (by modeling of the C-peptide response to oral glucose and by acute insulin response to intravenous glucose).

Results.—Insulin sensitivity was similar in weight gainers (top 20% of the distribution of BMI changes), weight losers (bottom 20%), and weight stable subjects across quartiles of baseline BMI. By multiple logistic or linear regression analyses controlling for center, age, sex, and baseline BMI, neither insulin sensitivity nor any β-cell function parameter showed an independent association with weight gain; this was true in normal glucose tolerance, impaired glucose tolerance, and whether subjects progressed to dysglycemia or not. Baseline BMI was significantly higher in gainers (26.1 ± 4.1 kg/m^2) and losers (26.6 ± 3.7 kg/m^2) than in weight stable subjects (24.8 ± 3.8 kg/m^2, $P < 0.0001$ for both gainers and losers). Baseline waist circumference (or equivalently, BMI or weight) was a positive, independent predictor of both weight gain and weight loss (odds ratio 1.48 [95% CI 1.12—1.97]) in men and (1.67 [1.28—2.12]) in women. In men only, better insulin sensitivity was an additional independent predictor of weight loss.

Conclusions.—Neither insulin sensitivity nor insulin secretion predicts spontaneous weight gain. Individuals who have attained a higher weight are prone to either gaining or losing weight regardless of their glucose tolerance.

▶ When uncontrolled, weight gain might result in obesity and ultimately in diabetes and cardiovascular disease. Thus, to identify risk factors for weight gain will help to prevent obesity. In contrast to other studies, that by Rebelos et al in an essentially healthy European cohort shows that body weight alone, and not insulin sensitivity, is a predictor of spontaneous weight changes. People with a higher body weight were more prone to gain or to lose weight than people with a lower body weight. This suggests that a stable weight protects against obesity and argues against a strict weight-reducing diet, which might result in yo-yo dieting and ultimately in obesity.

E. Oetjen, MD

Quantification of sleep behavior and of its impact on the cross-talk between the brain and peripheral metabolism

Hanlon EC, Van Cauter E (Univ of Chicago, IL)
Proc Natl Acad Sci U S A 108:15609-15616, 2011

Rates of obesity have been steadily increasing, along with disorders commonly associated with obesity, such as cardiovascular disease and type II diabetes. Simultaneously, average sleep times have progressively decreased. Recently, evidence from both laboratory and epidemiologic studies has suggested that insufficient sleep may stimulate overeating and thus play a role in the current epidemic of obesity and diabetes. In the human sleep laboratory it is now possible to carefully control sleep behavior and study the link between sleep duration and alterations in circulating hormones involved in feeding behavior, glucose metabolism, hunger, and appetite. This article focuses on the methodologies used in experimental protocols that have examined modifications produced by sleep restriction (or extension) compared with normal sleep. The findings provide evidence that sleep restriction does indeed impair glucose metabolism and alters the cross-talk between the periphery and the brain, favoring excessive food intake. A better understanding of the adverse effects of sleep restriction on the CNS control of hunger and appetite may have important implications for public health.

▶ It is obvious that our modern lifestyle is associated with increased risk of obesity and diabetes. It is not only the increased food intake and the decreased physical exertion but also loss of sleep that impair metabolism and contribute to obesity. The article by Hanlon and Van Cauter provides evidence that indeed the duration of sleep interferes with metabolism. However, more studies on the molecular and clinical basis are needed to elucidate how sleep and its quality interfere with satiety, hunger, and the peripheral metabolism.

E. Oetjen, MD

Incretin Effects on β-Cell Function, Replication, and Mass: The human perspective

Garber AJ (Baylor College of Medicine, Houston, TX)
Diabetes Care 34:S258-S263, 2011

Background.—Patients with type 2 diabetes show a progressive deterioration in β-cell function, having islet function levels at diagnosis that are often 50% of those shown by healthy controls and β-cell mass reduced as much as 60% from normal. As a result, patients must take multiple drugs and often eventually require insulin injections. Incretin hormones are released from the gastrointestinal tract after a meal and enhance glucose-dependent insulin secretion from the pancreas, helping to regulate glucose homeostasis in healthy subjects. These hormones, especially glucagon-like peptide (GLP)-1, offer protective effects to β-cells, such as reducing apoptosis and enhancing β-cell proliferation and neogenesis. GLP-1 receptor agonists such as exenatide and liraglutide may achieve durable glycemic control of diabetes while limiting the microvascular and macrovascular complications that often accompany type 2 diabetes.

Clinical Findings in Type 2 Diabetes.—Persons with type 2 diabetes experience a progressive decline in β-cell mass and function that begins well before they develop chronic hyperglycemia and are diagnosed with diabetes. Most current therapies focus on impaired glucose action or stimulate insulin secretion, even though the decline in β-cell mass and function is what causes most antidiabetic agents to fail. Some agents also accelerate β-cell failure and promote weight gain, further exacerbating the diabetes. Modifying β-cell loss and deterioration would target the primary defect.

Pancreatic β-cells secrete insulin at low levels between meals and higher levels after meals. Meal-related insulin secretion occurs in an immediate phase that reduces basal glucagon secretion and a second phase about 10 minutes later that is sustained until normal blood glucose levels are restored. Patients with type 2 diabetes have no or a severely blunted first phase, although fasting insulin levels can be higher than normal. A balance between cell replication, neogenesis, and apoptosis is needed to maintain β-cell mass. Patients with type 2 diabetes have levels of apoptosis that outweigh cell renewal processes and lose β-cell mass as a result.

Effects of Incretin Hormones.—The incretin hormones GLP-1 and glucose-dependent insulinotropic polypeptide (GIP) are secreted by the intestine in response to energy intake and glucose and may potentiate up to 70% of the meal-induced insulin response in healthy persons. This response is reduced by up to 50% in type 2 diabetes. Because pharmacologic GIP levels only marginally stimulate insulin secretion in type 2 diabetes, the focus has been on GLP-1 as a potential pharmacologic agent to manage type 2 diabetes. Infusing GLP-1 at pharmacologic levels (1 pmol/kg/min) increases late-phase insulin response to levels similar to those of healthy persons. GLP-1 improves tolerance in animal diabetic models at least in part because of changes in β-cell mass. However, animals and humans differ significantly in islet cell turnover and growth rates and capacities, so findings from animal studies cannot simply be extended to humans.

Liraglutide and exentide are GLP-1 receptor agonists associated with beneficial effects. Exenatide has a relatively short half-life and is given twice a day. Liraglutide given subcutaneously can be administered once daily. These agents lower A1C, improve other markers of glycemia, and exert direct and indirect effects on β-cell function, volume, and morphology. Both significantly increase β-cell mass and differentiation in rodents and reduce β-cell apoptosis in vitro, effectively protecting β-cell mass in type 2 diabetes.

Conclusions.—Deterioration in β-cell mass and function is critical in type 2 diabetes and must be addressed to alter the natural history of this disease. Incretin therapies offer promise as a way to target this primary defect.

▶ It is now generally accepted that there is a progressive loss of β-cell function and mass in type 2 diabetes. Therefore, a therapy that aims at preventing or at least retarding the deterioration of β-cells seems the most forward strategy. Agonists of the glucagon-like protein-1 (GLP-1) receptor or dipeptidyl-peptidase-4 inhibitors increase not only glucose-induced insulin secretion but also have been shown to exert β-cell protective effect in vitro and in rodents. This review article summarizes the arguments for a β-cell protective effect of GLP-1 receptor agonists in humans. It should be noted that this evidence has to be carefully evaluated because no direct measurement of β-cell mass in humans by noninvasive methods is available. Unfortunately, possible undesired side effects of GLP-1 agonists are not mentioned.

E. Oetjen, MD

Long-Term Persistence of Hormonal Adaptations to Weight Loss
Sumithran P, Prendergast LA, Delbridge E, et al (Univ of Melbourne, Victoria, Australia; La Trobe Univ, Melbourne, Victoria, Australia)
N Engl J Med 365:1597-1604, 2011

Background.—After weight loss, changes in the circulating levels of several peripheral hormones involved in the homeostatic regulation of body weight occur. Whether these changes are transient or persist over time may be important for an understanding of the reasons behind the high rate of weight regain after diet-induced weight loss.

Methods.—We enrolled 50 overweight or obese patients without diabetes in a 10-week weight-loss program for which a very-low-energy diet was prescribed. At baseline (before weight loss), at 10 weeks (after program completion), and at 62 weeks, we examined circulating levels of leptin, ghrelin, peptide YY, gastric inhibitory polypeptide, glucagon-like peptide 1, amylin, pancreatic polypeptide, cholecystokinin, and insulin and subjective ratings of appetite.

Results.—Weight loss (mean [$\pm$SE], 13.5 ± 0.5 kg) led to significant reductions in levels of leptin, peptide YY, cholecystokinin, insulin ($P<0.001$ for all comparisons), and amylin ($P = 0.002$) and to increases in levels of ghrelin ($P<0.001$), gastric inhibitory polypeptide ($P = 0.004$), and pancreatic polypeptide ($P = 0.008$). There was also a significant increase in subjective appetite ($P<0.001$). One year after the initial weight loss, there were still significant differences from baseline in the mean levels of leptin ($P<0.001$), peptide YY ($P<0.001$), cholecystokinin ($P=0.04$), insulin ($P = 0.01$), ghrelin ($P<0.001$), gastric inhibitory polypeptide ($P<0.001$), and pancreatic polypeptide ($P = 0.002$), as well as hunger ($P<0.001$).

Conclusions.—One year after initial weight reduction, levels of the circulating mediators of appetite that encourage weight regain after diet-induced weight loss do not revert to the levels recorded before weight loss. Long-term strategies to counteract this change may be needed to prevent obesity relapse. (Funded by the National Health and Medical Research Council and others; ClinicalTrials.gov number, NCT00870259.)

▶ Nearly everyone has already experienced it: it is much easier to lose weight than keep the reduced weight. This is especially strenuous for obese people. The study by Sumithran et al conducted in 50 obese people sheds light on some of the underlying reasons—namely, that the circulating mediators of appetite are still increased 1 year after diet-induced weight reduction. Thus, inhibiting the effects of these mediators might help to prevent weight gain and relapse into obesity. It remains to be investigated whether mediators of appetite are also increased in people with a body mass index between 25 and 30 kg/m^2 and how long this increase persists. In addition, the duration of the obese state should be considered.

E. Oetjen, MD

Prospective Associations of Vitamin D With β-Cell Function and Glycemia: The PROspective Metabolism and ISlet cell Evaluation (PROMISE) Cohort Study

Kayaniyil S, Retnakaran R, Harris SB, et al (Univ of Toronto, Ontario, Canada; Univ of Western Ontario, London, Ontario, Canada; et al)
Diabetes 60:2947-2953, 2011

Objective.—To examine the prospective associations of baseline vitamin D [25-hydroxyvitamin D; 25(OH)D] with insulin resistance (IR), β-cell function, and glucose homeostasis in subjects at risk for type 2 diabetes.

Research Design and Methods.—We followed 489 subjects, aged 50 ± 10 years, for 3 years. At baseline and follow-up, 75-g oral glucose tolerance tests (OGTTs) were administered. IR was measured using the Matsuda index (IS$_{OGTT}$) and the homeostasis model assessment of IR (HOMA-IR), β-cell function was determined using both the insulinogenic index divided by HOMA-IR (IGI/IR) and the insulin secretion sensitivity index-2 (ISSI-2), and glycemia was assessed using the area under the glucose curve (AUC$_{glucose}$). Regression models were adjusted for age, sex, ethnicity, season, and baseline value of the outcome variable, as well as baseline and change in physical activity, vitamin D supplement use, and BMI.

Results.—Multivariate linear regression analyses indicated no significant association of baseline 25(OH)D with follow-up IS$_{OGTT}$ or HOMA-IR. There were, however, significant positive associations of baseline 25(OH) D with follow-up IGI/IR (β = 0.005, P = 0.015) and ISSI-2 (β = 0.002, P = 0.023) and a significant inverse association of baseline 25(OH)D with follow-up AUC$_{glucose}$ (β = −0.001, P = 0.007). Progression to dysglycemia (impaired fasting glucose, impaired glucose tolerance, or type 2 diabetes) occurred in 116 subjects. Logistic regression analyses indicated a significant reduced risk of progression with higher baseline 25(OH)D (adjusted odds ratio 0.69 [95% CI 0.53−0.89]), but this association was not significant after additional adjustment for baseline and change in BMI (0.78 [0.59−1.02]).

Conclusions.—Higher baseline 25(OH)D independently predicted better β-cell function and lower $AUC_{glucose}$ at follow-up, supporting a potential role for vitamin D in type 2 diabetes etiology.

▶ It is controversially discussed whether a vitamin D deficiency is associated with the development of the metabolic syndrome and diabetes. In the PROspective Metabolism and Islet cell Evaluation (PROMISE) Cohort Study it was found that a higher baseline vitamin D level predicted a better β-cell function at a 3-year follow-up. It should be noted, that vitamin D levels were measured only at baseline and not at the follow-up and that β-cell function and insulin resistance were determined by oral glucose tolerance tests. However, this cohort consisted of approximately 500 subjects with high risk for diabetes. Clearly, more prospective studies will be needed to evaluate whether vitamin D supplement might at least retard the development of diabetes type 2.

E. Oetjen, MD

Noninvasive MRI of β-cell function using a Zn^{2+}-responsive contrast agent
Lubag AJM, De Leon-Rodriguez LM, Burgess SC, et al (Univ of Texas Southwestern Med Ctr, Dallas)
Proc Natl Acad Sci U S A 108:18400-18405, 2011

Elevation of postprandial glucose stimulates release of insulin from granules stored in pancreatic islet β-cells. We demonstrate here that divalent zinc ions coreleased with insulin from β-cells in response to high glucose are readily detected by MRI using the Zn^{2+}-responsive T_1 agent, GdDOTA-diBPEN. Image contrast was significantly enhanced in the mouse pancreas after injection of a bolus of glucose followed by a low dose of the Zn^{2+} sensor. Images of the pancreas were not enhanced by the agent in mice without addition of glucose to stimulate insulin release, nor were images enhanced in streptozotocin-treated mice with or without added glucose. These observations are consistent with MRI detection of Zn^{2+} released from β-cells only during glucose-stimulated insulin secretion. Images of mice fed a high-fat (60%) diet over a 12-wk period and subjected to this same imaging protocol showed a larger volume of contrast-enhanced pancreatic tissue, consistent with the expansion of pancreatic β-cell mass during fat accumulation and progression to type 2 diabetes. This MRI sensor offers the exciting potential for deep-tissue monitoring of β-cell function in vivo during development of type 2 diabetes or after implantation of islets in type I diabetic patients.

▶ The noninvasive imaging of beta cell mass and function in a living organism represents a promising method to evaluate an organism's risk to develop diabetes. Such a technique might be used to screen for prediabetic conditions in an early state and to then start the appropriate measures to prevent or at least retard loss of functional beta cell mass and diabetes. However, depiction of the pancreas and the beta cells within is hampered by its retroperitoneal location. In an elegant study, Lubag et al used a gadolinium-based zinc sensor to detect the mass and function of beta cells by MRI. Since zinc is secreted together with insulin on glucose stimulation, this method is suitable to detect time and amount of secreted insulin. It remains to be seen whether this technique is applicable to humans as well. In addition, an MRI-based technique is too expensive for a population-wide screening.

E. Oetjen, MD

Detection of β cell death in diabetes using differentially methylated circulating DNA
Akirav EM, Lebastchi J, Galvan EM, et al (Yale Univ School of Medicine, New Haven, CT; et al)
Proc Natl Acad Sci U S A 108:19018-19023, 2011

In diabetes mellitus, β cell destruction is largely silent and can be detected only after significant loss of insulin secretion capacity. We have developed a method for detecting β cell death in vivo by amplifying and measuring the proportion of insulin 1 DNA from β cells in the serum. By using primers that are specific for DNA methylation patterns in β cells, we have detected circulating copies of β cell-derived demethylated DNA in serum of mice by quantitative PCR. Accordingly, we have identified a relative increase of β cell-derived DNA after induction of diabetes with streptozotocin and during development of diabetes in nonobese diabetic mice. We have extended the use of this assay to measure β cell-derived insulin DNA in human tissues and serum. We found increased levels of demethylated insulin DNA in subjects with new-onset type 1 diabetes compared with age-matched control subjects. Our method provides a noninvasive approach for detecting β cell death in vivo that may be used to track the progression of diabetes and guide its treatment.

▶ Diabetes is not detected until fasting blood glucose levels are increased. At that point, approximately 50% of functional beta-cell mass is already destroyed, and thus the diagnosis often comes too late. An easy, reliable parameter to determine beta-cell death would help detect an early decline in beta-cell mass, allowing the physician to take appropriate measures to prevent or at least retard further deterioration. Akirav et al present a new assay to detect beta-cell death in the serum of patients with newly diagnosed type 1 diabetes. It would be interesting to see whether this assay is reliable in larger cohorts and in cohorts of patients in the prediabetic state or with diabetes type 2. It should be noted that at least in type 2 diabetes, a loss of beta-cell function such as disturbed insulin secretion kinetics often precedes beta-cell death.

E. Oetjen, MD

2 Lipoproteins and Atherosclerosis

Introduction

This year's section on Lipoproteins and Atherosclerosis offers up a variety of fascinating findings that lend considerable complexity to the decision making requisite to the clinical management of dyslipidemia in both the primary and secondary prevention settings. Many of these new studies will trigger and intensify furious debate about the role of specific therapies in the management of dyslipidemia, but also lend some reassurance about long-term safety and efficacy. In addition, there will be renewed focus on the need to address abnormalities in non-HDL-C, HDL-C, apoprotein B, and lipoprotein(a) in order to reduce residual risk.

A number of important analyses of statin trials help to clarify some nagging issues with these drugs. An issue that concerns the majority of clinicians is the observation that the statins as a drug class increase risk for type 2 diabetes mellitus. Preiss et al present a compelling analysis that compares patients treated with moderate dose and high dose statin therapy. They conclude that despite an increased signal for new onset diabetes, the benefits of statin therapy still outweigh the risks when comparing numbers needed to treat and numbers needed to harm. The Cholesterol Treatment Trialists Collaboration demonstrates in a meta-analysis of 175 000 patients enrolled in statin trials that statin therapy does not increase risk for any type of cancer. In a 6-year follow-up study of subjects enrolled in the Heart Protection Study, there was persistence of in-trial survival benefit with no increase in the detectable incidence of nonvascular morbidity or mortality. This is quite reassuring, especially now that many patients are about to enter one or two decades of statin therapy. Despite multiple negative randomized studies evaluating the impact of lipid-lowering therapy in patients with renal disease, the SHARP trial demonstrates a significant reduction in major cardiovascular events in patients with chronic kidney disease. Risk reduction in the study was proportional to magnitude of LDL-C reduction, suggesting that ezetimibe contributed to endpoint reductions. Flint and coworkers show that statin therapy reduces ischemic stroke mortality significantly; in contrast, discontinuing a statin for any reason during hospitalization for a stroke is significantly associated with increased mortality and poorer neurological outcomes. In addition, high-dose statin therapy in the setting of ischemic stroke outperformed moderate dose statin therapy.

Debate continues to rage over the role of HDL-C management in patients with dyslipidemia. The AIM HIGH trial was discontinued early due to futility and possible increased hazard from niacin therapy secondary to a trend for increased risk of ischemic stroke. The result was stunning, especially in view of the apparent benefit of niacin therapy in multiple smaller trials. The trial did not, however, disprove the HDL hypothesis. It does show that, among patients achieving the most stringent targets for LDL-C, non-HDL-C, and apoprotein B, the addition of high-dose niacin does not provide incremental benefit, at least over three years of follow-up. Work with the cholesterol ester transfer protein inhibitors continues. The newest entry for this drug class is evacetrapib. Nicholls and coworkers show that this drug is safe, well tolerated, and provides HDL-C elevation and LDL-C reduction on par with anacetrapib. All of these drugs will have to undergo testing in hard outcome trials before they will see the light of day in clinical practice. Haase and colleagues continue to make important contributions to our understanding of the molecular genetics of HDL. In an important new investigation, they show that, based on two large, well-defined cohorts from Copenhagen, Denmark, a low serum HDL-C stemming from a deficiency in lecithin cholesterol:acyltransferase does not increase risk for cardiovascular disease as expected. It is well known in the fields of endocrinology and cardiology that Asian patients with low HDL-C are at increased risk for premature multivessel coronary artery disease. In an important analysis by Huxley et al, it is shown that a low HDL-C in these patients incurs the same risk for coronary disease as a combination of either elevated LDL-C or triglyceride with low HDL-C. This constitutes a very important contribution to the management of dyslipidemia in Asian patients.

Quantifying the relative importance of atherogenic lipoproteins remains an area of major investigation. In an important meta-analysis of eight statin trials by Boekholdt et al, it is shown that patients on statin therapy with LDL-C < 100 mg/dL and non-HDL-C > 130 mg/dL have a higher risk for cardiovascular events than patients with LDL > 100 mg/dL but non-HDL-C < 130 mg/dL. Moreover, non-HDL-C reduction impacted risk more than the reductions in LDL-C or apoB. New data from the Women's Health Study show that among women in the lowest tertile for apoB, low HDL-C is no longer predictive of increased cardiovascular risk. In a post hoc analysis of patients given statin therapy in the JUPITER trial, among those achieving LDL-C < 70 mg/dL, non-HDL-C < 100 mg/dL, or apoB < 80 mg/dL, there was minimal residual risk attributable to triglycerides or other lipoproteins or apoproteins, results that are in line with AIM HIGH.

Metabolic syndrome is clearly associated with increased risk for diabetes and cardiovascular disease. Wong et al demonstrate that nonalcoholic fatty liver disease increases risk for coronary disease 2.3 fold. Analyses of patients enrolled in the placebo arm of the FIELD trial demonstrate that increased waist circumference was not associated with increased risk for cardiovascular events. The combination of high triglycerides and low HDL-C increased CV risk by 41% and an increasing number of metabolic syndrome components correlated with increased risk for CV events in the group without prior cardiovascular disease.

Finally, Sacks demonstrates that LDL particles enriched with apo CIII are significantly more atherogenic than those particles without apo CIII. It is well known that serum lipid concentrations generally correlate poorly with risk for ischemic stroke. Nasr et al show that serum lipoprotein(a) levels correlate highly with risk for obstructive disease in the carotid arteries in young adults. Finally, investigators from the Atherosclerosis Risk in Communities Study find that Lp(a) is at least as strong a risk factor for stroke in Blacks as it is in Whites.

Peter P. Toth, MD, PhD

Epidemiology and Diagnosis

Low-Density Lipoproteins Containing Apolipoprotein C-III and the Risk of Coronary Heart Disease

Mendivil CO, Rimm EB, Furtado J, et al (Harvard School of Public Health, Boston, MA)
Circulation 124:2065-2072, 2011

Background.—Low-density lipoprotein (LDL) that contains apolipoprotein (apo) C-III makes up only 10% to 20% of plasma LDL but has a markedly altered metabolism and proatherogenic effects on vascular cells.

Methods and Results.—We examined the association between plasma LDL with apoC-III and coronary heart disease in 320 women and 419 men initially free of cardiovascular disease who developed a fatal or nonfatal myocardial infarction during 10 to 14 years of follow-up and matched controls who remained free of coronary heart disease. Concentrations of LDL with apoC-III (measured as apoB in this fraction) were associated with risk of coronary heart disease in multivariable analysis that included the ratio of total cholesterol to high-density lipoprotein cholesterol, LDL cholesterol, apoB, triglycerides, or high-density lipoprotein cholesterol and other risk factors. In all models, the relative risks for the top versus bottom quintile of LDL with apoC-III were greater than those for LDL without apoC-III. When included in the same multivariable-adjusted model, the risk associated with LDL with apoC-III (relative risk for top versus bottom quintile, 2.38; 95% confidence interval, 1.54–3.68; P for trend <0.001) was significantly greater than that associated with LDL without apoC-III (relative risk for top versus bottom quintile, 1.25; 95% confidence interval, 0.76–2.05; P for trend=0.97; P for interaction <0.001). This divergence in association with coronary heart disease persisted even after adjustment for plasma triglycerides.

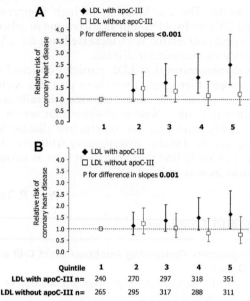

FIGURE 2.—Relative risk of coronary heart disease during follow-up in the complete study sample, mutually adjusting for apolipoprotein (apo) B in low-density lipoprotein (LDL) with and without apoC-III. Relative risks and 95% confidence intervals are given for each quintile vs the lowest quintile. **A**, The model was also adjusted for matching factors, presence or absence of a parental history of coronary heart disease before 60 years of age, alcohol intake, and personal history of hypertension. **B**, The model was adjusted for all variables in **A** plus personal history of diabetes mellitus and plasma triglycerides. Dark diamonds represent LDL with apoC-III; *P* for trend <0.001 in **A** and *P* for trend=0.07 in **B**. Light squares represent LDL without apoC-III; *P* for trend=0.97 in **A** and *P* for trend=0.22 in **B**. *P*<0.001 for difference in slopes in **A** and *P*=0.001 for difference in slopes in **B**. (Reprinted from Mendivil CO, Rimm EB, Furtado J, et al. Low-density lipoproteins containing apolipoprotein C-III and the risk of coronary heart disease. *Circulation.* 2011;124:2065-2072, with permission from American Heart Association, Inc.)

Conclusions.—The risk of coronary heart disease contributed by LDL appeared to result to a large extent from LDL that contains apoC-III (Fig 2, Table 2).

▶ Apoprotein (apo) CIII has diverse deleterious functions. It is carried in multiple lipoproteins, including very low-density lipoproteins (VLDLs), LDLS, chylomicrons, and high-density lipoprotein (HDLs). Its expression tends to be increased in the setting of insulin resistance.[1] ApoCIII potentiates hypertriglyceridemia by inhibiting lipoprotein lipase and blocking the ability of hepatic receptors to clear VLDL and its remnants. ApoCIII also appears to be directly atherogenic by stimulating endothelial expression of adhesion molecules,[2] activating nuclear factor kappa B,[3] and reducing endothelial nitric oxide production and promoting endothelial cell insulin resistance by inhibiting the tyrosine phosphorylation of insulin receptor substrate-1.[4]

Sacks et al compared the relationship between risk for cardiovascular events and serum levels of LDL particles containing apoCIII or containing no apoCIII. Serum was analyzed from 350 women in the Nurse's Health Study (NHS) and 425 men in the Health Professionals Follow-up Study (HPFS) who were initially

TABLE 2.—Relative Risks of Coronary Heart Disease During Follow-Up in the Complete Study Sample, According to the Quintile of Low-Density Lipoprotein Types (as Measured by the Apolipoprotein B Concentration in Each Fraction) or Apolipoprotein Concentrations at Baseline

	Quintile Categories					P for Trend[†]	P for Difference Between Sexes[‡]
	1	2	3	4	5		
LDL with apoC-III							
n	240	270	297	318	351		
Model 1*	1.00 (Ref)	1.38 (0.96–1.98)	1.71 (1.2–2.44)	2.12 (1.46–3.08)	2.58 (1.78–3.74)	<0.001	0.74
Model 2	1.00 (Ref)	1.32 (0.89–1.98)	1.65 (1.11–2.45)	1.99 (1.32–3.00)	2.41 (1.60–3.64)	<0.001	0.97
Model 3	1.00 (Ref)	1.28 (0.86–1.91)	1.57 (1.06–2.32)	1.87 (1.24–2.81)	2.23 (1.48–3.37)	<0.001	0.72
Model 4	1.00 (Ref)	1.16 (0.77–1.74)	1.35 (0.90–2.03)	1.50 (0.97–2.31)	1.64 (1.03–2.60)	<0.001	0.56
LDL without apoC-III							
n	265	295	317	288	311		
Model 1	1.00 (Ref)	1.4 (0.98–2.00)	1.60 (1.11–2.32)	1.38 (0.94–2.03)	1.72 (1.14–2.61)	0.06	0.09
Model 2	1.00 (Ref)	1.58 (1.05–2.38)	1.58 (1.04–2.40)	1.46 (0.95–2.25)	1.78 (1.11–2.84)	0.12	0.053
Model 3	1.00 (Ref)	1.58 (1.06–2.36)	1.57 (1.04–2.38)	1.49 (0.97–2.28)	1.72 (1.08–2.75)	0.13	0.039
Model 4	1.00 (Ref)	1.53 (1.02–2.31)	1.45 (0.96–2.21)	1.36 (0.88–2.10)	1.44 (0.89–2.32)	0.29	0.032
ApoC-III in LDL							
n	274	270	282	308	342		
Model 1	1.00 (Ref)	1.03 (0.72–1.47)	1.16 (0.81–1.67)	1.56 (1.07–2.29)	2.10 (1.41–3.14)	<0.001	0.88
Model 2	1.00 (Ref)	1.1 (0.75–1.63)	1.25 (0.84–1.84)	1.53 (1.01–2.32)	2.19 (1.42–3.38)	<0.001	0.65
Model 3	1.00 (Ref)	1.03 (0.69–1.53)	1.15 (0.77–1.71)	1.45 (0.95–2.21)	1.97 (1.26–3.06)	0.002	0.50
Model 4	1.00 (Ref)	0.98 (0.66–1.46)	0.96 (0.64–1.46)	1.15 (0.74–1.80)	1.33 (0.81–2.20)	0.004	0.43
Total plasma apoC-III							
n	279	296	285	286	330		
Model 1	1.00 (Ref)	1.21 (0.85–1.72)	1.11 (0.78–1.58)	1.15 (0.79–1.67)	1.60 (1.09–2.37)	0.016	0.23
Model 2	1.00 (Ref)	1.17 (0.80–1.71)	1.11 (0.76–1.64)	1.12 (0.75–1.68)	1.62 (1.06–2.48)	0.023	0.36
Model 3	1.00 (Ref)	1.18 (0.80–1.75)	1.12 (0.76–1.66)	1.11 (0.73–1.68)	1.48 (0.96–2.28)	0.085	0.40
Model 4	1.00 (Ref)	1.01 (0.68–1.51)	0.90 (0.6–1.36)	0.79 (0.50–1.24)	0.96 (0.60–1.56)	0.45	0.18

LDL indicates low-density lipoprotein; apo, apolipoproteins. Relative risks and 95% confidence intervals are given for each quintile compared with the lowest quintile of each apolipoprotein measurement. The group of women included 320 cases and 320 controls with 14 years of follow-up. The group of men included 419 cases and 419 controls with 10 years of follow-up. Quintiles and median values of apolipoprotein levels are based on values in controls. For each relative risk, quintile 1 served as the reference group. Matching factors were: age, smoking status, and the month of blood sampling. Among women, data were also adjusted for fasting status at the time of blood sampling.

*Model 1 is conditioned only on matching factors. Model 2 is also adjusted for the presence or absence of a parental history of coronary heart disease before 60 years of age, alcohol intake, and personal history of hypertension. Model 3 is adjusted for all variables in model 2 plus body mass index and personal history of diabetes mellitus. Model 4 is adjusted for all variables in model 3 plus plasma triglycerides.

[†]P values for trend are based on the median levels of apolipoproteins in quintiles of the controls.

[‡]Calculated as the P for the interaction between sex and median apolipoprotein levels in quintiles of the controls.

free of cardiovascular disease but who during the follow-up period either died from cardiovascular causes or sustained a nonfatal myocardial infarction. Compared with patients in the first quintile, those in the highest quintile of LDL-apoCIII or LDL without apoCIII had significant increases in risk for CHD with relative risk of 2.58 and 1.76, respectively. The augmented risk associated with LDL with apoCIII was similar for patients in both the NHS and HPFS, with no apparent gender effect. Increased apoCIII correlated with multiple features of insulin resistance, including high triglycerides, low HDL-C, hypertension, and diabetes mellitus. LDL with apoCIII remained a risk factor for CHD even after controlling for other risk factors (Table 2), including family history of CHD, diabetes mellitus, and triglycerides (Fig 2). Interestingly, LDL with apoCIII was not a significant risk factor in this model.

These results are intriguing, although they are unlikely to influence the next iteration of guidelines for the management of dyslipidemia. They are of great interest as they add to our current understanding about the enormous complexity of lipoprotein metabolism and its relationship to atherosclerosis. Our understanding of the relationship between LDL particles and atherogenesis remains somewhat rudimentary. There are no current recommendations for the routine measurement of apoCIII. At minimum, however, it is likely that among patients with increased LDL-apoCIII, relieving insulin resistance through aggressive lifestyle modification would likely impact serum availability of apoCIII. Much more work will have to be done before this information can become a part of daily clinical practice.

P. P. Toth, MD, PhD

References

1. Cohn JS, Patterson BW, Uffelman KD, Davignon J, Steiner G. Rate of production of plasma and very-low-density lipoprotein (VLDL) apolipoprotein C-III is strongly related to the concentration and level of production of VLDL triglyceride in male subjects with different body weights and levels of insulin sensitivity. *J Clin Endocrinol Metab.* 2004;89:3949-3955.
2. Kawakami A, Aikawa M, Alcaide P, Luscinskas FW, Libby P, Sacks FM. Apolipoprotein CIII induces expression of vascular cell adhesion molecule-1 in vascular endothelial cells and increases adhesion of monocytic cells. *Circulation.* 2006;114:681-687.
3. Sharif O, Bolshakov VN, Raines S, Newham P, Perkins ND. Transcriptional profiling of the LPS induced NF-kappaB response in macrophages. *BMC Immunol.* 2007;8:1.
4. Kawakami A, Osaka M, Tani M, et al. Apolipoprotein CIII links hyperlipidemia with vascular endothelial cell dysfunction. *Circulation.* 2008;118:731-742.

Isolated Low Levels of High-Density Lipoprotein Cholesterol Are Associated with an Increased Risk of Coronary Heart Disease: An Individual Participant Data Meta-Analysis of 23 Studies in the Asia-Pacific Region
Huxley RR, for the Asia Pacific Cohort Studies Collaboration and the Obesity in Asia Collaboration (Univ of Sydney, Australia; et al)
Circulation 124:2056-2064, 2011

Background.—Previous studies have suggested that there is a novel dyslipidemic profile consisting of isolated low high-density lipoprotein cholesterol (HDL-C) level that is associated with increased risk of coronary heart disease, and that this trait may be especially prevalent in Asian populations.

Methods and Results.—Individual participant data from 220 060 participants (87% Asian) in 37 studies from the Asia-Pacific region were included. Low HDL-C (HDL <1.03 mmol/L in men and <1.30 mmol/L in women) was seen among 33.1% (95% confidence interval [CI], 32.9−33.3) of Asians versus 27.0% (95% CI, 26.5−27.5) of non-Asians (*P*<0.001). The prevalence of low HDL-C in the absence of other lipid abnormalities (isolated low HDL-C) was higher in Asians compared with non-Asians: 22.4% (95% CI, 22.2−22.5) versus 14.5% (95% CI, 14.1−14.9), respectively (*P*<0.001). During 6.8 years of follow-up, there were 574 coronary heart disease and 739 stroke events. There was an inverse relationship between low HDL-C with coronary heart disease in all individuals (hazard ratio, 1.57; 95% CI, 1.31−1.87). In Asians, isolated low levels of HDL-C were as strongly associated with coronary heart disease risk as low levels of HDL-C combined with other lipid abnormalities (hazard ratio, 1.67 [95% CI, 1.27−2.19] versus 1.63 [95% CI, 1.24−2.15], respectively). There was no association between low HDL-C and stroke risk in this population (hazard ratio, 0.95 [95% CI, 0.78 to 1.17] with nonisolated low HDL-C and 0.81 [95% CI, 0.67−1.00] with isolated low HDL-C).

Conclusion.—Isolated low HDL-C is a novel lipid phenotype that appears to be more prevalent among Asian populations, in whom it is associated with increased coronary risk. Further investigation into this type of dyslipidemia is warranted (Figs 1 and 2).

▶ There is a well-known inverse relationship between risk for coronary heart disease (CHD) and serum levels of high-density lipoprotein cholesterol (HDL-C) that is remarkably consistent in men and women and in all racial and ethnic groups yet evaluated.[1-4] Among Asian populations, isolated low HDL-C

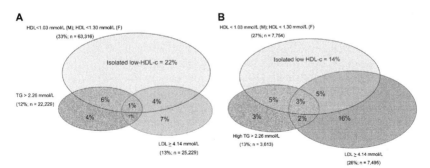

FIGURE 1.—**A** and **B**, Prevalence of lipid phenotypes in adult Asian populations (**A**; n=191 317) and adult populations from Australia and New Zealand (**B**; n=28 743). HDL indicates high-density lipoprotein; HDL-C, HDL cholesterol; LDL, low-density lipoprotein; and TG, triglycerides. (Reprinted from Huxley RR, for the Asia Pacific Cohort Studies Collaboration and the Obesity in Asia Collaboration. Isolated low levels of high-density lipoprotein cholesterol are associated with an increased risk of coronary heart disease: an individual participant data meta-analysis of 23 studies in the asia-pacific region. *Circulation.* 2011;124:2056-2064, Copyright 2011, with permission from American Heart Association, Inc.)

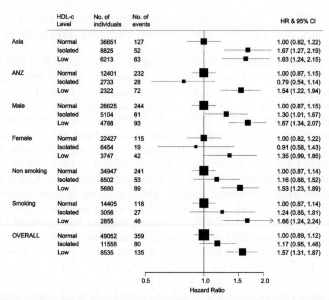

HDL-c Level	No. of individuals	No. of events	HR & 95% CI
Asia			
Normal	36651	127	1.00 (0.82, 1.22)
Isolated	8825	52	1.67 (1.27, 2.19)
Low	6213	63	1.63 (1.24, 2.15)
ANZ			
Normal	12401	232	1.00 (0.87, 1.15)
Isolated	2733	28	0.79 (0.54, 1.14)
Low	2322	72	1.54 (1.22, 1.94)
Male			
Normal	26625	244	1.00 (0.87, 1.15)
Isolated	5104	61	1.30 (1.01, 1.67)
Low	4788	93	1.67 (1.34, 2.07)
Female			
Normal	22427	115	1.00 (0.82, 1.22)
Isolated	6454	19	0.91 (0.58, 1.43)
Low	3747	42	1.35 (0.99, 1.85)
Non smoking			
Normal	34947	241	1.00 (0.87, 1.14)
Isolated	8502	53	1.16 (0.88, 1.52)
Low	5680	89	1.53 (1.23, 1.89)
Smoking			
Normal	14405	118	1.00 (0.87, 1.14)
Isolated	3056	27	1.24 (0.85, 1.81)
Low	2855	46	1.66 (1.24, 2.24)
OVERALL			
Normal	49052	359	1.00 (0.89, 1.12)
Isolated	11558	80	1.17 (0.95, 1.46)
Low	8535	135	1.57 (1.31, 1.87)

0.5   1.0   1.5   2.0
Hazard Ratio

FIGURE 2.—Adjusted hazard ratios (HRs) and 95% confidence intervals (CIs) for coronary heart disease associated with high-density lipoprotein cholesterol levels (HDL-C) by region (Asia vs Australia/New Zealand [ANZ]), sex, and smoking status (current vs not) from studies included in the Asia Pacific Cohort Studies Collaboration. Normal HDL-C means normal levels of HDL-C; isolated, isolated low levels of HDL-C; and low, low levels of HDL-C and high LDL-C and/or high triglycerides. The 3 groups are mutually exclusive. P for regional, sex, and smoking interaction=0.016, 0.04, and 0.95, respectively. (Reprinted from Huxley RR, for the Asia Pacific Cohort Studies Collaboration and the Obesity in Asia Collaboration. Isolated low levels of high-density lipoprotein cholesterol are associated with an increased risk of coronary heart disease: an individual participant data meta-analysis of 23 studies in the asia-pacific region. *Circulation.* 2011;124:2056-2064, Copyright 2011, with permission from American Heart Association, Inc.)

(meaning low-density lipoprotein (LDL)-C and triglycerides are "normal" based on risk stratification) appears to be particularly prevalent. This poses a difficult challenge, as no randomized, placebo-controlled trial has specifically targeted a cohort of patients with this phenotype. In the primary prevention trial, AFCAPs/TexCAPs, the use of lovastatin incurred a 3-fold higher reduction in risk for CHD-related events in patients with HDL-C less than 40 mg/dL compared with those with HDL-C greater than 40 mg/dL. This was, however, a post-hoc finding and must be considered hypothesis generating.

The study by Huxley and coworkers carefully evaluates the prevalence of low HDL-C in Asian populations and also estimates the impact of both isolated low HDL-C and low HDL-C combined with either elevated LDL-C or triglycerides. Patients (220 000) were included from the Asia Pacific Cohort Studies Collaboration and the Obesity in Asia Collaboration. Patients were defined as Asian if they lived in mainland China, Hong Kong, India, Japan, Korea, the Philippines, Singapore, South Korea, Taiwan, or Thailand. The incidence of isolated low HDL-C was significantly higher among Asians than non-Asians (patients living in Australia/New Zealand) at 22% and 14%, respectively. Of interest, the incidence of elevated LDL-C was also twice as high in Asians compared with non-Asians (26.1 vs 13.4%, respectively). The specific distribution of lipid abnormalities is shown in Fig 1. In Asians, isolated low HDL-C was as strongly associated with CHD risk as low HDL-C combined with either elevated LDL-C or triglyceride (hazard ratio, 1.67 [95% confidence interval (CI), 1.27−2.19] vs 1.63 [95% CI, 1.24−2.15], respectively) (Fig 2). The risk of CHD in patients with isolated low HDL-C was 20% higher than in those with normal HDL-C levels. Low HDL-C did not predict risk for stroke, a common finding in studies around the world.

This patient-level analysis is the first to quantify the prevalence of low HDL-C in patients living in a large number of Asian countries. Importantly, it also quantifies the excess risk attributable to an isolated low HDL-C and shows that among Asian peoples, an isolated low HDL-C incurs a level of risk identical to that of patients with combined dyslipidemia. There is urgent need to conduct a prospective, randomized study of patients with isolated low HDL-C to help determine if pharmacologic intervention in the primary prevention setting impacts risk for CHD-related events. In the meantime, close consideration should be given to the use of a statin in these patients because multiple post-hoc analyses have found that patients with low baseline HDL-C tend to derive somewhat greater benefit than patients with normal levels of HDL-C.

P. P. Toth, MD, PhD

References

1. Steyn K, Sliwa K, Hawken S, et al. Risk factors associated with myocardial infarction in Africa: the INTERHEART Africa study. *Circulation.* 2005;112:3554-3561.
2. Yusuf S, Hawken S, Ounpuu S, et al. Effect of potentially modifiable risk factors associated with myocardial infarction in 52 countries (the INTERHEART study): case-control study. *Lancet.* 2004;364:937-952.
3. Castelli WP. Cholesterol and lipids in the risk of coronary artery disease—the Framingham Heart Study. *Can J Cardiol.* 1988;4:5A-10A.
4. Assmann G, Cullen P, Schulte H. The Münster Heart Study (PROCAM). Results of follow-up at 8 years. *Eur Heart J.* 1998;19:A2-A11.

Association of High-Density Lipoprotein Cholesterol With Incident Cardiovascular Events in Women, by Low-Density Lipoprotein Cholesterol and Apolipoprotein B100 Levels: A Cohort Study

Mora S, Buring JE, Ridker PM, et al (Brigham and Women's Hosp, Boston, MA; Merck & Co, North Wales, PA)
Ann Intern Med 155:742-750, 2011

Background.—Prior studies have found inverse associations between high-density lipoprotein cholesterol (HDL-C) or apolipoprotein A-I levels and cardiovascular disease (CVD). Whether this observation is consistent across low-density lipoprotein cholesterol (LDL-C) levels or total atherogenic particle burden (apolipoprotein B100) is less well-studied, particularly in women.

Objective.—To determine the association between HDL-C or apolipoprotein A-I level and CVD across a range of LDL-C and apolipoprotein B100 values.

Design.—Prospective cohort study.

Setting.—The Women's Health Study, a cohort of U.S. female health professionals.

Participants.—26 861 initially healthy women, aged 45 years or older at study entry (1992–1995), who were followed for a mean of approximately 11 years.

Measurements.—Baseline lipids were measured directly, and apolipoproteins were measured with immunoassays. Outcomes were incident total CVD ($n = 929$), coronary events ($n = 602$), and stroke ($n = 319$).

Results.—In multivariable analyses, HDL-C and apolipoprotein A-I levels were inversely associated with CVD and coronary events but not stroke. Adjusted coronary hazard ratios for decreasing quintiles of HDL-C were 1.00 (reference), 1.23 (95% CI, 0.85 to 1.78), 1.42 (CI, 0.98 to 2.06), 1.90 (CI, 1.33 to 2.71), and 2.19 (CI, 1.51 to 3.19) (P for linear trend < 0.001); corresponding hazard ratios for apolipoprotein A-I were 1.00 (reference), 0.98 (CI, 0.71 to 1.35), 1.02 (CI, 0.72 to 1.44), 1.37 (CI, 0.98 to 1.90), and 1.58 (CI, 1.14 to 2.20) (P for linear trend = 0.005). Consistent inverse associations were found for HDL-C with coronary events across a range of LDL-C values, including among women with low LDL-C levels. No associations were noted for HDL-C or apolipoprotein A-I among women with low apolipoprotein B100 values (<0.90 g/L).

Limitation.—Participants were at low risk for CVD, the number of events in the lowest apolipoprotein B100 stratum was small, only a single baseline measurement was obtained, and residual confounding may have occurred.

Conclusion.—Consistent inverse associations were found for HDL-C with incident coronary events among women with a range of LDL-C values. Among women with low total atherogenic particle burden (apolipoprotein B100 level <0.90 g/L), few events occurred and no associations were seen.

Primary Funding Source.—Merck & Co. and the National Heart, Lung, and Blood Institute and National Cancer Institute, National Institutes of Health (Tables 2-4).

▶ The relation between high-density lipoprotein cholesterol (HDL-C) and risk for cardiovascular events is remarkably consistent in prospective observational cohorts followed across the world. There is an inverse relation between risk for myocardial infarction (MI) and coronary mortality in both men and women and people of all racial and ethnic groups.[1-3] This relation does not, however, appear to hold for ischemic stroke.[4] Given the apparent cardiovascular benefit of high serum levels of HDL-C, a large number of therapeutic approaches to raise serum levels of HDL-C are being developed. On the heels of the AIM-HIGH trial[5] comes an important new analysis from the Women's Health Study (WHS), which may help to explain at least in part why niacin therapy failed to provide incremental risk reduction in patients whose atherogenic lipoprotein burden was already treated to the most stringent levels advised by the National Cholesterol Education Program.

TABLE 2.—Association of HDL-C and Apolipoprotein A-I With Cardiovascular Outcomes

Outcome*	>1.60 mmol/L (>61.6 mg/dL)	1.37–1.60 mmol/L (52.8–61.6 mg/dL)	HDL-C Quintile 1.20–1.36 mmol/L (46.2–52.7 mg/dL)	1.03–1.19 mmol/L (39.6–46.1 mg/dL)	≤1.02 mmol/L (≤39.5 mg/dL)	P Value for Linear Trend
Total CVD						
Event rate per 1000 PYs (95% CI)	2.03 (1.74–2.36)	2.38 (2.03–2.79)	2.98 (2.55–3.48)	3.93 (3.42–4.52)	5.57 (4.93–6.29)	
HR (95% CI)						
Age-adjusted	1.0 (reference)	1.21 (0.97–1.51)	1.58 (1.27–1.96)	2.01 (1.63–2.48)	2.86 (2.35–3.49)	<0.001
Model 1[†]	1.0 (reference)	1.16 (0.90–1.48)	1.48 (1.16–1.89)	1.63 (1.28–2.07)	2.33 (1.86–2.93)	<0.001
Model 2[‡]	1.0 (reference)	1.13 (0.85–1.48)	1.29 (0.98–1.71)	1.47 (1.11–1.93)	1.69 (1.27–2.26)	<0.001
CHD[§]						
Event rate per 1000 PYs (95% CI)	1.12 (0.91–1.37)	1.40 (1.14–1.72)	1.86 (1.53–2.26)	2.70 (2.29–3.20)	4.02 (3.48–4.64)	
HR (95% CI)						
Age-adjusted	1.0 (reference)	1.29 (0.96–1.72)	1.77 (1.33–2.36)	2.51 (1.92–3.28)	3.75 (2.92–4.83)	<0.001
Model 1[†]	1.0 (reference)	1.31 (0.94–1.81)	1.72 (1.25–2.36)	2.08 (1.53–2.83)	3.01 (2.24–4.04)	<0.001
Model 2[‡]	1.0 (reference)	1.23 (0.85–1.78)	1.42 (0.98–2.06)	1.90 (1.33–2.71)	2.19 (1.51–3.19)	<0.001
Stroke						
Event rate per 1000 PYs (95% CI)	1.02 (0.82–1.26)	0.90 (0.69–1.16)	1.02 (0.78–1.33)	0.97 (0.73–1.28)	1.62 (1.29–2.02)	
HR (95% CI)						
Age-adjusted	1.0 (reference)	0.91 (0.65–1.28)	1.08 (0.76–1.52)	0.98 (0.69–1.40)	1.64 (1.20–2.24)	0.011
Model 1[†]	1.0 (reference)	0.83 (0.57–1.23)	0.98 (0.66–1.44)	0.80 (0.53–1.21)	1.38 (0.97–1.98)	0.22
Model 2[‡]	1.0 (reference)	0.89 (0.58–1.35)	1.03 (0.67–1.59)	0.83 (0.52–1.32)	1.21 (0.76–1.93)	0.68

Outcome*	>1.60 g/L	1.46–1.60 g/L	Apolipoprotein A-I Quintile 1.35–1.46 g/L	1.24–1.35 g/L	≤1.24 g/L	P Value for Linear Trend
Total CVD						
Event rate per 1000 PYs (95% CI)	2.62 (2.32–2.96)	2.72 (2.33–3.18)	2.87 (2.43–3.39)	3.90 (3.36–4.54)	4.64 (4.04–5.34)	
HR (95% CI)						
Age-adjusted	1.0 (reference)	1.11 (0.91–1.36)	1.19 (0.97–1.46)	1.69 (1.40–2.05)	2.11 (1.75–2.54)	<0.001
Model 1[†]	1.0 (reference)	1.17 (0.94–1.45)	1.05 (0.83–1.33)	1.58 (1.27–1.96)	1.80 (1.45–2.23)	<0.001
Model 2[‡]	1.0 (reference)	1.10 (0.86–1.40)	0.99 (0.75–1.30)	1.40 (1.09–1.81)	1.36 (1.04–1.78)	0.011
CHD[§]						
Event rate per 1000 PYs (95% CI)	1.59 (1.37–1.86)	1.61 (1.31–1.97)	1.91 (1.56–2.34)	2.50 (2.08–3.02)	3.39 (2.88–4.00)	
HR (95% CI)						
Age-adjusted	1.0 (reference)	1.07 (0.83–1.39)	1.30 (1.00–1.67)	1.77 (1.39–2.25)	2.50 (2.00–3.14)	<0.001

(Continued)

TABLE 2.—(Continued)

| | Apolipoprotein A-I Quintile | | | | | |
	>1.60 g/L	1.46–1.60 g/L	1.35–1.46 g/L	1.24–1.35 g/L	≤1.24 g/L	
Model 1[†]	1.0 (reference)	1.11 (0.84–1.47)	1.12 (0.84–1.51)	1.68 (1.28–2.20)	2.09 (1.61–2.71)	<0.001
Model 2[‡]	1.0 (reference)	0.98 (0.71–1.35)	1.02 (0.72–1.44)	1.37 (0.98–1.90)	1.58 (1.14–2.20)	0.005
Stroke						
Event rate per 1000 PYs (95% CI)						
HR (95% CI)						
Age-adjusted	1.12 (0.94–1.35)	1.07 (0.83–1.37)	0.76 (0.55–1.05)	1.15 (0.88–1.52)	1.27 (0.97–1.66)	0.195
Model 1[†]	1.0 (reference)	1.02 (0.75–1.40)	0.73 (0.51–1.06)	1.17 (0.84–1.62)	1.35 (0.97–1.86)	0.64
Model 2[‡]	1.0 (reference)	1.15 (0.82–1.51)	0.73 (0.45–1.18)	1.20 (0.78–1.83)	1.01 (0.64–1.60)	0.93

CHD = coronary heart disease; CVD = cardiovascular disease; HDL-C = high-density lipoprotein cholesterol; HR = hazard ratio; PY = person-year.

*Based on 929 total CVD events, 602 CHD events, and 319 stroke events among 26 861 participants.

†Adjusted for age, race, randomized treatment assignment, smoking status, blood pressure, antihypertensive medication use, fasting status, alcohol use, and family history.

‡Adjusted for the covariates in model 1 plus postmenopausal status, postmenopausal hormone use, body mass index, exercise, diabetes mellitus, high-sensitivity C-reactive protein level, triglyceride level, and low-density lipoprotein cholesterol level.

§Comprising myocardial infarction, coronary revascularization, and deaths from CHD.

TABLE 3.—Association of HDL-C With CHD Events, by LDL-C Tertile*

LDL-C Tertile†	HDL-C Quintile					P Value for Linear Trend
	>1.60 mmol/L (>61.6 mg/dL)	1.37–1.60 mmol/L (52.8–61.6 mg/dL)	1.20–1.36 mmol/L (46.2–52.7 mg/dL)	1.03–1.19 mmol/L (39.6–46.1 mg/dL)	≤1.02 mmol/L (≤39.5 mg/dL)	
Lowest						
CHD event rate per 1000 PYs (95% CI)	0.62 (0.40–0.97)	0.85 (0.54–1.35)	0.77 (0.44–1.35)	1.68 (1.13–2.51)	2.49 (1.93–3.49)	
HR (95% CI)						
Model 1‡	1.0 (reference)	1.48 (0.75–2.95)	1.36 (0.63–2.91)	1.99 (1.00–3.95)	3.22 (1.75–5.92)	<0.001
Model 2§	1.0 (reference)	1.78 (0.77–4.08)	0.98 (0.33–2.84)	2.30 (0.99–5.34)	2.71 (1.14–6.46)	0.031
Middle						
CHD event rate per 1000 PYs (95% CI)	1.16 (0.81–1.65)	1.19 (0.81–1.75)	1.80 (1.28–2.54)	2.38 (1.75–3.25)	4.13 (3.22–5.28)	
HR (95% CI)						
Model 1‡	1.0 (reference)	1.28 (0.71–2.30)	1.97 (1.12–3.44)	2.01 (1.14–3.55)	3.72 (2.22–6.24)	<0.001
Model 2§	1.0 (reference)	1.06 (0.55–2.03)	1.46 (0.77–2.77)	1.98 (1.06–3.69)	2.22 (1.16–4.24)	0.006
Highest						
CHD event rate per 1000 PYs (95% CI)	1.73 (1.27–2.36)	2.14 (1.61–2.86)	2.76 (2.12–3.60)	3.75 (2.97–4.72)	5.59 (4.49–6.96)	
HR (95% CI)						
Model 1‡	1.0 (reference)	1.16 (0.72–1.86)	1.51 (0.95–2.39)	1.94 (1.25–3.02)	2.41 (1.54–3.76)	<0.001
Model 2§	1.0 (reference)	1.13 (0.67–1.91)	1.44 (0.86–2.41)	1.74 (1.04–2.90)	1.75 (1.01–3.04)	0.016

CHD = coronary heart disease; HDL-C = high-density lipoprotein cholesterol; HR = hazard ratio; LDL-C = low-density lipoprotein cholesterol; PY = person-year.

*"CHD events" comprise myocardial infarction, coronary revascularization, and deaths from CHD.

†Lowest tertile, LDL-C level <2.80 mmol/L (<108 mg/dL) (mean, 2.31 mmol/L [89 mg/dL]); middle tertile, 2.80–3.50 mmol/L (108–135 mg/dL) (mean, 3.13 mmol/L [121 mg/dL]); and highest tertile, >3.50 mmol/L (>135 mg/dL) (mean, 4.17 mmol/L [161 mg/dL]). Based on 117 CHD events among 8965 participants in the lowest LDL-C tertile, 192 events among 8948 participants in the middle tertile, and 293 events among 8948 participants in the highest tertile.

‡Adjusted for age, race, randomized treatment assignment, smoking status, blood pressure, antihypertensive medication use, fasting status, alcohol use, and family history.

§Adjusted for the covariates in model 1 plus postmenopausal status, postmenopausal hormone use, body mass index, exercise, diabetes mellitus, high-sensitivity C-reactive protein level, triglyceride level, and LDL-C level.

TABLE 4.—Association of HDL-C With CHD Events, by Apolipoprotein B100 Tertile*

Apolipoprotein B100 Tertile†	HDL-C Quintile					P Value for Linear Trend
	>1.60 mmol/L (>61.6 mg/dL)	1.37–1.60 mmol/L (52.8–61.6 mg/dL)	1.20–1.36 mmol/L (46.2–52.7 mg/dL)	1.03–1.19 mmol/L (39.6–46.1 mg/dL)	≤1.02 mmol/L (≤39.5 mg/dL)	
Lowest						
CHD event rate per 1000 PYs (95% CI)	0.76 (0.53–1.09)	0.63 (0.38–1.04)	0.62 (0.33–1.15)	1.16 (0.69–1.95)	1.10 (0.57–2.11)	
HR (95% CI)						
Model 1‡	1.0 (reference)	1.07 (0.56–2.04)	1.01 (0.48–2.12)	1.20 (0.57–2.54)	1.31 (0.58–2.98)	0.54
Model 2§	1.0 (reference)	1.16 (0.56–2.40)	0.95 (0.39–2.35)	0.95 (0.38–2.34)	0.53 (0.15–1.94)	0.56
Middle						
CHD event rate per 1000 PYs (95% CI)	0.84 (0.55–1.28)	1.54 (1.11–2.15)	1.90 (1.37–2.65)	2.22 (1.61–3.06)	3.13 (2.34–4.19)	
HR (95% CI)						
Model 1‡	1.0 (reference)	2.35 (1.26–4.39)	3.02 (1.61–5.65)	2.22 (1.14–4.35)	4.51 (2.43–8.35)	<0.001
Model 2§	1.0 (reference)	2.11 (1.05–4.22)	2.24 (1.08–4.66)	2.54 (1.21–5.33)	3.92 (1.86–8.26)	<0.001
Highest						
CHD event rate per 1000 PYs (95% CI)	2.60 (1.88–3.59)	2.25 (1.65–3.06)	2.85 (2.19–3.71)	3.95 (3.19–4.88)	5.56 (4.69–6.59)	
HR (95% CI)						
Model 1‡	1.0 (reference)	0.82 (0.50–1.35)	1.11 (0.70–1.76)	1.59 (1.03–2.43)	1.93 (1.28–2.92)	<0.001
Model 2§	1.0 (reference)	0.75 (0.43–1.32)	1.02 (0.61–1.72)	1.45 (0.89–2.36)	1.37 (0.83–2.27)	<0.001

CHD = coronary heart disease; HDL-C = high-density lipoprotein cholesterol; HR = hazard ratio; PY = person-year.

**"CHD events" comprise myocardial infarction, coronary revascularization, and deaths from CHD.

†Lowest tertile, apolipoprotein B100 level <0.90 g/L (mean, 0.75 g/L); middle tertile, 0.90 –1.13 g/L (mean, 1.01 g/L); and highest tertile, >1.13 g/L (mean, 1.34 g/L). Based on 78 CHD events among 8989 participants in the lowest apolipoprotein B100 tertile, 174 events among 8940 participants in the middle tertile, and 350 events among 8932 participants in the highest tertile.

‡Adjusted for age, race, randomized treatment assignment, smoking status, antihypertensive medication use, fasting status, alcohol use, and family history.

§Adjusted for the covariates in model 1 plus postmenopausal status, postmenopausal hormone use, body mass index, exercise, diabetes mellitus, high-sensitivity C-reactive protein level, triglyceride level, and low-density lipoprotein cholesterol level.

The WHS is a completed randomized, double-blind, placebo-controlled trial of low-dose aspirin and vitamin E in the primary prevention of cardiovascular disease (CVD) and cancer in apparently healthy low-risk female health care professionals, aged 45 years or older, who were free of self-reported CVD and cancer at study entry (1992 to 1995). In this analysis by Mora and coworkers, the cohort is evaluated for the relation between HDL-C/ apoprotein (apo) AI across the range of low-density lipoprotein cholesterol (LDL-C)/apo B levels and risk of developing incident cardiovascular events. The group (26 861) was followed over 11 years.

The relation between quintiles of HDL-C and apo AI and risk for cardiovascular events followed a familiar theme: high levels were associated with less risk for coronary heart disease (CHD) and CVD related events, while low levels were associated with high risk (Table 2). HDL-C and apo AI levels did not correlate with risk for stroke. The relation held across tertiles of LDL-C (Table 3). The association between HDL-C and CHD/CVD also held for the middle and highest tertiles of apo B, but not the lowest tertile (Table 4).

These findings confirm the long-standing relation between HDL-C and apo AI and risk for CVD/CHD, but demonstrate them in the largest cohort of women to date. They also confirm that HDL-C and apo AI correlate poorly with risk for ischemic stroke. Of great interest is the observation that the relationship between HDL-C and risk for CVD/CHD drops out in the lowest tertile of apo B. This suggests that at the lowest levels of atherogenic lipoprotein burden (for which apo B is a measure as it includes very low-density lipoprotein (VLDL), VLDL remnants, intermediate-density lipoproteins, LDL, and Lp(a)), HDL-C is no longer predictive of risk. This is consistent with the core findings of AIM-HIGH study.

P. P. Toth, MD, PhD

References

1. Castelli WP. Cholesterol and lipids in the risk of coronary artery disease—the Framingham heart study. *Can J Cardiol.* 1988;4:5A-10A.
2. Toth PP. High-density lipoprotein: epidemiology, metabolism, and antiatherogenic effects. *Dis Mon.* 2001;47:365-416.
3. Steyn K, Sliwa K, Hawken S, et al. Risk factors associated with myocardial infarction in Africa: the INTERHEART Africa study. *Circulation.* 2005;112:3554-3561.
4. Sacco RL, Benson RT, Kargman DE, et al. High-density lipoprotein cholesterol and ischemic stroke in the elderly: the northern manhattan stroke study. *JAMA.* 2001;285:2729-2735.
5. AIM-HIGH Investigators, Boden WE, Probstfield JL, Anderson T, et al. Niacin in patients with low HDL cholesterol levels receiving intensive statin therapy. *N Engl J Med.* 2011;365:2255-2267.

Associations Between Lipoprotein(a) Levels and Cardiovascular Outcomes in Black and White Subjects: The Atherosclerosis Risk in Communities (ARIC) Study

Virani SS, Brautbar A, Davis BC, et al (Michael E. DeBakey Veterans Affairs Med Ctr Health Services Res and Development Ctr of Excellence, Houston, TX; Baylor College of Medicine, Houston, TX; Univ of Texas Health Science Ctr at Houston; et al)
Circulation 125:241-249, 2012

Background.—On the basis of studies with limited statistical power, lipoprotein(a) [Lp(a)] is not considered a risk factor for cardiovascular disease (CVD) in blacks. We evaluated associations between Lp(a) and incident CVD events in blacks and whites in the Atherosclerosis Risk in Communities (ARIC) study.

Methods and Results.—Plasma Lp(a) was measured in blacks (n=3467) and whites (n=9851). Hazards ratios (HRs) for incident CVD events (coronary heart disease and ischemic strokes) were calculated. Lp(a) levels were higher with wider interindividual variation in blacks (median [interquartile range], 12.8 [7.1−21.7] mg/dL) than whites (4.3 [1.7−9.5] mg/dL; $P<0.0001$). At 20 years of follow-up, 676 CVD events occurred in blacks, and 1821 events occurred in whites. Adjusted HRs (95% confidence interval) per race-specific 1-SD−greater log-transformed Lp(a) were 1.13 (1.04−1.23) for incident CVD, 1.11 (1.00−1.22) for incident coronary heart disease, and 1.21 (1.06−1.39) for ischemic strokes in blacks. For whites, the respective HRs (95% confidence intervals) were 1.09 (1.04−1.15), 1.10 (1.05−1.16), and 1.07 (0.97−1.19). Quintile analyses showed that risk for incident CVD was graded but statistically significant only for the highest compared with the lowest quintile (HR [95% confidence interval], 1.35 [1.06−1.74] for blacks and 1.27 [1.10−1.47] for whites). Similar results were obtained with the use of Lp(a) cutoffs of ≤10 mg/dL, >10 to ≤20 mg/dL, >20 to ≤30 mg/dL, and >30 mg/dL.

Conclusions.—Lp(a) levels were positively associated with CVD events. Associations were at least as strong, with a larger range of Lp(a) concentrations, in blacks compared with whites (Tables 3-6).

▶ Lipoprotein (a) [Lp(a)] is highly atherogenic and is a recognized risk factor for developing atherosclerotic disease.[1] Lp(a) comprises a low-density lipoprotein particle conjugated with apoprotein(a). The evidence favoring Lp(a) as a risk factor for coronary artery disease was examined for white patients.[2,3] To date there has been no clear, convincing evidence that Lp(a) is atherogenic in black patients.[4] Despite having no prospective randomized clinical trials to show that reducing Lp(a) impacts risk for future cardiovascular events, it is important to determine more precisely whether Lp(a) contributes to risk in blacks.

The Atherosclerosis Risk in Communities (ARIC) study examined a prospective epidemiologic cohort of 15 792 white and black participants aged 45 to 64 living in 4 communities in the United States. This study evaluated the impact of

TABLE 3.—Hazard Ratios* for Incident CVD Events for Race-Specific Lipoprotein(a) Quintiles (Blacks)

Incident Events	Quintile 1 0.1–≤6.1 mg/dL	Quintile 2 >6.1–≤10.3 mg/dL	Hazard Ratio (95% CI); No. of Events Quintile 3 >10.3–≤15.8 mg/dL	Quintile 4 >15.8–≤24 mg/dL	Quintile 5 >24 mg/dL	P for Linear Trend
Blacks						
CVD	Reference; 122	1.008 (0.78–1.31); 115	1.21 (0.95–1.55); 142	1.10 (0.85–1.41); 131	1.35 (1.06–1.74); 166	0.0004
CHD	Reference; 87	1.03 (0.76–1.39); 82	1.24 (0.92–1.66); 104	1.07 (0.79–1.44); 93	1.27 (0.94–1.71); 115	0.009
Ischemic strokes	Reference; 49	0.95 (0.63–1.43); 45	1.21 (0.82–1.78); 57	1.09 (0.73–1.63); 53	1.60 (1.10–2.34); 79	0.0004

CVD indicates cardiovascular disease; CI, confidence interval; and CHD, coronary heart disease.
*Adjusted for age, gender, smoking, systolic blood pressure, antihypertensive medication use, diabetes mellitus, low-density lipoprotein cholesterol, high-density lipoprotein cholesterol, and triglycerides.

TABLE 4.—Hazard Ratios* for Incident CVD Events for Race-Specific Lipoprotein(a) Quintiles (Whites)

Incident Events	Quintile 1 0.1–≤1.5 mg/dL	Quintile 2 >1.5–≤3.1 mg/dL	Quintile 3 >3.1–≤6.0 mg/dL	Quintile 4 >6.0–≤13.5 mg/dL	Quintile 5 >13.5 mg/dL	P for Linear Trend
			Hazard Ratio (95% CI); No. of Events			
Whites						
CVD	Reference; 383	0.94 (0.81–1.09); 327	1.01 (0.87–1.17); 339	1.05 (0.90–1.22); 363	1.27 (1.10–1.47); 409	0.001
CHD	Reference; 330	0.91 (0.78–1.08); 274	0.99 (0.84–1.16); 285	1.09 (0.93–1.28); 322	1.28 (1.10–1.50); 353	0.002
Ischemic strokes	Reference; 77	1.03 (0.74–1.44); 72	1.17 (0.85–1.62); 81	0.87 (0.62–1.23); 64	1.27 (0.92–1.76); 86	0.25

CVD indicates cardiovascular disease; CI, confidence interval; and CHD, coronary heart disease.
*Adjusted for age, gender, smoking, systolic blood pressure, antihypertensive medication use, diabetes mellitus, low-density lipoprotein cholesterol, high-density lipoprotein cholesterol, and triglycerides.

TABLE 5.—Hazard Ratios for Incident CVD Events per SD Increase* in Log-Transformed Lipoprotein(a) Levels

| | Hazard Ratio (95% CI) | | |
Incident Events	Model 1	Model 2	Model 3
Blacks			
CVD	1.17 (1.07–1.23)	1.18 (1.09–1.28)	1.13 (1.04–1.23)
CHD	1.17 (1.06–1.28)	1.17 (1.07–1.29)	1.11 (1.00–1.22)
Ischemic strokes	1.21 (1.06–1.37)	1.20 (1.06–1.37)	1.21 (1.06–1.39)
Whites			
CVD	1.09 (1.04–1.14)	1.12 (1.07–1.18)	1.09 (1.04–1.15)
CHD	1.10 (1.05–1.16)	1.13 (1.08–1.19)	1.10 (1.05–1.16)
Ischemic strokes	1.06 (0.96–1.18)	1.09 (0.99–1.21)	1.07 (0.97–1.19)

CVD indicates cardiovascular disease; CI, confidence interval; and CHD, coronary heart disease. Model 1 is adjusted for age and gender; model 2, adjusted for model 1 plus smoking, systolic blood pressure, antihypertensive medication use, and diabetes mellitus; and model 3, adjusted for model 2 plus low-density lipoprotein cholesterol, high-density lipoprotein cholesterol, and triglycerides.

*Race-specific SD of log lipoprotein(a) levels=0.90 for blacks and 1.15 for whites.

Lp(a) levels on risk for incident cardiovascular events in the ARIC cohort. Mean Lp(a) levels were higher for blacks than for whites and correlated with cardiovascular risk in both racial groups (Tables 3 and 4). The hazard ratios for risk of incident events (including cardiovascular disease, coronary heart disease, and ischemic stroke), adjusted according to 3 models, were significant for blacks, and the effect size per standard deviation increase in Lp(a) was at least as high as those for whites (Table 5). The hazard ratios for incident cardiovascular events per 10 mg/dL increase in Lp(a) escalated in a dose-response manner, with the trend for rising serum level of Lp(a) being statistically highly significant for blacks (Table 6).

This evaluation of the ARIC data is the first to demonstrate the clinical significance of Lp(a) on risk for cardiovascular events in blacks. This study is an important addition to the literature examining the relationship of specific risk factors for cardiovascular disease in blacks. Although no therapy has yet been developed to specifically inhibit Lp(a) biosynthesis, elevated Lp(a) can be used to assess risk and help determine low-density lipoprotein cholesterol and non-high-density lipoprotein cholesterol targets in patients at risk for cardiovascular events. There is great need for the development of drugs that can specifically inhibit the production of Lp(a), so we can determine in a prospective fashion whether therapeutic Lp(a) reduction will beneficially impact risk for cardiovascular events.

P. P. Toth, MD, PhD

References

1. Davidson MH, Ballantyne CM, Jacobson TA, et al. Clinical utility of inflammatory markers and advanced lipoprotein testing: advice from an expert panel of lipid specialists. *J Clin Lipidol.* 2011;5:338-367.
2. Kamstrup PR, Tybjaerg-Hansen A, Steffensen R, Nordestgaard BG. Genetically elevated lipoprotein(a) and increased risk of myocardial infarction. *JAMA.* 2009; 301:2331-2339.

TABLE 6.—Hazard Ratios* for Incident CVD Events per 10-mg/dL Increase in Lipoprotein(a)

Incident Events	≤10 mg/dL	Hazard Ratio (95% CI); No. of Events			P for Linear Trend
		>10–≤20 mg/dL	>20–≤30 mg/dL	>30 mg/dL	
Blacks					
CVD	Reference; 228	1.08 (0.89–1.30); 217	1.16 (0.92–1.46); 120	1.58 (1.24–2.01); 111	<0.0001
CHD	Reference; 164	1.06 (0.85–1.32); 155	1.17 (0.89–1.53); 88	1.33 (1.00–1.78); 74	0.008
Ischemic strokes	Reference; 90	1.14 (0.85–1.54); 89	1.15 (0.80–1.64); 49	2.12 (1.48–3.03); 55	<0.0001
Whites					
CVD	Reference; 1265	1.25 (1.11–1.41); 340	1.27 (1.06–1.51); 137	1.42 (1.12–1.79); 79	0.014
CHD	Reference; 1078	1.29 (1.13–1.47); 300	1.35 (1.12–1.63); 124	1.35 (1.04–1.75); 62	0.14
Ischemic strokes	Reference; 270	1.05 (0.79–1.39); 61	1.11 (0.74–1.67); 27	1.65 (1.04–2.61); 22	0.014

CVD indicates cardiovascular disease; CI, confidence interval; and CHD, coronary heart disease.
*Adjusted for age, gender, smoking, systolic blood pressure, antihypertensive medication use, diabetes mellitus, low-density lipoprotein cholesterol, high-density lipoprotein cholesterol, and triglycerides.

3. Clarke R, Peden JF, Hopewell JC, et al. Genetic variants associated with Lp(a) lipoprotein level and coronary disease. *N Engl J Med.* 2009;361:2518-2528.
4. Moliterno DJ, Jokinen EV, Miserez AR, et al. No association between plasma lipoprotein(a) concentrations and the presence or absence of coronary atherosclerosis in African-Americans. *Arterioscler Thromb Vasc Biol.* 1995;15:850-855.

LCAT, HDL Cholesterol and Ischemic Cardiovascular Disease: A Mendelian Randomization Study of HDL Cholesterol in 54,500 Individuals

Haase CL, Tybjærg-Hansen A, Qayyum AA, et al (Univ of Copenhagen, Denmark)
J Clin Endocrinol Metab 97:E248-E256, 2012

Background.—Epidemiologically, high-density lipoprotein (HDL) cholesterol levels associate inversely with risk of ischemic cardiovascular disease. Whether this is a causal relation is unclear.

Methods.—We studied 10,281 participants in the Copenhagen City Heart Study (CCHS) and 50,523 participants in the Copenhagen General Population Study (CGPS), of which 991 and 1,693 participants, respectively, had developed myocardial infarction (MI) by August 2010. Participants in the CCHS were genotyped for all six variants identified by resequencing lecithin-cholesterol acyltransferase in 380 individuals. One variant, S208T (rs4986970, allele frequency 4%), associated with HDL cholesterol levels in both the CCHS and the CGPS was used to study causality of HDL cholesterol using instrumental variable analysis.

Results.—Epidemiologically, in the CCHS, a 13% (0.21 mmol/liter) decrease in plasma HDL cholesterol levels was associated with an 18% increase in risk of MI. S208T associated with a 13% (0.21 mmol/liter) decrease in HDL cholesterol levels but not with increased risk of MI or other ischemic end points. The causal odds ratio for MI for a 50% reduction in plasma HDL cholesterol due to S208T genotype in both studies combined was 0.49 (0.11–2.16), whereas the hazard ratio for MI for a 50% reduction in plasma HDL cholesterol in the CCHS was 2.11 (1.70–2.62) ($P_{comparison} = 0.03$).

Conclusion.—Low plasma HDL cholesterol levels robustly associated with increased risk of MI but genetically decreased HDL cholesterol did not. This may suggest that low HDL cholesterol levels per se do not cause MI.

▶ Although a number of post-hoc analyses of randomized, clinical trials[1,2] with lipid-modifying medications and meta-analyses[3-5] suggest that increasing high-density lipoprotein (HDL)-C contributes to overall cardiovascular risk reduction, there is as yet no convincing evidence that this is in fact the case. In light of the results of such clinical trials as ILLUMINATE (Investigation of Lipid Level Management to Understand its Impact in Atherosclerotic Events)[6] and AIM-HIGH (Atherothrombosis Intervention in Metabolic Syndrome With Low HDL/High Triglycerides: Impact on Global Health Outcomes),[7] the efficacy of HDL-C increasing as a therapeutic strategy has been called into some question.

This, however, is far from settled, and works with numerous agents designed to impact HDL metabolism are in development.

Danish investigators have found that common polymorphisms in apoprotein AI that are causal for high serum levels of HDL-C are not associated with reduced risk for coronary heart disease. In fact, the increased levels of HDL-C have a neutral effect on cardiovascular risk.[8] Haase and coworkers extend these investigations by probing the impact of a loss of function polymorphism (S208 T) of lecithin cholesterol: acyltransferase on risk for CHD in the Copenhagen City heart Study and the Copenhagen General Population Study. The investigators confirm that a 13% reduction in HDL-C in these populations is associated with an increase in risk for CHD by 18%. In this study, S208 T was in Hardy-Weinberg equilibrium and was associated with significant reductions in serum HDL-C. Reductions in HDL-C attributable to S208 T had no impact on the hazard ratio for cardiovascular disease (CVD) events (including myocardial infarction and stroke) (Fig 1 in the original article). The authors conclude that, based on the totality of evidence from these studies in Denmark and elsewhere, HDL-C does not impact risk. Rather, when HDL-C is low, its impact on risk is confounded by an increase of triglycerides and atherogenic lipoproteins, which are the true modifiers of risk.

The molecular cardiovascular genetic studies out of Copenhagen certainly call into question whether HDL-C elevation will be a viable therapeutic alternative for reducing residual risk in patients already treated with a statin. A large number of clinical trials are underway with a variety of drug classes to further probe and test this approach. In the meantime, low HDL-C is most certainly a marker of risk; whether it should be a target of therapy will be determined at some point in the future.

P. P. Toth, MD, PhD

References

1. Secondary prevention by raising HDL cholesterol and reducing triglycerides in patients with coronary artery disease: the Bezafibrate Infarction Prevention (BIP) study. *Circulation.* 2000;102:21-27.
2. Cui Y, Watson DJ, Girman CJ, et al. Effects of increasing high-density lipoprotein cholesterol and decreasing low-density lipoprotein cholesterol on the incidence of first acute coronary events (from the Air Force/Texas Coronary Atherosclerosis Prevention Study). *Am J Cardiol.* 2009;104:829-834.
3. Ballantyne CM, Raichlen JS, Nicholls SJ, et al. Effect of rosuvastatin therapy on coronary artery stenoses assessed by quantitative coronary angiography: a study to evaluate the effect of rosuvastatin on intravascular ultrasound-derived coronary atheroma burden. *Circulation.* 2008;117:2458-2466.
4. Nicholls SJ, Tuzcu EM, Sipahi I, et al. Statins, high-density lipoprotein cholesterol, and regression of coronary atherosclerosis. *JAMA.* 2007;297:499-508.
5. Alsheikh-Ali AA, Kuvin JT, Karas RH. High-density lipoprotein cholesterol in the cardiovascular equation: does the "good" still count? *Atherosclerosis.* 2005;180: 217-223.
6. Barter PJ, Caulfield M, Eriksson M, et al. Effects of torcetrapib in patients at high risk for coronary events. *N Engl J Med.* 2007;357:2109-2122.
7. Boden WE, Probstfield JL, Anderson T, et al. Niacin in patients with low HDL cholesterol levels receiving intensive statin therapy. *N Engl J Med.* 2011;365: 2255-2267.

8. Haase CL, Tybjærg-Hansen A, Grande P, Frikke-Schmidt R. Genetically elevated apolipoprotein A-I, high-density lipoprotein cholesterol levels, and risk of ischemic heart disease. *J Clin Endocrinol Metab.* 2010;95:E500-E510.

Metabolic Syndrome

Impact of metabolic syndrome and its components on cardiovascular disease event rates in 4900 patients with type 2 diabetes assigned to placebo in the field randomised trial

Scott R, for The FIELD Study Investigators (Christchurch Hosp, New Zealand; et al)
Cardiovasc Diabetol 10:102, 2011

Background.—Patients with the metabolic syndrome are more likely to develop type 2 diabetes and may have an increased risk of cardiovascular disease (CVD) events. We aimed to establish whether CVD event rates were influenced by the metabolic syndrome as defined by the World Health Organisation (WHO), the National Cholesterol Education Program (NCEP) Adult Treatment Panel III (ATP III) and the International Diabetes Federation (IDF) and to determine which component(s) of the metabolic

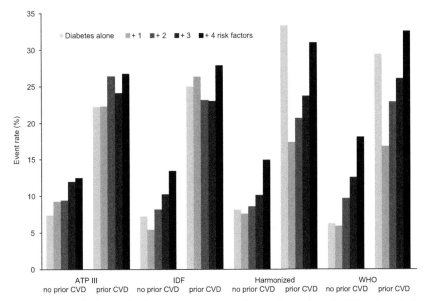

FIGURE 1.—Cardiovascular disease event rates according to the number of additional metabolic syndrome components (risk factors) at baseline in relation to the ATPIII, IDF, harmonized, and WHO categories in patients allocated to placebo without ($n = 3837$) or with ($n = 1063$) prior cardiovascular disease. Apparent high event rates in the groups with no additional risk factors by the harmonized and WHO definitions are an artifact of low patient numbers. (Reprinted from Scott R, for The FIELD Study Investigators. Impact of metabolic syndrome and its components on cardiovascular disease event rates in 4900 patients with type 2 diabetes assigned to placebo in the field randomised trial. *Cardiovasc Diabetol.* 2011;10:102, with permission from licensee BioMed Central Ltd.)

syndrome (MS) conferred the highest cardiovascular risk in in 4900 patients with type 2 diabetes allocated to placebo in the Fenofibrate Intervention and Event Lowering in Diabetes (FIELD) trial. *Research Design and Methods.*—We determined the influence of MS variables, as defined by NCEP ATPIII, IDF and WHO, on CVD risk over 5 years, after adjustment for CVD, sex, HbA1$_c$, creatinine, and age, and interactions between the MS variables in a Cox proportional-hazards model. *Results.*—About 80% had hypertension, and about half had other features of the metabolic syndrome (IDF, ATPIII). There was no difference in the prevalence of metabolic syndrome variables between those with and without CVD at study entry. The WHO definition identified those at higher CVD risk across both sexes, all ages, and in those without prior CVD, while the ATPIII definition predicted risk only in those aged over 65 years and in men but not in women. Patients meeting the IDF definition did not have higher risk than those without IDF MS. CVD risk was strongly influenced by prior CVD, sex, age (particularly in women), baseline HbA1$_c$, renal dysfunction, hypertension, and dyslipidemia (low HDL-c, triglycerides >1.7 mmol/L). The combination of low HDL-c and marked hypertriglyceridemia (>2.3 mmol/L) increased CVD risk by 41%. Baseline

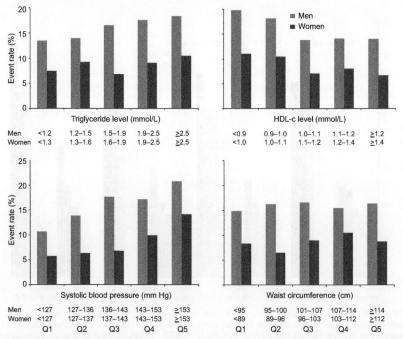

FIGURE 2.—Cardiovascular disease event rates according to quintiles of baseline triglycerides, HDL-c, systolic blood pressure, and waist circumference in men and women allocated to placebo. (Reprinted from Scott R, for The FIELD Study Investigators. Impact of metabolic syndrome and its components on cardiovascular disease event rates in 4900 patients with type 2 diabetes assigned to placebo in the field randomised trial. *Cardiovasc Diabetol.* 2011;10:102, with permission from licensee BioMed Central Ltd.)

systolic blood pressure increased risk by 16% per 10 mmHg in those with no prior CVD, but had no effect in those with CVD. In those without prior CVD, increasing numbers of metabolic syndrome variables (excluding waist) escalated risk.

Conclusion.—Absence of the metabolic syndrome (by the WHO definition) identifies diabetes patients without prior CVD, who have a lower risk of future CVD events. Hypertension and dyslipidemia increase risk (Figs 1, 2, Tables 1, 3).

▶ Metabolic syndrome identifies a group of patients with features of insulin resistance (visceral obesity, dyslipidemia, elevated blood pressure, and hyperglycemia) who have elevated risk for both diabetes mellitus and cardiovascular disease. A variety of definitions of metabolic syndrome have been put forth by several organizations, including the National Cholesterol Education Program

TABLE 1.—Prevalence of Features of Metabolic Syndrome at Baseline in Patients Assigned to Placebo in the FIELD Study (Points of Difference in Criteria are Shown in Bold)

Feature of Metabolic Syndrome	Men (n = 3067)	Women (n = 1833)	All Patients (n = 4900)
ATPIII criteria (any 3)			
Diabetes or impaired fasting glucose	100	100	100
High waist measurement (**M >102 cm, F >88 cm**)	54.5	80.6	64.3
Hypertension history or BP ≥130/85 mmHg	82.2	85.8	83.6
High triglycerides (≥ 1.7 mmol/L)	50.0	54.1	51.5
Low HDL cholesterol (M <1.03 mmol/L, F <1.29 mmol/L)	54.8	66.2	59.1
Metabolic syndrome according to ATPIII	78.3	90.3	82.8
IDF criteria (waist + any 2)			
Diabetes or impaired fasting glucose	100	100	100
High waist measurement (**M ≥94 cm, F ≥80 cm**)	83.9	95.0	88.0
Hypertension history or BP ≥130/85 mmHg	82.2	85.8	83.6
High triglycerides (≥1.7 mmol/L)	50.0	54.1	51.5
Low HDL cholesterol (M <1.03 mmol/L, F <1.29 mmol/L)	54.8	66.2	59.1
Metabolic syndrome according to IDF	80.5	92.5	85.0
Harmonized criteria (any 3)			
Diabetes or impaired fasting glucose	100	100	100
High waist measurement (M ≥94 cm, F ≥80 cm)	83.9	95.0	88.0
Hypertension history or BP ≥130/85 mmHg	82.2	85.8	83.6
High triglycerides (≥ 1.7 mmol/L)	50.0	54.1	51.5
Low HDL cholesterol (M < 1.03 mmol/L, F <1.29 mmol/L)	54.8	66.2	59.1
Metabolic syndrome according to harmonized definition	87.6	94.7	90.3
WHO criteria (diabetes + any 2)			
Diabetes or impaired fasting glucose	100	100	100
High waist-hip ratio (M > 0.9, F >0.85) or BMI >30	88.5	80.5	85.5
Hypertension history or blood pressure ≥140/90 mmHg	68.5	73.3	70.3
High triglycerides (≥ 1.7 mmol/L) and/or low HDL-c (M < 0.9 mmol/L, F < 1.0 mmol/L)	58.9	59.0	58.9
Microalbuminuria (urine albumin/creatinine ≥ 3.4 mg/mmol)	23.6	20.8	22.6
Metabolic syndrome according to WHO	82.6	80.7	81.9

* IDF criteria for hypertension, high triglyceride, and low HDL-c are the same as those for ATPIII.
† Harmonized criteria are the same as for IDF except metabolic syndrome does not require high waist measurement.
‡ Ethnic and sex-specific cut-offs for waist circumference define high risk in the harmonized definition. This analysis, for a population mainly of European origin, used the "Caucasian" waist cut-off.
  FIELD, Fenofibrate Intervention and Event Lowering in Diabetes; ATPIII, Adult Treatment Panel III; M, male; F, female; BP, blood pressure; IDF, International Diabetes Federation; WHO, World Health HDL-c, high-density lipoprotein cholesterol

TABLE 3.—Cox Regression Model* for the Effect of Continuous Variables, Including
Features of the Metabolic Syndrome as Defined by ATPIII, on the Risk of Total CVD Events
in Patients Assigned to Placebo in the FIELD Study

Variable[†]	Hazard Ratio (95% CI)	P
Predictive variable		
Female (at 62 years)	0.70 (0.55-0.88)	0.003
Age (per 10 years): male	1.21 (1.06-1.39)	< 0.001
Age (per 10 years): female	1.74 (1.38-2.19)	
Prior CVD (at 140 mmHg SBP, 6.85% HbA_{1c})	2.14 (1.81-2.53)	< 0.001
Hemoglobin A_{1c} (per 1%): no prior CVD	1.18 (1.10-1.26)	< 0.001
Hemoglobin A_{1c} (per 1%): prior CVD	1.03 (0.95-1.13)	
Creatinine (per 20 μmol/L)	1.21 (1.09-1.35)	< 0.001
Metabolic syndrome variable[‡]		
Waist -hip ratio (per 0.1)	1.03 (0.91-1.17)	0.60
Systolic BP (per 10 mmHg): no prior CVD	1.16 (1.09-1.24)	< 0.001
Systolic BP (per 10 mmHg): prior CVD	1.01 (0.94-1.09)	
Triglycerides (per 0.5 mmol/L)	1.03 (0.99-1.07)	0.19
HDL-c (per 0.1 mmol/L)	0.94 (0.90-0.97)	< 0.001
Urine albumin-creatinine ratio (per doubling)	1.06 (1.02-1.10)	0.002

ATPIII, Adult Treatment Panel III; CVD, cardiovascular disease; FIELD, Fenofibrate Intervention and Event Lowering in
Diabetes; BP, blood pressure; HDL-c, high-density lipoprotein cholesterol.
*Cox proportional-hazards assumptions were met.
[†]All variables were centered at medians. Standard deviations for distributions of the continuous variables were: age, 6.9
years; HbA_{1c}, 1.35%; creatinine, 15.8 μmol/L; waist, 13 cm; systolic BP, 15 mmHg; triglycerides, 0.88 mmol/L; HDL-c,
0.26 mmol/L.
[‡]Corrected for age, sex, prior CVD, baseline HbA_{1c} and creatinine.

(NCEP),[1] the International Diabetes Federation (IDF),[2] and the World Health
Organization (WHO),[3] and a harmonized set attempts to integrate definitions
by a number of organizations.[4] Although the NCEP did not define the metabolic
syndrome (MS) as a coronary heart disease risk equivalent, it has been assumed
that as the number of components of MS increases, risk increases continuously.

Scott et al evaluate the impact of MS and its various components on risk for
cardiovascular disease (CVD) in the placebo group of the Fenofibrate Intervention and Event Lowering in Diabetes (FIELD)[5] study. The majority of patients
met criteria for MS, with prevalence rates varying according to gender and definition (NCEP, WHO, IDF, or harmonized) (Table 1). The WHO definition emerged
as the most discriminatory definition for predicting future CVD. Reductions in
high-density lipoprotein (HDL)-C and increases in systolic blood pressure and
urine albumin to creatinine ratio were associated with significant increases in
risk for CVD (Table 3). Interestingly, waist circumference did not correlate with
increased CVD risk. The combination of low HDL-C and hypertriglyceridemia
(> 2.3 mmol/L) increased CVD risk by 41%. Among participants without prior
CVD, increasing numbers of components of the metabolic syndrome were associated with increased risk for CVD, while among patients with prior CVD, an
increase in number of components of MS was not associated with a clear increase
in risk for CVD (Fig 1). Increasing triglycerides correlated with increased CVD risk
in men but not women (Fig 2).

These data call into question the sensitivity of the NCEP definition of MS. The
WHO definition appears to have been most predictive in this study. Importantly,

waist circumference did not predict risk in either gender; triglycerides were also not an independent predictor of CVD in women. Of particular interest is the finding that among participants with established CVD, the number of components of MS was poorly predictive of cardiovascular events. This calls into question whether patients with CVD and multiple poorly controlled components of MS are truly very high risk.[6,7] This study certainly calls the adequacy of the current NCEP definition for MS into question and suggests that the WHO definition is most highly predictive. Given the implications for patient care, these are issues that warrant urgent further clarification and definition.

P. P. Toth, MD, PhD

References

1. Expert Panel on Detection, Evaluation, and Treatment of High Blood Cholesterol in Adults. Executive summary of the third report of the National Cholesterol Education Program (NCEP) expert panel on detection, evaluation, and treatment of high blood cholesterol in adults (adult treatment panel III). *JAMA*. 2001;285: 2486-2497.
2. Alberti KG, Zimmet P, Shaw J. The metabolic syndrome—a new worldwide definition. *Lancet*. 2005;366:1059-1062.
3. Alberti KG, Zimmet PZ. Definition, diagnosis and classification of diabetes mellitus and its complications. Part 1: diagnosis and classification of diabetes mellitus provisional report of a WHO consultation. *Diabet Med*. 1998;15:539-553.
4. Alberti KG, Eckel RH, Grundy SM, et al. Harmonizing the metabolic syndrome: a joint interim statement of the International Diabetes Federation Task Force on Epidemiology and Prevention; National Heart, Lung, and Blood Institute; American Heart Association; World Heart Federation; International Atherosclerosis Society; and International Association for the Study of Obesity. *Circulation*. 2009;120: 1640-1645.
5. Keech A, Simes RJ, Barter P, et al. Effects of long-term fenofibrate therapy on cardiovascular events in 9795 people with type 2 diabetes mellitus (the FIELD study): randomised controlled trial. *Lancet*. 2005;366:1849-1861.
6. Grundy SM, Brewer HB Jr, Cleeman JI, Smith SC Jr, Lenfant C. Definition of metabolic syndrome: report of the National Heart, Lung, and Blood Institute/American Heart Association conference on scientific issues related to definition. *Circulation*. 2004;109:433-438.
7. Grundy SM, Cleeman JI, Merz CN, et al. Implications of recent clinical trials for the National Cholesterol Education Program Adult Treatment Panel III guidelines. *Circulation*. 2004;110:227-239.

Coronary artery disease and cardiovascular outcomes in patients with non-alcoholic fatty liver disease

Wong VW-S, Wong GL-H, Yip GW-K, et al (The Chinese Univ of Hong Kong)
Gut 60:1721-1727, 2011

Objective.—Non-alcoholic fatty liver disease (NAFLD) is the hepatic manifestation of metabolic syndrome and is associated with cardiovascular risk. The aim of this study was to determine the role of fatty liver in predicting coronary artery disease and clinical outcomes in patients undergoing coronary angiogram.

Methods.—This was a prospective cohort study carried out in a University hospital. Consecutive patients who underwent coronary angiogram had ultrasound screening for fatty liver. Significant cardiovascular disease was defined as ≥50% stenosis in at least one coronary artery. The primary outcome was a composite end point comprising cardiovascular deaths, non-fatal myocardial infarction and the need for further coronary intervention during prospective follow-up.

Results.—Among 612 recruited patients, 356 (58.2%) had fatty liver by ultrasonography, 318 (52.0%) had elevated serum alanine aminotransferase and 465 (76.0%) had significant coronary artery disease. Coronary artery disease occurred in 84.6% of patients with fatty liver and 64.1% of those without fatty liver (p<0.001). After adjusting for demographic and metabolic factors, fatty liver (adjusted OR 2.31; 95% CI 1.46 to 3.64) and alanine aminotransferase level (adjusted OR 1.01; 95% CI 1.00 to 1.02) remained independently associated with coronary artery disease. At a mean follow-up of 87 ± 22 weeks, 30 (10.0%) patients with fatty liver and 18 (11.0%) patients without fatty liver reached the composite clinical end point (p=0.79).

Conclusions.—In patients with clinical indications for coronary angiogram, fatty liver is associated with coronary artery disease independently of other metabolic factors. However, fatty liver cannot predict cardiovascular mortality and morbidity in patients with established coronary artery disease (Tables 1 and 2).

▶ The metabolic syndrome as defined by the National Cholesterol Education Program has been a useful clinical construct for helping to identify patients at heightened risk for developing coronary artery disease (CAD) as well as diabetes mellitus.[1] Although not defined as a CAD risk equivalent, considerable evidence shows that the heightened risk for atherosclerotic disease is due to obesity, insulin resistance or hyperglycemia, dyslipidemia, hypertension, and heightened systemic inflammation. A frequent manifestation of insulin resistance is hepatic steatosis (ie, nonalcoholic fatty liver disease [NAFLD]). All forms of ectopic fat deposition are considered to be abnormal and pathogenic, including within the liver, pancreas, skeletal muscle, and pericardium or myocardium. NAFLD is associated with increased risk for both carotid atherosclerosis and CAD.[2-5] It has not been clear, however, whether NAFLD is an independent risk factor for CAD.

In this study, 612 patients, with and without NAFLD, who had clinical indications for coronary angiography were evaluated. NAFLD was documented by ultrasonography. Significant CAD was defined as a stenotic lesion that was at least 50% occlusive. Groups were not well matched by risk factor burden, metabolic features, and background pharmacologic therapies. A significant reason for this likely has to do with the fact that the 2 groups were mismatched for incidence of diabetes at 41% and 17% in the NAFLD and normal liver groups, respectively. Nevertheless, based on multivariate regression analysis, NAFLD was an independent predictor of significant CAD in all branches of the coronary tree, incurring an increased hazard for disease of 2.3-fold (95% confidence interval, 1.46–3.64;

TABLE 1.—Baseline Characteristics of Patients with and Without Fatty Liver

Characteristics	All	Fatty liver	No fatty liver	p Value
n	612	356	256	
Age (years)	63±11	63±10	63±12	0.61
Male gender, n (%)	433 (70.8)	264 (74.2)	169 (66.0)	0.029
Smoking, n (%)				0.23
Current smoker	194 (31.7)	122 (34.3)	72 (28.1)	
Ex-smoker	115 (18.8)	67 (18.8)	48 (18.8)	
Non-smoker	303 (49.5)	167 (46.9)	136 (53.1)	
Alcohol, n (%)				0.84
Current drinker	93 (15.2)	54 (15.2)	39 (15.2)	
Ex-drinker	30 (4.9)	19 (5.3)	11 (4.3)	
Non-drinker	489 (79.9)	283 (79.5)	206 (80.5)	
Diabetes, n (%)	191 (31.2)	147 (41.3)	44 (17.2)	<0.001
Hypertension, n (%)	401 (65.5)	252 (70.8)	149 (58.2)	0.001
Systolic blood pressure (mm Hg)	137±22	140±22	132±21	<0.001
Diastolic blood pressure (mm Hg)	75±13	77±13	72±13	<0.001
Body mass index (kg/m^2)	24.7±3.9	25.7±4.0	23.2±3.1	<0.001
Male	24.3±3.3	25.2±3.4	23.0±2.8	<0.001
Female	25.5±4.9	27.2±5.2	23.6±3.7	<0.001
Waist circumference (cm)	90±9	93±8	87±9	<0.001
Male	91±8	93±8	88±8	<0.001
Female	89±11	93±9	84±10	<0.001
Fasting glucose (mmol/l)	6.2±2.1	6.4±2.2	6.0±2.0	0.021
Total cholesterol (mmol/l)	4.5±1.2	4.5±1.3	4.5±1.1	0.66
HDL-cholesterol (mmol/l)	1.2±0.3	1.1±0.3	1.2±0.4	<0.001
LDL-cholesterol (mmol/l)	2.6±0.9	2.6±0.9	2.6±0.9	0.50
Triglycerides (mmol/l)	1.4 (1.0, 1.9)	1.4 (1.0, 2.1)	1.2 (0.9, 1.8)	0.001
Creatinine (μmol/l)	89 (76, 105)	91 (78, 107)	87 (74, 104)	0.033
Alanine aminotransferase (IU/l)	26 (19, 40)	28 (19, 44)	24 (18, 38)	0.052
Drugs, n (%)				
Aspirin	523 (85.5)	323 (90.7)	200 (78.1)	<0.001
Clopidogrel	377 (61.6)	242 (68.0)	135 (52.7)	<0.001
β-Blockers	423 (69.1)	267 (75.0)	156 (60.9)	<0.001
Calcium channel blockers	133 (21.7)	87 (24.4)	46 (18.0)	0.056
ACE inhibitors	310 (50.7)	192 (53.9)	118 (46.1)	0.056
Angiotensin receptor antagonists	32 (5.2)	20 (5.6)	12 (4.7)	0.61
Statins	399 (65.2)	252 (70.8)	147 (57.4)	0.001
Metformin	77 (12.6)	62 (17.4)	15 (5.9)	<0.001
Thiazolidinedione	13 (2.1)	10 (2.8)	3 (1.2)	0.26
Sulfonylurea	111 (18.1)	83 (23.3)	28 (10.9)	<0.001
Insulin	25 (4.1)	19 (5.3)	6 (2.3)	0.065
Indication of coronary angiogram, n (%)				<0.001
Acute coronary syndrome or myocardial infarction	279 (45.6)	167 (46.9)	112 (43.8)	
Stable angina	273 (44.6)	173 (48.6)	100 (39.1)	
Valvular heart disease	46 (7.5)	10 (2.8)	36 (14.1)	
Others	14 (2.3)	6 (1.7)	8 (3.1)	
Follow-up duration (weeks)	87±22	89±19	85±25	0.055

Continuous variables were expressed as mean ± SD or median (IQR).
ACE, angiotensin-converting enzyme; HDL, high-density lipoprotein; LDL, low-density lipoprotein.

P < .001). NAFLD did not, however, predict risk for cardiovascular events (myocardial infarction, stroke, or death), possibly because of small sample size and relatively short duration of mean follow-up (87 weeks).

This study certainly introduces important implications and widens the toxicity associated with NAFLD. Larger studies will be needed to help confirm whether

TABLE 2.—Coronary Angiogram Findings of Patients with and Without Fatty Liver

Parameters	Fatty Liver	No Fatty Liver	p Value
Left main stem stenosis (%)	0 (0, 0)	0 (0, 0)	0.17
Left main stem steatosis ≥50%, n (%)	29 (8.1)	22 (8.6)	0.84
Left anterior descending artery stenosis (%)	80 (30, 90)	50 (0, 80)	<0.001
Left anterior descending artery stenosis ≥50%, n (%)	232 (65.2)	135 (52.7)	0.002
Left circumflex artery stenosis (%)	50 (0, 90)	0 (0, 70)	<0.001
Left circumflex artery stenosis ≥50%, n (%)	176 (49.4)	88 (34.4)	<0.001
Right coronary artery stenosis (%)	50 (0, 90)	20 (0, 80)	<0.001
Right coronary artery stenosis ≥50%, n (%)	188 (52.8)	95 (37.1)	<0.001
Stenosis ≥50% in any coronary artery, n (%)	301 (84.6)	164 (64.1)	<0.001
Triple vessel disease, n (%)	100 (28.1)	60 (23.4)	0.20

The percentage stenosis of each coronary artery with respect to its diameter was expressed as the median (IQR).

NAFLD should be considered a CAD risk factor and count in CAD risk scoring paradigms used around the world. At minimum, it can be stated that the finding that NAFLD increases risk for significant CAD makes sense and helps to identify patients with diabetes mellitus or metabolic syndrome who have higher CAD risk than their counterparts who do not have NAFLD. It will be important to determine if patients who successfully achieve resorption of intrahepatic fat through lifestyle modification and pharmacologic intervention also experience a reduction in risk for CAD or regression of coronary atherosclerotic plaques.

P. P. Toth, MD, PhD

References

1. Expert Panel on Detection, Evaluation, and Treatment of High Blood Cholesterol in Adults. Executive summary of the third report of the National Cholesterol Education Program (ncep) expert panel on detection, evaluation, and treatment of high blood cholesterol in adults (adult treatment panel III). *JAMA.* 2001;285: 2486-2497.
2. Villanova N, Moscatiello S, Ramilli S, et al. Endothelial dysfunction and cardiovascular risk profile in nonalcoholic fatty liver disease. *Hepatology.* 2005;42: 473-480.
3. Mirbagheri SA, Rashidi A, Abdi S, Saedi D, Abouzari M. Liver: an alarm for the heart? *Liver Int.* 2007;27:891-894.
4. McKimmie RL, Daniel KR, Carr JJ, et al. Hepatic steatosis and subclinical cardiovascular disease in a cohort enriched for type 2 diabetes: the Diabetes Heart Study. *Am J Gastroenterol.* 2008;103:3029-3035.
5. Assy N, Djibre A, Farah R, Grosovski M, Marmor A. Presence of coronary plaques in patients with nonalcoholic fatty liver disease. *Radiology.* 2010;254:393-400.

Effect of Metabolic Syndrome on Coronary Artery Stenosis and Plaque Characteristics as Assessed with 64–Detector Row Cardiac CT

Lim S, Shin H, Lee Y, et al (Seoul Natl Univ College of Medicine and Seoul Natl Univ Bundang Hosp, Seongnam City, Gyeonggi-do, South Korea; Johns Hopkins Bloomberg School of Public Health, Baltimore, MD)
Radiology 261:437-445, 2011

Purpose.—To investigate the prevalence and severity of subclinical coronary atherosclerosis and plaque characteristics in asymptomatic subjects according to the presence or absence of metabolic syndrome (MS) with multidetector computed tomography (CT).

Materials and Methods.—This study was approved and the requirement for informed patient consent was waived by the local institutional review board. Degree of coronary artery stenosis, multivessel involvement, and plaque characteristics, as well as coronary artery calcium score (CACS), were assessed with 64–detector row CT in 3000 age- and sex-matched asymptomatic individuals (mean age, 50.2 years ± 8.9 [standard deviation]; age range, 30–79 years). Anthropometric and metabolic profiles were also measured. Multivariate logistic regression analyses were performed to identify variables related to coronary atherosclerosis and plaque types.

Results.—Subjects with MS had significant coronary artery stenosis (>50% stenosis), multivessel involvement, more positive remodeling, more atherosclerotic coronary segments, and higher CACS than subjects without MS ($P < .01$ for all). Mixed and noncalcified plaques were also more prominent in subjects with MS than in those without MS (14.2% ± 4.4 vs 7.6% ± 3.1 and 13.1% ± 4.3 vs 7.3% ± 2.8, respectively; $P < .01$ for both). After adjustment for confounding factors, MS was strongly associated with significant coronary artery stenosis, multivessel involvement, and mixed plaque.

Conclusion.—Multidetector CT is useful in the early diagnosis and evaluation of subclinical coronary atherosclerosis in asymptomatic patients with MS; however, future prospective studies are needed to address the clinical implications of these findings (Tables 1 and 2).

▶ The metabolic syndrome (MS) represents a cluster of important risk factors for coronary artery disease (CAD). This study compared the results of 64-detector row coronary CT angiography in 3000 asymptomatic age- (mean 50.2 years) and sex-matched Asian patients with and without MS. The patients with MS had a significantly larger burden of cardiovascular risk factor compared to those without MS (Table 1). Among both men and women, the patients with MS had significantly greater plaque burden, evidence of significant stenosis (greater than 50%), a higher incidence of multivessel disease, and higher coronary artery calcium scores (Table 2). In men, both calcified and noncalcified plaque burden was higher among patients with MS compared to those without. In women only, noncalcified plaque occurred more frequently in the MS group compared to the group without MS.

TABLE 1.—Comparison of Clinical and Biochemical Characteristics According to MS

Characteristic	Men (n = 1500)			Women (n = 1500)		
	Non-MS Group (n = 1000)	MS Group (n = 500)	P Value	Non-MS Group (n = 1000)	MS Group (n = 500)	P Value
Age (y)	49.6 ± 9.0	50.2 ± 8.9	NS	49.7 ± 9.6	50.7 ± 6.5	NS
BMI (kg/m^2)	24.4 ± 2.3	26.7 ± 2.4	<.01	22.7 ± 2.6	25.1 ± 2.5	<.05
Waist circumference (cm)	86.0 ± 6.5	93.2 ± 5.9	<.01	79.5 ± 7.8	87.0 ± 6.5	<.01
SBP (mm Hg)	115.3 ± 12.6	127.8 ± 14.5	<.01	110.8 ± 13.8	126.5 ± 13.8	<.01
Diastolic blood pressure (mm Hg)	75.9 ± 9.8	84.7 ± 9.7	<.01	67.3 ± 11.2	76.6 ± 11.4	<.01
Fasting glucose level (mg/dL)*	95.5 ± 20.1	122.4 ± 42.1	<.01	89.7 ± 13.4	111.2 ± 30.0	<.01
Hemoglobin A1c level (%)†	5.7 ± 0.6	6.4 ± 1.2	<.01	5.6 ± 0.5	6.4 ± 1.1	<.01
Total cholesterol level (mg/dL)‡	204.9 ± 32.1	216.8 ± 38.4	<.05	200.4 ± 35.7	221.6 ± 36.9	<.01
Triglyceride level (mg/dL)§	137.6 ± 79.9	231.6 ± 132.6	<.01	85.4 ± 36.9	186.5 ± 77.5	<.01
High-density lipoprotein cholesterol level (mg/dL)‡	47.8 ± 12.6	41.7 ± 11.5	<.01	57.3 ± 14.2	49.4 ± 11.4	<.01
LDL cholesterol level (mg/dL)‡	120.6 ± 30.0	124.5 ± 33.2	<.01	116.1 ± 32.7	126.9 ± 35.5	<.01
Creatinine level (mg/dL)∥	1.2 ± 0.1	1.2 ± 0.1	NS	0.9 ± 0.1	1.0 ± 0.1	NS
hsCRP level (mg/dL)#	0.14 ± 0.36	0.23 ± 0.47	<.01	0.09 ± 0.21	0.18 ± 0.22	<.01
Framingham risk score	2.8 ± 2.6	8.5 ± 2.7	<.01	0.7 ± 5.7	6.7 ± 3.4	<.01
Current smoker (%)	37.7	46.6	<.01	5.1	7.2	NS
Current drinker (%)	42.3	51.2	<.01	17.7	21.8	NS
Hypertension (%)	18.0	71.6	<.01	12.4	69.8	<.01
Diabetes mellitus (%)	6.5	41.2	<.01	5.7	37.2	<.01
Dyslipidemia (%)	13.4	34.4	<.01	9.0	21.6	<.01
Family history of premature CAD (%)	12.7	17.2	<.01	11.3	18.6	<.01

Note.—Unless otherwise indicated, data are mean ± standard deviation. NS = not significant, SBP = systolic blood pressure.
*To convert to SI units (millimoles per liter), multiply by 0.05551.
†To convert to SI units (proportion of total hemoglobin), multiply by 0.01.
‡To convert to SI units (millimoles per liter), multiply by 0.02586.
§To convert to SI units (millimoles per liter), multiply by 0.01129.
∥To convert to SI units (micromoles per liter), multiply by 88.4.
#To convert to SI units (nanomoles per liter), multiply by 9.524.

TABLE 2.—Comparison of Cardiac CT Findings According to MS

Finding	Men (*n* = 1500)			Women (*n* = 1500)		
	Non-MS Group (*n* = 1000)	MS Group (*n* = 500)	*P* Value	Non-MS Group (*n* = 1000)	MS Group (*n* = 500)	*P* Value
Atherosclerotic coronary segments (any plaque)	24.7	38.9	<.01	8.7	20.8	<.01
Plaque type						
Calcified	9.9	18.7	.007	4.5	6.3	NS
Noncalcified	11.8	17.6	.021	1.3	2.2	<.05
Mixed	9.7	18.2	<.01	5.4	10.1	<.01
Significant coronary artery stenosis	7.7	14.2	<.01	2.9	6.4	<.01
Multivessel disease	1.5	4.4	<.01	1.3	2.6	<.01
Positive remodeling	5.5	7.4	<.01	2.3	4.6	<.01
CACS*	20.1 ± 4.7	42.8 ± 16.3	<.01	5.7 ± 2.5	18.3 ± 7.8	<.01

Note.—Unless otherwise indicated, data are percentages. NS = not significant.
*Data are mean ± standard deviation.

This important study in a large group of asymptomatic patients clearly demonstrates that MS is associated with increased risk for subclinical coronary disease in both men and women. Of concern is the observation that the burden of noncalcified plaque is increased by MS in both genders. This type of plaque will not be detected by screening procedures for coronary artery calcium. Non-calcified plaque is also believed to be associated with less stable plaque that is more prone to rupture and induce acute coronary events.[1] Another particularly concerning finding in this study is the 3-fold and 2-fold heightened risk for multivessel disease in men and women, respectively. These results certainly support continued screening for, and treatment of, the various components of the MS to reduce the risk for coronary disease in both men and women.

P. P. Toth, MD, PhD

Reference

1. Libby P. Act local, act global: inflammation and the multiplicity of "vulnerable" coronary plaques. *J Am Coll Cardiol.* 2005;45:1600-1602.

Pharmacologic Therapy

Statin Use in Outpatients With Obstructive Coronary Artery Disease

Arnold SV, Spertus JA, Tang F, et al (Saint Luke's Mid America Heart Inst, Kansas City, MO; et al)
Circulation 124:2405-2410, 2011

Background.—Clinical trials have shown that statin therapy reduces cardiovascular morbidity and mortality in patients with coronary artery disease (CAD), even among patients with low-density lipoprotein cholesterol levels <100 mg/dL. We sought to determine the extent to which patients with obstructive CAD in routine outpatient care are treated with statins, nonstatins, or no lipid-lowering therapy.

Methods and Results.—Within the American College of Cardiology's Practice Innovation and Clinical Excellence (PINNACLE) outpatient registry, we examined rates of treatment with statin and nonstatin medications in 38 775 outpatients with obstructive CAD (history of myocardial infarction or coronary revascularization) and without documented contraindications to statin therapy. Among these patients, 30 160 (77.8%) were prescribed statins, 2042 (5.3%) were treated only with nonstatin lipid-lowering medications, and 6573 (17.0%) were untreated. Lack of medical insurance was associated with no statin treatment, and male sex, coexisting hypertension, and a recent coronary revascularization were associated with statin treatment. Among those not on any lipid-lowering therapy, low-density lipoprotein cholesterol levels were available for 51.2% (3365/6573). Among these untreated patients, low-density lipoprotein cholesterol levels were <100 mg/dL in 1794 patients (53.3%) and <100 mg/dL in 1571 patients (46.7%).

Conclusions.—Despite robust clinical trial evidence, a substantial number of patients with obstructive CAD remain untreated with statins. A small proportion were treated with nonstatin therapy, and 1 in 6 patients was simply untreated; half of the untreated patients had low-density lipoprotein cholesterol values <100 mg/dL. These findings illustrate important opportunities to improve lipid management in outpatients with obstructive CAD (Figs 3 and 4).

▶ In the secondary prevention setting, particularly in patients with a history of myocardial infarction or coronary revascularization, statin therapy is recommended for the lowering of atherogenic lipoprotein burden.[1] Statins have been found to reduce risk irrespective of baseline low-density lipoprotein (LDL)-C level.[2-4] Among patients presenting with an acute coronary syndrome or patients about to undergo either emergent or planned percutaneous coronary intervention (PCI),

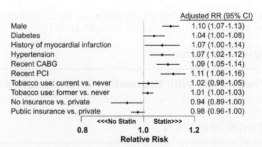

FIGURE 3.—Patient factors associated with statin therapy among patients with obstructive coronary artery disease in a multivariable model. Age and body mass index were included as nonlinear terms in the model with the use of cubic splines (Figures I and II in the online-only Data Supplement). CABG indicates coronary artery bypass graft surgery; PCI, percutaneous coronary intervention; RR, relative risk; and CI, confidence interval. (Reprinted from Arnold SV, Spertus JA, Tang F, et al. Statin use in outpatients with obstructive coronary artery disease. *Circulation.* 2011;124:2405-2410, with permission from American Heart Association, Inc.)

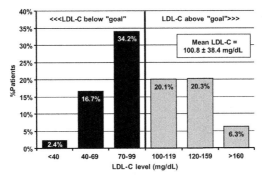

FIGURE 4.—Distribution of low-density lipoprotein cholesterol (LDL-C) levels among patients with obstructive coronary artery disease untreated with any lipid-lowering medications. (Reprinted from Arnold SV, Spertus JA, Tang F, et al. Statin use in outpatients with obstructive coronary artery disease. *Circulation.* 2011;124:2405-2410, with permission from American Heart Association, Inc.)

it is standard of care to initiate statin therapy without regard to baseline LDL-C given its benefit on cardiovascular morbidity and mortality.

In this important evaluation of statin usage among patients with a history of obstructive coronary artery disease (CAD), Arnold and coworkers extract data on 38 775 patients from the American College of Cardiology's Practice Innovation and Clinical Excellence (PINNACLE) outpatient registry. They found that although 78% of patients were treated with a statin, 17% were not. Six percent of patients received a nonstatin lipid-lowering medication. A lack of health insurance correlated with statins not having been prescribed. Male gender, history of myocardial infarction, coronary artery bypass grafting, PCI, and being hypertensive or diabetic all correlated with the initiation of statin therapy (Fig 3). Among patients not prescribed a statin, one-half had LDL-C levels greater than 100 mg/dL (Fig 4).

Unfortunately, despite guidelines by multiple specialty societies and the National Cholesterol Education Program, statin therapy is still not prescribed to 1 in 6 patients with a history of obstructive CAD. There is little doubt that some of the patients not prescribed a statin may have been intolerant of the medication, refused to take the medication, could not afford it, or had another reason for not taking it. It is unlikely that the managing physician simply did not prescribe a statin in these high-risk patients without a reason. This is an area that warrants serious additional investigation, as the cost of statin therapy has certainly decreased enough to make it affordable to virtually anyone who requires it. Statin therapy is highly efficacious and cost effective in this patient group, and strong efforts to initiate and continue therapy should be a high clinical priority.

P. P. Toth, MD, PhD

References

1. Grundy SM, Cleeman JI, Merz CN, et al. Implications of recent clinical trials for the National Cholesterol Education Program Adult Treatment Panel III guidelines. *Circulation.* 2004;110:227-239.

2. Heart Protection Study Collaborative Group. MRC/BHF Heart Protection Study of cholesterol lowering with simvastatin in 20,536 high-risk individuals: a randomised placebo-controlled trial. *Lancet.* 2002;360:7-22.
3. Sever PS, Dahlöf B, Poulter NR, et al. Prevention of coronary and stroke events with atorvastatin in hypertensive patients who have average or lower-than-average cholesterol concentrations, in the Anglo-Scandinavian Cardiac Outcomes Trial—Lipid Lowering Arm (ASCOT-LLA): a multicentre randomised controlled trial. *Lancet.* 2003;361:1149-1158.
4. Ridker PM, Danielson E, Fonseca FA, et al. Rosuvastatin to prevent vascular events in men and women with elevated C-reactive protein. *N Engl J Med.* 2008;359:2195-2207.

On-Treatment Non–High-Density Lipoprotein Cholesterol, Apolipoprotein B, Triglycerides, and Lipid Ratios in Relation to Residual Vascular Risk After Treatment With Potent Statin Therapy: JUPITER (Justification for the Use of Statins in Prevention: An Intervention Trial Evaluating Rosuvastatin)

Mora S, Glynn RJ, Boekholdt SM, et al (Brigham and Women's Hosp, Boston, MA; Harvard School of Public Health, Boston, MA; et al)
J Am Coll Cardiol 59:1521-1528, 2012

Objectives.—The goal of this study was to determine whether residual risk after high-dose statin therapy for primary prevention individuals with reduced levels of low-density lipoprotein cholesterol (LDL-C) is related to on-treatment apolipoprotein B, non–high-density lipoprotein cholesterol (non–HDL-C), trigylcerides, or lipid ratios, and how they compare with on-treatment LDL-C.

Background.—Guidelines focus on LDL-C as the primary target of therapy, yet residual risk for cardiovascular disease (CVD) among statin-treated individuals remains high and not fully explained.

Methods.—Participants in the randomized placebo-controlled JUPITER (Justification for the Use of Statins in Prevention: An Intervention Trial Evaluating Rosuvastatin) trial were adults without diabetes or CVD, with baseline LDL-C levels <130 mg/dl, high-sensitivity C-reactive protein levels ≥2 mg/l, and triglyceride concentrations <500 mg/dl. Individuals allocated to receive rosuvastatin 20 mg daily with baseline and on-treatment lipids and lipoproteins were examined in relation to the primary endpoint of incident CVD (nonfatal myocardial infarction or stroke, hospitalization for unstable angina, arterial revascularization, or cardiovascular death).

Results.—Using separate multivariate Cox models, statistically significant associations of a similar magnitude with residual risk of CVD were found for on-treatment LDL-C, non–HDL-C, apolipoprotein B, total cholesterol/HDL-C, LDL-C/HDL-C, and apolipoprotein B/A-I. The respective adjusted standardized hazard ratios (95% confidence intervals) for each of these measures were 1.31 (1.09 to 1.56), 1.25 (1.04 to 1.50), 1.27 (1.06 to 1.53), 1.22 (1.03 to 1.44), 1.29 (1.09 to 1.52), and 1.27 (1.09 to 1.49). The overall residual risk and the risk associated with these measures decreased among participants achieving on-treatment

LDL-C ≤70 mg/dl, on-treatment non–HDL-C ≤100 mg/dl, or on-treatment apolipoprotein B ≤80 mg/dl. In contrast, on-treatment triglycerides showed no association with CVD.

Conclusions.—In this primary prevention trial of nondiabetic individuals with low LDL-C and elevated high-sensitivity C-reactive protein, on-treatment LDL-C was as valuable as non–HDL-C, apolipoprotein B, or ratios in predicting residual risk. (JUPITER—Crestor 20 mg Versus Placebo in Prevention of Cardiovascular [CV] Events; NCT00239681) (Tables 1 and 4).

▶ Debate continues over which lipoprotein fraction or apoprotein best describes risk for cardiovascular disease. Low-density lipoprotein cholesterol (LDL-C) has been defined as the primary target of therapy in dyslipidemia management based on a large number of clinical trials. However, arguments have also been advanced suggesting that non-high-density lipoprotein cholesterol (HDL-C), apoprotein B (apo B), or LDL particle number be designated the primary target of therapy.[1-3]

In a post hoc analysis of the Justification for the Use of Statins in Primary Prevention: An Intervention Trial Evaluating Rosuvastatin (JUPITER) trial (a primary prevention trial in patients with high-sensitivity C-reactive protein greater than 2.0 g/L and LDL-C less than 130 mg/dL treated with either rosuvastatin 20 mg or placebo), these authors evaluated the impact of on-treatment apo B, non-HDL-C, lipid ratios, and triglycerides on residual risk in patients treated to a low LDL-C. The participants treated with rosuvastatin achieved very low levels of atherogenic indices (LDL-C 55 mg/dL, non-HDL-C 76 mg/dL, apo B 66 mg/dL, and TC/HDL-C ratio 2.5) (Table 1). Neither HDL-C nor apoprotein AI (apo AI) levels were predictive of residual risk in the JUPITER cohort. Among patients achieving LDL-C less than 100 mg/dL or non-HDL-C less than 130 mg/dL, standardized adjusted hazard ratios for first cardiovascular disease event or death were approximately equal for LDL-C, non-HDL-C, apo B, TC/HDL-C, and apo B/apo

TABLE 1.—Lipids, Apolipoproteins, and Ratios Among 7,832 Rosuvastatin-Treated Individuals With Baseline and 1-Year Measures of All Lipid Variables Examined

Variables	Baseline	Year 1	Change	p Value
Lipids (mg/dl)				
TC	186 (169, 200)	133 (116, 155)	−50 (−67, −27)	<0.0001
LDL-C	108 (94, 119)	55 (44, 71)	−50 (−63, −29)	<0.0001
Non–HDL-C	134 (118, 147)	76 (64, 96)	−54 (−70, −31)	<0.0001
Triglycerides	118 (85, 169)	99 (74, 137)	−17 (−48, 5)	<0.0001
HDL-C	49 (40, 60)	52 (43, 64)	3 (−2, 8)	<0.0001
Apolipoproteins (mg/dl)				
Apolipoprotein A-I	163 (144, 185)	165 (145, 188)	2 (−12, 16)	<0.0001
Apolipoprotein B	109 (95, 122)	66 (56, 81)	−41 (−54, −24)	<0.0001
Ratios				
TC/HDL-C	3.67 (3.06, 4.41)	2.50 (2.10, 3.05)	−1.11 (−1.65, −0.61)	<0.0001
LDL-C/HDL-C	2.14 (1.69, 2.64)	1.05 (0.78, 1.46)	−1.02 (−1.44, −0.57)	<0.0001
Apolipoprotein B/A-I	0.66 (0.55, 0.80)	0.40 (0.32, 0.52)	−0.25 (−0.35, −0.14)	<0.0001

Values are median (25th, 75th percentile).
HDL-C = high-density lipoprotein cholesterol; LDL-C = low-density lipoprotein cholesterol; TC = total cholesterol.

TABLE 4.—Risk of First CVD Event or Death for Standardized On-Treatment Lipids, Apolipoproteins, and Ratios According to Subgroups

Variable	CVD Standardized HR_adjusted (95% CI)	p Value	CVD/Death Standardized HR_adjusted (95% CI)	p Value
LDL-C ≤100 mg/dl (no. CVD/no. CVD or death/total N: 86/140/6,970)				
LDL-C	1.70 (1.22–2.36)	0.002	1.47 (1.13–1.91)	0.004
Non–HDL-C	1.31 (0.97–1.79)	0.08	1.34 (1.05–1.71)	0.02
Apolipoprotein B	1.40 (1.05–1.86)	0.02	1.35 (1.08–1.70)	0.009
TC/HD-C	1.15 (0.90–1.48)	0.26	1.18 (0.97–1.42)	0.10
LDL-C/HDL-C	1.43 (1.09–1.88)	0.01	1.34 (1.07–1.67)	0.01
Apolipoprotein B/A-I	1.31 (1.07–1.61)	0.009	1.30 (1.12–1.51)	0.001
LDL-C ≤70 mg/dl (no. CVD/no. CVD or death/total N: 61/103/5,793)				
LDL-C	0.96 (0.56–1.73)	0.96	0.88 (0.58–1.36)	0.57
Non–HDL-C	0.66 (0.39–1.12)	0.13	0.85 (0.57–1.28)	0.44
Apolipoprotein B	0.88 (0.56–1.37)	0.56	1.00 (0.71–1.40)	0.96
TC/HDL-C	0.92 (0.61–1.37)	0.67	1.05 (0.79–1.40)	0.73
LDL-C/HDL-C	1.17 (0.72–1.89)	0.52	1.15 (0.80–1.66)	0.46
Apolipoprotein B/A-I	1.18 (0.86–1.62)	0.31	1.24 (1.01–1.53)	0.04
Non–HDL-C ≤130 mg/dl (no. CVD/no. CVD or death/total N: 87/141/7,035)				
LDL-C	1.58 (1.18–2.13)	0.002	1.37 (1.08–1.74)	0.01
Non–HDL-C	1.36 (0.99–1.88)	0.06	1.36 (1.06–1.76)	0.02
Apolipoprotein B	1.40 (1.04–1.87)	0.03	1.35 (1.07–1.70)	0.01
TC/HDL-C	1.15 (0.87–1.53)	0.33	1.20 (0.97–1.49)	0.10
LDL-C/HDL-C	1.41 (1.07–1.86)	0.02	1.32 (1.05–1.65)	0.02
Apolipoprotein B/A-I	1.29 (1.05–1.60)	0.02	1.29 (1.11–1.51)	0.001
Non–HDL-C ≤100 mg/dl (no. CVD/no. CVD or death/total N: 70/114/6,108)				
LDL-C	1.26 (0.79–2.01)	0.33	1.11 (0.77–1.59)	0.58
Non–HDL-C	0.98 (0.59–1.62)	0.93	1.05 (0.71–1.57)	0.79
Apolipoprotein B	1.14 (0.74–1.73)	0.56	1.10 (0.79–1.53)	0.58
TC/HDL-C	1.05 (0.71–1.56)	0.79	1.12 (0.83–1.50)	0.45
LDL/HDL-C	1.29 (0.85–1.97)	0.24	1.22 (0.88–1.70)	0.24
Apolipoprotein B/A-I	1.23 (0.93–1.63)	0.14	1.26 (1.03–1.52)	0.02
Apolipoprotein B ≤90 mg/dl (no. CVD/no. CVD or death/total N: 76/125/6,511)				
LDL-C	1.44 (0.98–2.11)	0.06	1.25 (0.92–1.69)	0.15
Non–HDL-C	1.12 (0.74–1.69)	0.60	1.23 (0.89–1.68)	0.21
Apolipoprotein B	1.29 (0.86–1.91)	0.22	1.30 (0.96–1.78)	0.09
TC/HDL-C	1.03 (0.73–1.47)	0.86	1.14 (0.88–1.48)	0.34
LDL-C/HDL-C	1.31 (0.90–1.89)	0.16	1.24 (0.93–1.66)	0.14
Apolipoprotein B/A-I	1.23 (0.94–1.60)	0.12	1.28 (1.06–1.53)	0.009
Apolipoprotein B ≤80 mg/dl (no. CVD/no. CVD or death/total N: 66/107/5,798)				
LDL-C	1.38 (0.86–2.23)	0.18	1.15 (0.80–1.67)	0.45
Non–HDL-C	1.05 (0.62–1.76)	0.86	1.08 (0.72–1.62)	0.72
Apolipoprotein B	1.27 (0.77–2.09)	0.36	1.18 (0.80–1.75)	0.41
Total/HDL-C	0.96 (0.62–1.47)	0.84	1.05 (0.76–1.44)	0.78
LDL-C/HDL-C	1.20 (0.76–1.92)	0.44	1.15 (0.80–1.65)	0.45
Apolipoprotein B/A–I	1.18 (0.85–1.63)	0.32	1.22 (0.98–1.51)	0.08

Standardized HRs were adjusted for sex, age, smoking status, family history of premature atherosclerosis, body mass index, systolic blood pressure, and fasting glucose.
Abbreviations as in Tables 1 and 2.

AI (Table 4). Triglycerides had no predictivity. Among patients achieving an LDL less than 70 mg/dL, non-HDL-C less than 100 mg/dL, or apo B less than 80 mg/dL, there appears to be minimal residual risk attributable to other lipoprotein/apoprotein measures (Table 4).

In this very interesting analysis, neither triglycerides nor HDL-C contributed significantly to residual risk. Once LDL-C was reduced to less than 70 mg/dL, or non-HDL-C or apo B were decreased below 100 mg/dL and 80 mg/dL, respectively, the contributions of other lipid fractions to residual risk were no longer significant. These findings are consistent with the findings of AIM-HIGH study.[4] These results will have to be tested in a prospective, randomized study before they can be regarded as definitive. Moreover, because JUPITER evaluated a very specific type of patient in the primary prevention setting, these findings may also not be generalizable to all patients in primary prevention. Evidence is mounting, however, that aggressive reduction in atherogenic lipoprotein mass appears to significantly attenuate the need to reduce triglycerides or raise HDL-C in the average patient at risk.

P. P. Toth, MD, PhD

References

1. Robinson JG. Are you targeting non—high-density lipoprotein cholesterol? *J Am Coll Cardiol.* 2009;55:42-44.
2. Sniderman A, Williams K, de Graaf J. Non-HDL C equals apolipoprotein B: except when it does not! *Curr Opin Lipidol.* 2010;21:518-524.
3. Cromwell WC, Otvos JD. Low-density lipoprotein particle number and risk for cardiovascular disease. *Curr Atheroscler Rep.* 2004;6:381-387.
4. AIM-HIGH Investigators, Boden WE, Probstfield JL, Anderson T, et al. Niacin in patients with low HDL cholesterol levels receiving intensive statin therapy. *N Engl J Med.* 2011;365:2255-2267.

Association of LDL Cholesterol, Non—HDL Cholesterol, and Apolipoprotein B Levels With Risk of Cardiovascular Events Among Patients Treated With Statins: A Meta-analysis

Boekholdt SM, Arsenault BJ, Mora S, et al (Academic Med Ctr, Amsterdam, the Netherlands; Brigham and Women's Hosp, Boston, MA; et al)
JAMA 307:1302-1309, 2012

Context.—The associations of low-density lipoprotein cholesterol (LDL-C), non—high-density lipoprotein cholesterol (non—HDL-C), and apolipoprotein B (apoB) levels with the risk of cardiovascular events among patients treated with statin therapy have not been reliably documented.

Objective.—To evaluate the relative strength of the associations of LDL-C, non—HDL-C, and apoB with cardiovascular risk among patients treated with statin therapy.

Design.—Meta-analysis of individual patient data from randomized controlled statin trials in which conventional lipids and apolipoproteins were determined in all study participants at baseline and at 1-year follow-up.

Data Sources.—Relevant trials were identified by a literature search updated through December 31, 2011. Investigators were contacted and individual patient data were requested and obtained for 62154 patients enrolled in 8 trials published between 1994 and 2008.

Data Extraction.—Hazard ratios (HRs) and corresponding 95% CIs for risk of major cardiovascular events adjusted for established risk factors by 1-SD increase in LDL-C, non—HDL-C, and apoB.

Results.—Among 38 153 patients allocated to statin therapy, 158 fatal myocardial infarctions, 1678 nonfatal myocardial infarctions, 615 fatal events from other coronary artery disease, 2806 hospitalizations for unstable angina, and 1029 fatal or nonfatal strokes occurred during follow-up. The adjusted HRs for major cardiovascular events per 1-SD increase were 1.13 (95% CI, 1.10-1.17) for LDL-C, 1.16 (95% CI, 1.12-1.19) for non—HDL-C, and 1.14 (95% CI, 1.11-1.18) for apoB. These HRs were significantly higher for non—HDL-C than LDL-C (*P* = .002) and apoB (*P* = .02). There was no significant difference between apoB and LDL-C (*P* = .21).

Conclusion.—Among statin-treated patients, on-treatment levels of LDL-C, non—HDL-C, and apoB were each associated with risk of future major cardiovascular events, but the strength of this association was greater for non—HDL-C than for LDL-C and apoB (Table 1).

▶ Apoprotein B100 (apoB) is the primary apoprotein constituent of atherogenic lipoproteins, including very low-density lipoproteins (VLDL) and their remnants, intermediate-density lipoproteins, low-density lipoproteins (LDL), and lipoprotein (a). Non—high-density lipoprotein (non-HDL; defined as total cholesterol minus HDL) is a surrogate of apoB, as it includes all atherogenic lipoproteins. According to the National Cholesterol Education Program's Third Adult Treatment Panel (ATPIII), risk-stratified levels of LDL are the primary target of therapy in patients with dyslipidemia. ATPIII also recommended that among patients with baseline fasting triglycerides that exceed 200 mg/dL, risk-stratified non-HDL levels be the secondary target of therapy. Considerable debate has been raging for years about whether LDL-C, non—HDL-C, or apoB should be the primary target of therapy when treating patients who have dyslipidemia so as to maximize risk reduction for cardiovascular events.[1,2]

Boekholdt et al reassess this issue by performing a meta-analysis on patient level data from 8 major statin trials. A 1-standard-deviation increase in serum levels of LDL-C, non—HDL-C, and apoB resulted in hazard ratios of 1.13, 1.16, and 1.14, respectively (Table 1). Statin-induced changes in LDL-C, non—HDL-C, and apoB were responsible for 50%, 64%, and 54% of the total effect of statin therapy. The proportion of treatment effect by statin therapy was greater for non—HDL-C than either LDL-C (*P* < .001) or apoB (*P* < .007). Consequently, non—HDL-C had a stronger association of risk for cardiovascular events than either LDL-C or apoB, and non—HDL-C reduction with statin therapy was therapeutically more efficacious than reductions in LDL-C or apoB. Of great practical interest is the finding that patients whose LDL-C is less than 100 mg/dL but whose non—HDL-C is greater than 130 mg/dL have significantly greater risk than those whose LDL-C is greater than 100 mg/dL but non—HDL-C is less than 130 mg/dL (Fig 1 in the original article).

While this debate cannot be considered definitely settled, these findings provide strong support for the conclusion that non—HDL-C is a better predictor of risk than is either LDL-C or apoB. Another issue that supports the use of non—HDL-C for managing risk is the fact that its calculation is mathematically trivial, and it can be determined from any standard lipid profile without incurring

TABLE 1.—Lipid and Apolipoprotein Levels and Risk of Major Cardiovascular Events in Statin-Treated Patients[a]

	Quartiles[b]				P Value[c]	Per 1-SD Increase	P Value
	1	2	3	4			
LDL-C							
Mean, mg/dL	49	74	97	129			
Range, mg/dL	<62	62-85	86-108	≥109			
Event rate, %	7.3	14.2	17.1	17.9			
Events/total[d]	697/9538	1360/9573	1616/9478	1714/9564			
Hazard ratio (95% CI)[e]	1 [Reference]	1.06 (0.97-1.17)	1.15 (1.05-1.27)	1.26 (1.14-1.39)	<.001	1.13 (1.10-1.17)	<.001
Non–HDL-C							
Mean, mg/dL	69	98	124	161			
Range, mg/dL	<85	85-112	113-137	>137			
Event rate, %	7.3	14.2	16.4	18.7			
Events/total[d]	701/9659	1340/9404	1568/9564	1778/9526			
Hazard ratio (95% CI)[e]	1 [Reference]	1.12 (1.02-1.24)	1.17 (1.06-1.28)	1.42 (1.29-1.56)	<.001	1.16 (1.12-1.19)	<.001
Apolipoprotein B							
Mean, mg/dL	60	80	97	127			
Range, mg/dL	<70	71-90	91-108	≥109			
Event rate, %	8.6	12.9	15.5	19.7			
Events/total[d]	856/9998	1166/9038	1489/9582	1876/9535			
Hazard ratio (95% CI)[e]	1 [Reference]	1.05 (0.96-1.16)	1.12 (1.03-1.23)	1.33 (1.22-1.45)	<.001	1.14 (1.11-1.18)	<.001

Abbreviations: HDL-C, high-density lipoprotein cholesterol; LDL-C, low-density lipoprotein cholesterol.
[a]Analyses were based only on study participants allocated to statin therapy.
[b]Analyses were performed by quartiles of lipid or apolipoprotein B levels using those in the bottom quartile as reference, and also by SD.
[c]P values for linear trend across quartiles of lipids or apolipoproteins.
[d]Indicates number of events/total number of study participants.
[e]Proportional hazard models were adjusted for sex, age, smoking, diabetes mellitus, systolic blood pressure, and trial.

additional cost to patients or second-party payers. These data also support expansion of non—HDL-C treatment to all patients, not just those with baseline triglycerides that exceed 200 mg/dL.

P. P. Toth, MD, PhD

References

1. Sniderman A, Williams K, de Graaf J. Non-HDL C equals apolipoprotein B: except when it does not! *Curr Opin Lipidol.* 2010;21:518-524.
2. Robinson JG. Are you targeting non-high-density lipoprotein cholesterol? *J Am Coll Cardiol.* 2009;55:42-44.

The effects of lowering LDL cholesterol with simvastatin plus ezetimibe in patients with chronic kidney disease (Study of Heart and Renal Protection): a randomised placebo-controlled trial
Baigent C, on behalf of the SHARP Investigators (Univ of Oxford, UK; et al)
Lancet 377:2181-2192, 2011

Background.—Lowering LDL cholesterol with statin regimens reduces the risk of myocardial infarction, ischaemic stroke, and the need for coronary revascularisation in people without kidney disease, but its effects in people with moderate-to-severe kidney disease are uncertain. The SHARP trial aimed to assess the efficacy and safety of the combination of simvastatin plus ezetimibe in such patients.

Methods.—This randomised double-blind trial included 9270 patients with chronic kidney disease (3023 on dialysis and 6247 not) with no known history of myocardial infarction or coronary revascularisation. Patients were randomly assigned to simvastatin 20 mg plus ezetimibe 10 mg daily versus matching placebo. The key prespecified outcome was first major atherosclerotic event (non-fatal myocardial infarction or coronary death, non-haemorrhagic stroke, or any arterial revascularisation procedure). All analyses were by intention to treat. This trial is registered at ClinicalTrials.gov, NCT00125593, and ISRCTN54137607.

Findings.—4650 patients were assigned to receive simvastatin plus ezetimibe and 4620 to placebo. Allocation to simvastatin plus ezetimibe yielded an average LDL cholesterol difference of $0·85$ mmol/L (SE $0·02$; with about two-thirds compliance) during a median follow-up of $4·9$ years and produced a 17% proportional reduction in major atherosclerotic events (526 [11·3%] simvastatin plus ezetimibe *vs* 619 [13·4%] placebo; rate ratio [RR] $0·83$, 95% CI $0·74—0·94$; log-rank $p=0·0021$). Non-significantly fewer patients allocated to simvastatin plus ezetimibe had a non-fatal myocardial infarction or died from coronary heart disease (213 [4·6%] *vs* 230 [5·0%]; RR $0·92$, 95% CI $0·76—1·11$; $p=0·37$) and there were significant reductions in non-haemorrhagic stroke (131 [2·8%] *vs* 174 [3·8%]; RR $0·75$, 95% CI $0·60—0·94$; $p=0·01$) and arterial revascularisation procedures (284 [6·1%] *vs* 352 [7·6%]; RR $0·79$, 95% CI $0·68—0·93$; $p=0·0036$). After weighting for subgroup-specific reductions in LDL cholesterol, there was no good evidence that the proportional effects on major atherosclerotic events differed from the summary rate ratio in any subgroup examined, and, in particular, they were similar in patients on dialysis and those who were not. The excess risk of myopathy was only two per 10 000 patients per year of treatment with this combination (9 [0·2%] *vs* 5 [0·1%]). There was no evidence of excess risks of hepatitis (21 [0·5%] *vs* 18 [0·4%]), gallstones (106 [2·3%] *vs* 106 [2·3%]), or cancer (438 [9·4%] *vs* 439 [9·5%], *p*=0·89) and there was no significant excess of death from any non-vascular cause (668 [14·4%] *vs* 612 [13·2%], *p*=0·13).

Interpretation.—Reduction of LDL cholesterol with simvastatin 20 mg plus ezetimibe 10 mg daily safely reduced the incidence of major atherosclerotic events in a wide range of patients with advanced chronic kidney disease (Figs 2, 3, and 5).

▶ Chronic kidney disease (CKD) is highly prevalent and is associated with an increase in risk not only for the development of end-stage renal disease, but also for cardiovascular morbidity and mortality.[1,2] As renal filtration capacity progressively declines, risk for cardiovascular disease increases significantly. Two previous studies to evaluate the efficacy of statin therapy for reducing risk of cardiovascular events in patients who receive hemodialysis showed trends for benefit but were unable to achieve statistical significance.[3,4] Another trial to test the benefit of statin therapy in patients who had undergone previous renal transplantation was also negative for significant cardiovascular risk reduction.[5] Given the significant prevalence of dyslipidemia in patients with CKD and

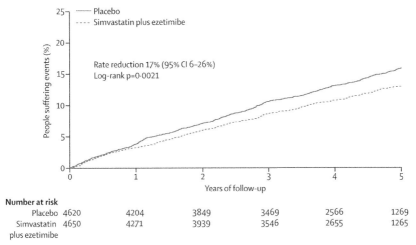

FIGURE 2.—Life-table plot of effects of allocation to simvastatin plus ezetimibe versus placebo on major atherosclerotic events. Numbers remaining at risk of a first major atherosclerotic event at the beginning of each year are shown for both treatment groups. (Reprinted from Baigent C, on behalf of the SHARP Investigators. The effects of lowering LDL cholesterol with simvastatin plus ezetimibe in patients with chronic kidney disease (Study of Heart and Renal Protection): a randomised placebo-controlled trial. *Lancet.* 2011;377:2181-2192, © 2011, with permission from Elsevier.)

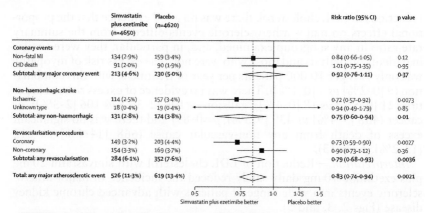

FIGURE 3.—Major atherosclerotic events subdivided by type. MI=myocardial infarction. CHD=coronary heart disease. (Reprinted from Baigent C, on behalf of the SHARP Investigators. The effects of lowering LDL cholesterol with simvastatin plus ezetimibe in patients with chronic kidney disease (Study of Heart and Renal Protection): a randomised placebo-controlled trial. *Lancet.* 2011;377:2181-2192, © 2011, with permission from Elsevier.)

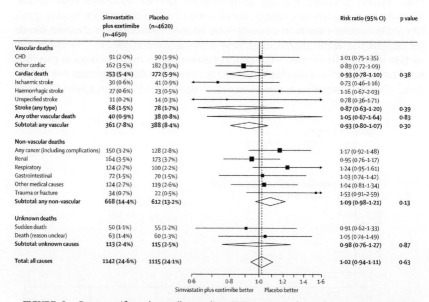

FIGURE 5.—Cause-specific and overall mortality. CHD=coronary heart disease. (Reprinted from Baigent C, on behalf of the SHARP Investigators. The effects of lowering LDL cholesterol with simvastatin plus ezetimibe in patients with chronic kidney disease (Study of Heart and Renal Protection): a randomised placebo-controlled trial. *Lancet.* 2011;377:2181-2192, © 2011, with permission from Elsevier.)

the heightened risk for cardiovascular morbidity and mortality that this condition entails, it remains a high clinical priority to make attempts to reduce this risk.

The Study of Heart and Renal Protection (SHARP) evaluated the potential benefit of treating patients with CKD with or without dialysis with a combination of simvastatin and ezetimibe to reduce risk for acute cardiovascular events. Because simvastatin has a significant dependence on renal elimination, the dose of this drug was kept fixed at 20 mg so as to reduce risk for adverse events. The simvastatin was used in combination with ezetimibe and compared to placebo in 9270 patients followed for approximately 5 years. Lipid-lowering therapy was associated with a statistically significant ($P = .0021$) 17% reduction in risk for acute atherosclerotic events (Fig 2). There was a trend for a 16% reduction in risk for nonfatal myocardial infarction (MI), a significant 28% reduction in risk of ischemic stroke, and a 27% reduction in need for coronary revascularization (Fig 3). Patients who received dialysis showed a trend for benefit, but this did not achieve statistical significance. Similarly, there was no significant reduction in risk for coronary or all-cause mortality (Fig 5). The study size was not large enough to detect a reduction in coronary mortality, because only 24% of deaths in the study were definitely attributed to cardiac etiologies. There was no excess risk for cancer attributable to combination lipid-lowering therapy.

SHARP is an important clinical trial. It is the first trial to demonstrate significant impact on risk for atherosclerotic events in patients with CKD. Therapy was shown to be safe and well tolerated. Although nonfatal MI and coronary mortality were not reduced, important other endpoints, such as ischemic stroke and coronary revascularization, were. In addition, the authors showed that the magnitude of risk reduction in the primary composite endpoint was proportional to the magnitude of low-density lipoprotein cholesterol (LDL-C) reduction, suggesting that ezetimibe contributed to overall risk reduction. LDL-C lowering should be an important component of risk management in patients with CKD.

P. P. Toth, MD, PhD

References

1. Matsushita K, van der Velde M, Astor BC, et al. Association of estimated glomerular filtration rate and albuminuria with all-cause and cardiovascular mortality in general population cohorts: a collaborative meta-analysis. *Lancet.* 2010;375: 2073-2081.
2. Foley RN, Parfrey PS, Sarnak MJ. Clinical epidemiology of cardiovascular disease in chronic renal disease. *Am J Kidney Dis.* 1998;325:S112-S119.
3. Wanner C, Krane V, März W, et al. Atorvastatin in patients with type 2 diabetes mellitus undergoing hemodialysis. *N Engl J Med.* 2005;353:238-248.
4. Fellström BC, Jardine AG, Schmieder RE, et al. Rosuvastatin and cardiovascular events in patients undergoing hemodialysis. *N Engl J Med.* 2009;360:1395-1407.
5. Holdaas H, Fellström B, Jardine AG, et al. Effect of fluvastatin on cardiac outcomes in renal transplant recipients: a multicentre, randomised, placebo-controlled trial. *Lancet.* 2003;361:2024-2031.

High-density lipoprotein cholesterol as a predictor of clinical outcomes in patients achieving low-density lipoprotein cholesterol targets with statins after percutaneous coronary intervention

Seo SM, Catholic University of Korea, Percutaneous Coronary Intervention Registry investigators (Catholic Univ of Korea, Seoul; et al)
Heart 97:1943-1950, 2011

Background.—A low level of high-density lipoprotein cholesterol (HDL-C) is strongly associated with cardiovascular events. However, the significance of HDLC after statin therapy on the outcome of patients who have undergone percutaneous coronary intervention (PCI) with drug eluting stents (DES) is unclear.

Objectives.—To investigate the significance of HDL-C after statin therapy on cardiovascular events in patients with coronary artery disease after DES implantation.

Methods.—Patients who underwent PCI with DES from January 2004 to December 2009 were prospectively enrolled. The follow-up lipid panel of 2693 patients (median lab follow-up duration 225 days) who had continued using statins after PCI and who attained low-density lipoprotein cholesterol (LDL-C) <100 mg/dl was analysed. Major adverse cardiac events (MACE), including all-cause death, non-fatal myocardial infarction, and target vessel revascularisation according to follow-up HDL-C level (40 mg/dl for men or 50 mg/dl for women) were compared with the use of propensity scores matching.

Results.—Median follow-up duration was 832 days. 1585 (58.9%) patients had low follow-up HDL-C and 1108 had high follow-up HDL-C. The low follow-up HDL-C group had significantly higher rates of MACE. Low follow-up HDL-C was a significant independent predictor of MACE (adjusted HR 1.404, 95% CI 1.111 to 1.774, $p=0.004$). In further analysis with propensity scores matching, overall findings were consistent.

Conclusions.—Raising HDL-C levels may be a subsequent goal after achieving target LDL-C levels in patients with DES implantation (Fig 2).

▶ The high-density lipoproteins (HDLs) have a highly diverse proteasome, which confers a wide range of functionality to these particles, such as a capacity to engage in reverse cholesterol transport, antagonize lipoprotein oxidation, inhibit platelet activation, and participate in immunity.[1,2] The HDLs also appear to play an important role in endothelial cell health and viability, as they reverse many features of endothelial cell dysfunction, such as downregulating adhesion molecule expression, normalizing the ratio of tissue plasminogen activator to plasminogen activator inhibitor-1, and promoting nitric production and release, among other effects.[3] In patients with coronary artery disease, there is evidence that the functionality of the HDLs is compromised, which may facilitate disease progression.[4] Among patients undergoing coronary revascularization with drug-eluting stents (DES), a low HDL-C was an independent predictor of risk for reinfarction and death and need for repeat vascularization.[5] Seo and coworkers evaluated the impact of a low serum HDL-C (< 40 mg/dL in men

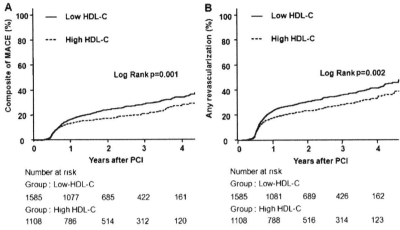

FIGURE 2.—Kaplane—Meier curves in all study populations. (A) Kaplane—Meier curves for major adverse cardiac events (MACE) in the all-study population with low follow-up high-density lipoprotein cholesterol (HDL-C) (solid line) versus high follow-up HDL-C (dashed line). (B) Kaplane—Meier curves for any revascularisation in the all-study population with low follow-up HDL-C (solid line) versus high follow-up HDL-C (dashed line). PCI, percutaneous coronary intervention. (Reprinted from Seo SM, Catholic University of Korea, Percutaneous Coronary Intervention Registry investigators. High-density lipoprotein cholesterol as a predictor of clinical outcomes in patients achieving low-density lipoprotein cholesterol targets with statins after percutaneous coronary intervention. *Heart.* 2011;97:1943-1950, Copyright 2011, with permission from the BMJ Publishing Group Ltd.)

and < 50 mg/dL in women) on risk of major acute coronary events (MACE; nonfatal myocardial infarction, stroke, death, and need for revascularization) among 2693 Asian patients who have an low-density lipoprotein (LDL)-C less than 100 mg/dL and have undergone placement of a DES. Compared with patients with normal levels of HDL-C, those with a low level as defined above had a 40% higher risk of MACE (*P* = .004) and a 45% (*P* = .008) and 46% (*P* = .003) higher risk of requiring target lesion revascularization and target vessel revascularization, respectively (Fig 2).

Consistent with post-hoc analyses of statin trials, a low HDL-C remains an important predictor of risk for future cardiovascular events even in patients treated with statins whose LDL-C is at National Cholesterol Education Program target levels.[6,7] The placement of a DES in these patients may be particularly risk provoking, as HDL particles can modulate endothelial cell function, thereby possibly modulating the pace of re-endothelialization or neointimalization of coronary stents, although this is hypothetical and requires considerable investigation. How best to intervene in these patients, whether it is by more LDL-C/non—HDL-C lowering, or greater HDL-C elevation, is a subject that only prospective, randomized studies will be able to settle in a definitive manner.

P. P. Toth, MD, PhD

References

1. Heinecke JW. The HDL proteome: a marker—and perhaps mediator—of coronary artery disease. *J Lipid Res.* 2009;50:S167-S171.

2. Vaisar T, Pennathur S, Green PS, et al. Shotgun proteomics implicates protease inhibition and complement activation in the antiinflammatory properties of HDL. *J Clin Invest.* 2007;117:746-756.
3. Calabresi L, Gomaraschi M, Franceschini G. Endothelial protection by high-density lipoproteins: from bench to bedside. *Arterioscler Thromb Vasc Biol.* 2003;23: 1724-1731.
4. Ansell BJ, Fonarow GC, Fogelman AM. High-density lipoprotein: is it always atheroprotective? *Curr Atheroscler Rep.* 2006;8:405-411.
5. Wolfram RM, Brewer HB, Xue Z, et al. Impact of low high-density lipoproteins on in-hospital events and one-year clinical outcomes in patients with non-ST-elevation myocardial infarction acute coronary syndrome treated with drug-eluting stent implantation. *Am J Cardiol.* 2006;98:711-717.
6. Barter P, Gotto AM, LaRosa JC, et al. HDL cholesterol, very low levels of LDL cholesterol, and cardiovascular events. *N Engl J Med.* 2007;357:1301-1310.
7. Jafri H, Alsheikh-Ali AA, Karas RH. Meta-analysis: statin therapy does not alter the association between low levels of high-density lipoprotein cholesterol and increased cardiovascular risk. *Ann Intern Med.* 2010;153:800-808.

Effects of the CETP Inhibitor Evacetrapib Administered as Monotherapy or in Combination With Statins on HDL and LDL Cholesterol: A Randomized Controlled Trial

Nicholls SJ, Brewer HB, Kastelein JJP, et al (Cleveland Clinic, OH; Medstar Res Inst, Washington, DC; Academic Med Ctr, Amsterdam, the Netherlands; et al)

JAMA 306:2099-2109, 2011

Context.—Interest remains high in cholesteryl ester transfer protein (CETP) inhibitors as cardioprotective agents. Few studies have documented the efficacy and safety of CETP inhibitors in combination with commonly used statins.

Objective.—To examine the biochemical effects, safety, and tolerability of evacetrapib, as monotherapy and in combination with statins, in patients with dyslipidemia.

Design, Setting, and Participants.—Randomized controlled trial conducted among 398 patients with elevated low-density lipoprotein cholesterol (LDL-C) or low high-density lipoprotein cholesterol (HDL-C) levels from April 2010 to January 2011 at community and academic centers in the United States and Europe.

Interventions.—Following dietary lead-in, patients were randomly assigned to receive placebo (n=38); evacetrapib monotherapy, 30 mg/d (n=40), 100 mg/d (n=39), or 500 mg/d (n=42); or statin therapy (n=239) (simvastatin, 40 mg/d; atorvastatin, 20 mg/d; or rosuvastatin, 10 mg/d) with or without evacetrapib, 100 mg/d, for 12 weeks.

Main Outcome Measures.—The co–primary end points were percentage changes from baseline in HDL-C and LDL-C after 12 weeks of treatment.

Results.—The mean baseline HDL-C level was 55.1 (SD, 15.3) mg/dL and the mean baseline LDL-C level was 144.3 (SD, 26.6) mg/dL. As monotherapy, evacetrapib produced dose-dependent increases in HDL-C of 30.0 to 66.0 mg/dL (53.6% to 128.8%) compared with a decrease with placebo of -0.7 mg/dL (-3.0%; $P < .001$ for all compared with placebo) and decreases in LDL-C of -20.5 to -51.4 mg/dL (-13.6% to -35.9%) compared with an increase with placebo of 7.2 mg/dL (3.9%; $P < .001$ for all compared with placebo). In combination with statin therapy, evacetrapib, 100 mg/d, produced increases in HDL-C of 42.1 to 50.5 mg/dL (78.5% to 88.5%; $P < .001$ for all compared with statin monotherapy) and decreases in LDL-C of -67.1 to -75.8 mg/dL (-11.2% to -13.9%; $P < .001$ for all compared with statin monotherapy). Compared with evacetrapib monotherapy, the combination of statins and evacetrapib resulted in greater reductions in LDL-C ($P < .001$) but no greater increase in HDL-C ($P = .39$). Although the study was underpowered, no adverse effects were observed.

Conclusions.—Compared with placebo or statin monotherapy, evacetrapib as monotherapy or in combination with statins increased HDL-C levels and decreased LDL-C levels. The effects on cardiovascular outcomes require further investigation.

Trial Registration.—clinicaltrials.gov Identifier: NCT01105975 (Tables 3 and 5).

▶ Cholesterol ester transfer protein (CETP) inhibitors offer a particularly potent means by which to increase serum levels of high-density lipoprotein cholesterol (HDL-C). The CETP inhibitors inhibit the loading of HDL particles with triglyceride and apolipoprotein (apo) B containing particles with cholesterol ester. It is hypothesized that this may be antiatherogenic because: (1) as the triglyceride mass in HDL decreases, the HDL particle is less vulnerable to lipolysis and catabolism by hepatic lipase and (2) there will be less enrichment of the apo B fraction with cholesterol ester, perhaps rendering it less atherogenic. Concern with this class of therapeutic agent is driven by the fact that another member of this class, torcetrapib, was associated with increased risk for cardiovascular morbidity and mortality[1] and no impact on the progression of atherosclerotic disease in either the carotid[2] or coronary vasculature.[3] It is currently believed that the majority of the toxicity of torcetrapib arose from off-target toxicity, namely an increase in serum aldosterone, electrolyte disturbances, and blood pressure that could be substantial (> 15/10 mm Hg). Recent investigations with dalcetrapib and anacetrapib suggest no such toxicity associated with these agents.[4,5]

Evacetrapib is the third CETP inhibitor to go into phase 3 evaluation. Nicholls and coworkers found that Evacetrapib raises HDL-C (54-129%) and lowers LDL-C (13.6-35.9%) in a dose-dependent manner (Table 3). Triglycerides are impacted negligibly. There was also no safety signal associated with use of the drug either alone or in combination with a statin (Table 5). Specifically, there was no increased risk for liver or muscle toxicity, no increase in blood pressure, and no disturbance in serum electrolytes (sodium, potassium, bicarbonate). Serum aldosterone and salivary cortisol were unchanged compared with placebo.

These are promising data. It remains to be seen whether subtle or overt differences emerge between the 3 CETP inhibitors currently in development for

TABLE 3.—Change in Laboratory Measures (Monotherapy Evaluation)[a]

Measures	Placebo (n = 38)	30 mg/d (n = 40)	Evacetrapib 100 mg/d (n = 38)	500 mg/d (n = 40)
LDL-C, mg/dL				
Follow-up	153.3 (32.8)	124.4 (26.8)	114.8 (34.0)	87.4 (24.8)
Absolute change	7.2 (0 to 14.4)	−20.5 (−27.8 to −13.3)	−31.7 (−39.0 to −24.4)	−51.4 (−58.9 to −43.9)
Percentage change	3.9 (−1.0 to 8.9)	−13.6 (−18.6 to −8.7)	−22.3 (−27.3 to −17.3)	−35.9 (−41.1 to −30.7)
Relative change		−17.6 (−24.6 to −10.5)[b]	−26.2 (−33.2 to −19.2)[b]	−39.8 (−47.0 to −32.7)[b]
HDL-C, mg/dL				
Follow-up	51.6 (13.7)	87.1 (24.0)	108.6 (28.9)	126.1 (25.7)
Absolute change	−0.7 (−5.6 to 4.3)	30.0 (25.1 to 35.0)	50.9 (45.9 to 55.9)	66.0 (60.8 to 71.1)
Percentage change	−3.0 (−12.3 to 6.2)	53.6 (44.4 to 62.9)	94.6 (85.2 to 104.0)	128.8 (119.2 to 138.4)
Relative change		56.7 (43.6 to 69.8)[b]	97.6 (84.5 to 110.8)[b]	131.9 (118.5 to 145.2)[b]
Triglycerides, mg/dL, median (IQR)				
Follow-up, median (IQR)	121.3 (86.4 to 178.9)	106.3 (85.0 to 147.9)	113.4 (83.3 to 148.8)	94.8 (80.6 to 121.3)
Absolute change	−0.5 (−12.4 to 11.4)	−13.2 (−25.2 to −1.2)	−9.8 (−21.8 to 2.3)	−26.7 (−39.1 to −14.4)
Percentage change	9.3 (1.0 to 17.5)	−3.1 (−11.4 to 5.2)	−3.1 (−11.5 to 5.2)	−10.8 (−19.4 to −2.2)
Relative change		−12.4 (−24.1 to −0.6)	−12.4 (−24.2 to −0.6)	−20.1 (−32.0 to −8.2)[c]
CRP, mg/L[d]				
Follow-up, median (IQR)	1.8 (1.0 to 4.0)	1.7 (0.6 to 6.4)	1.2 (0.8 to 3.2)	1.7 (0.7 to 5.6)
Absolute change	−1.7 (−4.4 to 1.0)	0.9 (−1.7 to 3.6)	1.2 (−1.4 to 3.9)	0.9 (−1.6 to 3.5)
Percentage change	75.5 (5.9 to 145.1)	127.8 (58.7 to 196.9)	76.6 (7.2 to 146.0)	120.0 (53.5 to 186.4)
Relative change		52.3 (−45.5 to 150.1)	1.1 (−97.5 to 99.8)	44.5 (−51.5 to 140.5)

Abbreviations: CRP, C-reactive protein; HDL-C, high-density lipoprotein cholesterol; IQR, interquartile range; LDL-C, low-density lipoprotein cholesterol. SI conversions: To convert HDL-C and LDL-C to mmol/L, multiply by 0.0259; to convert triglycerides to mmol/L, multiply by 0.0113.

[a]Follow-up values are mean (SD) unless otherwise noted. Absolute changes are least-squares mean changes from baseline until follow-up visit 7 from analysis of covariance model (90% CI) unless otherwise noted. Percentage changes are least-squares mean percentage changes from baseline until follow-up visit 7 from analysis of covariance model (90% CI) unless otherwise noted. Relative changes are differences in percentage changes between placebo and evacetrapib counterpart.

[b]*P*<.001.

[c]*P*<.01.

[d]Last-observation-carried-forward data are applied in the analysis.

TABLE 5.—Safety Data[a]

Measures	Placebo (n = 38)	Evacetrapib 30 mg/d (n = 40)	Evacetrapib 100 mg/d (n = 38)	Evacetrapib 500 mg/d (n = 40)	Statin Monotherapy (n = 121)	Statin + Evacetrapib, 100 mg/d (n = 116)
Drug-related adverse events, No. (%)	7 (18.4)	8 (20.0)	5 (13.2)	10 (25.0)	22 (18.2)	31 (26.7)
Adverse events leading to discontinuation, No. (%)	1 (2.6)	2 (5.0)	1 (2.6)	5 (12.5)	3 (2.5)	9 (7.8)
Serious adverse events, No. (%)	0	0	0	1(2.5)	1 (0.8)	2 (1.7)
Drug-related serious adverse events, No. (%)	0	0	0	0	0	0
Elevation in systolic blood pressure ≥15 mm Hg, No. (%)[b]	4 (10.5)	9 (23.1)	5 (13.2)	8 (20.0)	23 (19.3)	25 (21.6)
Elevation in diastolic blood pressure ≥10 mm Hg, No. (%)[b]	10 (26.3)	7 (17.9)	9 (23.7)	11 (27.5)	30 (25.2)	23 (19.8)
Creatinine >ULN, No. (%)[b]	1 (2.6)	1 (2.6)	2 (5.2)	4 (10.0)	9 (7.6)	6 (5.2)
Creatine kinase >5× ULN, No. (%)[b]	1 (2.6)	0	0	0	2 (1.7)	2 (1.7)
Alanine aminotransferase >3× ULN, No. (%)[b]	0	0	0	0	0	1 (0.9)
Aldosterone, ng/dL[c]						
Baseline	8.30 (8.108)	7.71 (8.17)	5.97 (4.27)	6.73 (5.94)	7.67 (5.29)	6.99 (4.38)
Follow-up	6.54 (4.67)	6.87 (4.80)	7.77 (6.74)	6.76 (5.49)	6.34 (5.63)	6.82 (5.26)
Absolute change	-1.00 (-2.69 to 0.68)	-0.45 (-2.18 to 1.27)	0.96 (-0.75 to 2.67)	-0.30 (-2.06 to 1.45)	-1.12 (-2.11 to -0.13)	-0.45 (-1.48 to 0.58)
Percentage change	112.84 (14.94 to 210.74)	90.37 (-9.17 to 189.91)	69.84 (-29.07 to 168.74)	271.04 (169.64 to 372.44)	34.88 (-22.15 to 91.91)	30.93 (-27.60 to 89.46)
Relative change		-22.47 (-162.03 to 117.09)	-43.00 (-182.18 to 96.17)	158.20 (17.23 to 299.17)[d]		-3.95 (-85.65 to 77.75)
Salivary cortisol, µg/dL[c,e]						
Baseline	0.11 (0.12)	0.10 (0.12)	0.07 (0.07)	0.07 (0.06)	0.07 (0.06)	0.07 (0.08)
Follow-up	0.08 (0.12)	0.06 (0.05)	0.07 (0.05)	0.09 (0.09)	0.10 (0.16)	0.08 (0.09)
Absolute change	-0.003 (-0.05 to 0.04)	-0.03 (-0.08 to 0.02)	0.002 (-0.05 to 0.05)	0.004 (-0.05 to 0.06)	0.03 (0.001 to 0.05)	0.01 (-0.02 to 0.03)

(Continued)

TABLE 5.—(Continued)

Measures	Placebo (n = 38)	30 mg/d (n = 40)	Evacetrapib 100 mg/d (n = 38)	500 mg/d (n = 40)	Statin Monotherapy (n = 121)	Statin + Evacetrapib, 100 mg/d (n = 116)
Percentage change	6.53 (−68.79 to 81.86)	9.96 (−65.44 to 85.36)	109.05 (33.59 to 184.52)	63.11 (−20.79 to 147.01)	64.78 (22.04 to 107.51)	32.10 (−12.90 to 77.11)
Relative change		3.42 (−102.55 to 109.41)	102.52 (−4.13 to 209.18)	56.58 (−56.47 to 169.62)		−32.67 (−94.77 to 29.42)
Sodium, mEq/L[c]						
Baseline	142.32 (3.36)	141.65 (2.95)	141.92 (3.16)	141.28 (2.47)	141.45 (2.55)	141.28 (2.52)
Follow-up	142.03 (2.89)	141.89 (2.59)	142.09 (3.01)	142.00 (2.76)	142.48 (2.94)	142.18 (2.55)
Absolute change	0.11 (−0.70 to 0.92)	0.26 (−0.56 to 1.08)	0.27 (−0.55 to 1.10)	0.47 (−0.38 to 1.31)	0.83 (0.36 to 1.30)	0.62 (0.13 to 1.11)
Percentage change	0.11 (−0.46 to 0.68)	0.21 (−0.36 to 0.79)	0.23 (−0.35 to 0.80)	0.36 (−0.23 to 0.95)		0.45 (0.11 to 0.80)
Relative change		0.10 (−0.71 to 0.91)	0.11 (−0.70 to 0.92)	0.25 (−0.58 to 1.07)		−0.15 (−0.62 to 0.33)
Potassium, mEq/L[c]						
Baseline	2.87 (0.33)	3.90 (0.36)	3.86 (0.30)	3.80 (0.34)	3.91 (0.29)	3.92 (0.35)
Follow-up	3.84 (0.29)	3.91 (0.33)	3.96 (0.39)	3.86 (0.28)	3.92 (0.25)	3.88 (0.28)
Absolute change	−0.01 (−0.10 to 0.08)	0.03 (−0.06 to 0.12)	0.06 (−0.03 to 0.16)	0.02 (−0.07 to 0.12)	0.02 (−0.04 to 0.07)	−0.01 (−0.06 to 0.05)
Percentage change		1.39 (−1.04 to 3.81)	1.78 (−0.65 to 4.21)	0.94 (−1.57 to 3.44)	0.85 (−0.54 to 2.25)	0.35 (−1.11 to 1.81)
Relative change	0.21 (−2.19 to 2.61)	1.18 (−2.24 to 4.59)	1.57 (−1.85 to 4.99)	0.73 (−2.74 to 4.20)		−0.50 (−2.52 to 1.51)
Bicarbonate, mEq/L[c]						
Baseline	22.62 (3.59)	22.79 (3.00)	23.28 (2.93)	22.92 (3.09)	22.74 (3.34)	22.98 (3.02)
Follow-up	22.75 (3.25)	23.31 (2.46)	23.29 (2.76)	23.22 (3.26)	23.34 (3.09)	23.47 (2.48)
Absolute change	0.27 (−0.44 to 0.98)	0.41 (−0.31 to 1.12)	0.60 (−0.11 to 1.31)	0.51 (−0.23 to 1.25)	0.66 (0.25 to 1.06)	0.80 (0.38 to 1.23)
Percentage change	2.01 (−1.25 to 5.28)	2.50 (−0.80 to 5.79)	3.34 (0.06 to 6.62)	2.56 (−0.85 to 5.98)	4.03 (2.15 to 5.91)	4.59 (2.64 to 6.54)
Relative change		0.48 (−4.16 to 5.12)	1.33 (−3.29 to 5.95)	0.55 (−4.17 to 5.28)		0.56 (−2.15 to 3.27)

Abbreviation: ULN, upper limit of normal.

[a] The denominators shown are the intention-to-treat population for the individual treatment groups.

[b] Patients without a postbaseline measurement are excluded from the analysis.

[c] Baseline and follow-up data are mean (SD) unless otherwise indicated. Baseline is defined as the last nonmissing observation prior to the first dose of study medication. If the first dose date were unavailable, the treatment dispense date from the interactive voice response system was used. Follow-up is defined as the observation at visit 7 unless otherwise indicated. Absolute changes are least-squares mean changes from baseline until follow-up visit 7 from analysis of covariance model (95% CI) unless otherwise indicated. Percentage changes are least-squares mean percentage changes from baseline until follow-up visit 7 from analysis of covariance model (95% CI) unless otherwise indicated. Relative changes are differences in percentage changes between placebo and evacetrapib counterpart.

[d] $p < .05$.

[e] Follow-up is defined as the observation at visit 6. Absolute changes are least-squares means changes from baseline until follow-up visit 6 from analysis of covariance model (95% CI). Percentage changes are least-squares mean percentage changes from baseline until follow-up visit 6 from analysis of covariance model (95% CI).

reducing cardiovascular events or slowing rates or atherosclerosis progression. An important unknown in all of the trials testing the long-term efficacy of these drugs is how much CETP inhibition is enough and if there can there be too much. None of these drugs will gain approval without being able to show that they reduce risk of cardiovascular events against a background of statin therapy. Two trials with dalcetrapib and anacetrapib are already underway to test the impact of these drugs on residual risk in secondary prevention. If they work, they would most certainly be a welcome addition to the armamentarium of lipid-modifying drugs.

P. P. Toth, MD, PhD

References

1. Barter PJ, Caulfield M, Eriksson M, et al. Effects of torcetrapib in patients at high risk for coronary events. *N Engl J Med.* 2007;357:2109-2122.
2. Kastelein JJ, van Leuven SI, Burgess L, et al. Effect of torcetrapib on carotid athero-sclerosis in familial hypercholesterolemia. *N Engl J Med.* 2007;356:1620-1630.
3. Nissen SE, Tardif JC, Nicholls SJ, et al. Effect of torcetrapib on the progression of coronary atherosclerosis. *N Engl J Med.* 2007;356:1304-1316.
4. Stein EA, Roth EM, Rhyne JM, Burgess T, Kallend D, Robinson JG. Safety and tolerability of dalcetrapib (RO4607381/JTT-705): results from a 48-week trial. *Eur Heart J.* 2010;31:480-488.
5. Cannon CP, Shah S, Dansky HM, et al. Safety of anacetrapib in patients with or at high risk for coronary heart disease. *N Engl J Med.* 2010;363:2406-2415.

Niacin in Patients with Low HDL Cholesterol Levels Receiving Intensive Statin Therapy
The AIM-HIGH Investigators (Univ at Buffalo, NY; Univ of Washington, Seattle; Univ of Calgary and Libin Cardiovascular Inst, Calgary, Alberta, Canada; et al)
N Engl J Med 365:2255-2267, 2011

Background.—In patients with established cardiovascular disease, resi-dual cardiovascular risk persists despite the achievement of target low-density lipoprotein (LDL) cholesterol levels with statin therapy. It is unclear whether extended-release niacin added to simvastatin to raise low levels of high-density lipoprotein (HDL) cholesterol is superior to simvastatin alone in reducing such residual risk.

Methods.—We randomly assigned eligible patients to receive extended-release niacin, 1500 to 2000 mg per day, or matching placebo. All patients received simvastatin, 40 to 80 mg per day, plus ezetimibe, 10 mg per day, if needed, to maintain an LDL cholesterol level of 40 to 80 mg per deciliter (1.03 to 2.07 mmol per liter). The primary end point was the first event of the composite of death from coronary heart disease, nonfatal myocardial infarction, ischemic stroke, hospitalization for an acute coronary syndrome, or symptom-driven coronary or cerebral revascularization.

Results.—A total of 3414 patients were randomly assigned to receive niacin (1718) or placebo (1696). The trial was stopped after a mean follow-up period of 3 years owing to a lack of efficacy. At 2 years, niacin therapy had significantly increased the median HDL cholesterol level from 35 mg per deciliter (0.91 mmol per liter) to 42 mg per deciliter (1.08 mmol per liter), lowered the triglyceride level from 164 mg per deciliter (1.85 mmol per liter) to 122 mg per deciliter (1.38 mmol per liter), and lowered the LDL cholesterol level from 74 mg per deciliter (1.91 mmol per liter) to 62 mg per deciliter (1.60 mmol per liter). The primary end point occurred in 282 patients in the niacin group (16.4%) and in 274 patients in the placebo group (16.2%) (hazard ratio, 1.02; 95% confidence interval, 0.87 to 1.21; $P=0.79$ by the log-rank test).

Conclusions.—Among patients with atherosclerotic cardiovascular disease and LDL cholesterol levels of less than 70 mg per deciliter (1.81 mmol per liter), there was no incremental clinical benefit from the addition of niacin to statin therapy during a 36-month follow-up period, despite significant improvements in HDL cholesterol and triglyceride levels. (Funded by the National Heart, Lung, and Blood Institute and Abbott Laboratories; AIM-HIGH ClinicalTrials.gov number, NCT00120289.) (Tables 1 and 4).

► Nicotinic acid (niacin) is a broad-spectrum lipid-modifying agent that reduces atherogenic lipoprotein burden (very low-density lipoprotein, low-density lipoprotein [LDL], Lp[a]) and is currently the best drug available for raising serum levels of high-density lipoprotein (HDL)-C. It has demonstrable efficacy for reducing risk of cardiovascular events in patients with established coronary artery disease (CAD) when used as monotherapy.[1] In a number of smaller trials, the addition of niacin to other lipid-lowering medications such as statins[2,3] and fibrates[4,5] yielded relatively large reductions in risk for acute cardiovascular events. The High-Density Lipoprotein Atherosclerosis Treatment Study 2 (HATS) was of particular interest because patients in this secondary prevention trial experienced an average 89% relative risk reduction in the primary composite endpoint of the study (myocardial infarction [MI], stroke, death, and need for revascularization). Unfortunately, each treatment arm of the study contained only approximately 40 patients. While the magnitude of risk reduction was certainly impressive, it was of interest to ascertain whether such a large risk reduction could be confirmed in a larger cohort of patients.

The Atherothrombosis Intervention in Metabolic Syndrome with Low HDL/High Triglycerides: Impact on Global Health Outcomes (AIM-HIGH) trial evaluated whether extended-release niacin added to intensive statin therapy compared with statin therapy alone would lower the risk of cardiovascular events in patients with CAD and atherogenic dyslipidemia and low levels of HDL-C and elevated triglyceride levels. The study randomly assigned 3414 patients. The primary composite endpoint included MI, stroke, coronary death, need for coronary or cerebral revascularization, and hospitalization for acute coronary syndromes. The average baseline HDL-C was 35 mg/dL, LDL-C was 71 mg/dL, triglyceride was 161 mg/dL, and non—HDL-C was 106 mg/dL. The target LDL-C in this study was 40 to 80 mg/dL. The groups were well matched by demographic criteria (Table 1). Baseline statin therapy was in excess of 90% in both groups, and background therapy with β-blockers, angiotensin-converting enzyme inhibitors, and aspirin was high (Table 1). Approximately 20% and 10% of the patients

TABLE 1.—Baseline Demographic and Clinical Characteristics of the Study Patients*

Characteristic	Placebo Plus Statin (N = 1696)	Extended-Release Niacin Plus Statin (N = 1718)
Age		
Mean — yr	63.7 (8.7)	63.7 (8.8)
Distribution — no. (%)		
<65 yr	915 (54.0)	917 (53.4)
≥65 yr	781 (46.0)	801 (46.6)
Sex — no. (%)		
Female	251 (14.8)	253 (14.7)
Male	1445 (85.2)	1465 (85.3)
Race or ethnic group — no. (%)[†]		
White	1576 (92.9)	1572 (91.5)
Black	49 (2.9)	68 (4.0)
Asian	21 (1.2)	20 (1.2)
American Indian, Alaskan Native, or Aboriginal Canadian	11 (0.6)	11 (0.6)
Native Hawaiian or other Pacific Islander	5 (0.3)	7 (0.4)
Multiracial or other	33 (1.9)	40 (2.3)
Hispanic or non-Hispanic ethnic group — no. (%)[†]		
Non-Hispanic	1619 (95.5)	1654 (96.3)
Hispanic	77 (4.5)	63 (3.7)
Presenting history or diagnosis — no. (%)		
History of myocardial infarction	955 (56.3)	968 (56.3)
CABG	627 (37.0)	600 (34.9)
PCI	1044 (61.6)	1057 (61.5)
Stroke or cerebrovascular disease	362 (21.3)	358 (20.8)
Peripheral vascular disease	231 (13.6)	234 (13.6)
Metabolic syndrome	1353 (79.8)	1414 (82.3)
History of hypertension	1189 (70.1)	1250 (72.8)
History of diabetes	570 (33.6)	588 (34.2)
Laboratory values in patients with history of diabetes		
Glucose — mg/dl	126.4±27.1	126.9±26.9
Glycated hemoglobin — %	6.68±0.85	6.70±0.88
Insulin — μU/ml	25.63±31.09	25.32±29.23
Concomitant medications — no. (%)		
Statin		
Use at baseline	1601 (94.4)	1595 (92.8)
Duration of prior statin therapy[‡]		
<1 yr	190 (11.2)	202 (11.8)
1–5 yr	629 (37.1)	627 (36.5)
>5 yr	684 (40.3)	669 (38.9)
Previous use of niacin or Niaspan[§]	338 (19.9)	324 (18.9)
Beta-blocker	1342 (79.1)	1377 (80.2)
ACE inhibitor or ARB	1271 (74.9)	1258 (73.2)
Aspirin or other antiplatelet or anticoagulant agent	1654 (97.5)	1680 (97.8)

*Plus—minus values are means ±SD. There were no significant differences between the treatment groups at baseline in any of the baseline characteristics. To convert the values for glucose to millimoles per liter, multiply by 0.05551. ACE denotes angiotensin-converting enzyme, ARB angiotensin II—receptor blocker, CABG coronary-artery bypass grafting, and PCI percutaneous coronary intervention.
[†]Race or ethnic group was self-reported.
[‡]The duration of prior statin therapy was not ascertained in 204 patients (6.0%).
[§]Niacin and other lipid-modifying drugs except statins and ezetimibe were discontinued 30 days before enrollment.

in the placebo and niacin groups, respectively, were also receiving adjuvant ezetimibe therapy to facilitate LDL-C goal attainment.

The addition of niacin to aggressive statin plus ezetimibe therapy did not beneficially impact any major cardiovascular outcome (Table 4). The Kaplan-Meier

TABLE 4.—Primary, Secondary, and Tertiary End Points

End Point	Placebo Plus Statin (N = 1696)	Extended-Release Niacin Plus Statin (N = 1718)	Hazard Ratio with Niacin (95% CI)	P Value*
	Number of Patients (Percent)			
Primary end point: death from coronary heart disease, nonfatal myocardial infarction, ischemic stroke, hospitalization for acute coronary syndrome, or symptom-driven coronary or cerebral revascularization	274 (16.2)	282 (16.4)	1.02 (0.87–1.21)	0.80
Individual primary-end-point events				
Death from coronary heart disease	26 (1.5)	20 (1.2)		
Nonfatal myocardial infarction	80 (4.7)	92 (5.4)		
Ischemic stroke	15 (0.9)	27 (1.6)		
Hospitalization for acute coronary syndrome	67 (4.0)	63 (3.7)		
Symptom-driven coronary or cerebral revascularization	86 (5.1)	80 (4.7)		
Secondary end points				
Death from coronary heart disease, nonfatal myocardial infarction, high-risk acute coronary syndrome, or ischemic stroke	158 (9.3)	171 (10.0)	1.08 (0.87–1.34)	0.49
Death from coronary heart disease, nonfatal myocardial infarction, or ischemic stroke	138 (8.1)	156 (9.1)	1.13 (0.90–1.42)	0.30
All deaths from cardiovascular causes	38 (2.2)	45 (2.6)	1.17 (0.76–1.80)	0.47
Tertiary end points†				
Death from coronary heart disease	34 (2.0)	38 (2.2)	1.10 (0.69–1.75)	0.68
Death from any cause	82 (4.8)	96 (5.6)	1.16 (0.87–1.56)	0.32
Nonfatal myocardial infarction	93 (5.5)	104 (6.1)	1.11 (0.84–1.47)	0.46
Hospitalizations for acute coronary syndrome	82 (4.8)	72 (4.2)	0.87 (0.63–1.19)	0.38
Symptom-driven coronary or cerebral revascularizations	168 (9.9)	167 (9.7)	0.99 (0.80–1.22)	0.90
Ischemic stroke‡	18 (1.1)	29 (1.7)	1.61 (0.89–2.90)	0.11
Ischemic stroke or stroke of uncertain origin	18 (1.1)	30 (1.7)	1.67 (0.93–2.99)	0.09

*The P value is for the superiority of niacin therapy over placebo, adjusted for sex and history of diabetes, with the use of a Cox proportional-hazards model to estimate the Wald statistic.

†The tertiary end point included all events, rather than just those that occurred as the first study event (which are listed in the category of individual primary-end-point events).

‡Three strokes in the niacin group were detected during a blinded re-review, after the database was locked, of cases of transient ischemic attack; these three events are not included in these analyses.

survival curves are essentially superimposable for the entire 3-year duration of the study. This is despite the fact that niacin increased HDL-C by 7 mg/dL (this was dampened by a 3-mg/dL increase in the placebo group relative to baseline), decreased triglycerides to 122 mg/dL, and decreased LDL-C to 65 mg/dL. The National Heart Lung and Blood Institute terminated the study due to futility as well as the possibility for harm because of a small, statistically nonsignificant trend for an increase in risk for ischemic stroke (29 vs 18 patients, $P = .11$). These findings most certainly did not reproduce the results of the HATS trial. However, in HATS, baseline LDL-C was 124 mg/dL, and combination statin/niacin therapy was compared with placebo. In AIM-HIGH, the baseline LDL-C was dramatically lower, and patients were aggressively treated with statin therapy or combination therapy (statin/ezetimibe). Apo B and non—HDL-C were also stringently controlled at 80 mg/dL and 106 mg/dL, respectively. The most likely explanation for these results is that: (1) niacin does not provide incremental risk reduction in patients with atherogenic dyslipidemia when the atherogenic lipoprotein burden of a patient with CAD is this stringently controlled and (2) increasing HDL-C with a net difference between groups of 4 mg/dL did not appear to impact risk for events when other lipids were already well controlled. Some caution is urged when applying these results to direct patient care, as the average AIM-HIGH patient likely represents less than 12% of patients with CAD. The lipids of the large majority of patients with CAD are not nearly this well controlled. The increased signal for ischemic stroke is somewhat puzzling, especially given the fact that stroke risk was reduced by niacin in the Coronary Drug Project.[1] Had the study been allowed to proceed longer, we could have perhaps gleaned a more precise quantitative assessment of stroke risk in response to niacin therapy.

The results of the Heart Protection Study-2: Treatment of HDL to Reduce the Incidence of Vascular Events (HPS2-THRIVE) are eagerly awaited to either affirm or nuance the findings of AIM-HIGH. HPS-2 THRIVE has enrolled more than 25 000 patients with a broad range of entry lipid parameters to help further define the role of niacin adjuvant therapy in patients with a variety of dyslipidemias, not just those with "atherogenic dyslipidemia." A large number of post-hoc analyses are expected from AIM-HIGH. One that will be of particular interest is to determine if niacin was beneficial in the patients in the lowest tertile for baseline HDL-C or the highest tertile for baseline triglycerides.

P. P. Toth, MD, PhD

References

1. Clofibrate and niacin in coronary heart disease. *JAMA.* 1975;231:360-381.
2. Brown BG, Zhao XQ, Chait A, et al. Simvastatin and niacin, antioxidant vitamins, or the combination for the prevention of coronary disease. *N Engl J Med.* 2001; 345:1583-1592.
3. Brown G, Albers JJ, Fisher LD, et al. Regression of coronary artery disease as a result of intensive lipid-lowering therapy in men with high levels of apolipoprotein B. *N Engl J Med.* 1990;323:1289-1298.
4. Whitney EJ, Krasuski RA, Personius BE, et al. A randomized trial of a strategy for increasing high-density lipoprotein cholesterol levels: effects on progression of coronary heart disease and clinical events. *Ann Intern Med.* 2005;142:95-104.

5. Carlson LA, Rosenhamer G. Reduction of mortality in the Stockholm Ischaemic Heart Disease Secondary Prevention Study by combined treatment with clofibrate and nicotinic acid. *Acta Med Scand.* 1988;223:405-418.

Statin Safety

Lack of Effect of Lowering LDL Cholesterol on Cancer: Meta-Analysis of Individual Data from 175,000 People in 27 Randomised Trials of Statin Therapy

Cholesterol Treatment Trialists' (CTT) Collaboration (Clinical Trial Service Unit and Epidemiological Studies Unit (CTSU), Oxford, UK; Univ College Cork, Ireland; New York Univ Med Ctr; et al)

PLoS One 7:e29849, 2012

Background.—Statin therapy reduces the risk of occlusive vascular events, but uncertainty remains about potential effects on cancer. We sought to provide a detailed assessment of any effects on cancer of lowering LDL cholesterol (LDL-C) with a statin using individual patient records from 175,000 patients in 27 large-scale statin trials.

Methods and Findings.—Individual records of 134,537 participants in 22 randomised trials of statin versus control (median duration 4.8 years)

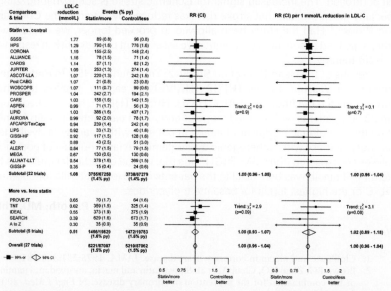

FIGURE 1.—Effects of statin therapy on cancer incidence in each study. In the left panel, unweighted rate ratios (RRs) are plotted for each trial of the comparison of first event rates between randomly allocated treatment groups, along with their 99% confidence intervals (CIs). Trials are ordered according to the absolute reduction in LDL cholesterol at 1 year within each type of trial comparison (statin versus control and more versus less statin). In the right panel, rate ratios are weighted per 1 mmol/L LDL cholesterol difference at 1 year. Totals and subtotals, together with their 95% CIs, are indicated by open diamonds. (Reprinted from Cholesterol Treatment Trialists' (CTT) Collaboration. Lack of effect of lowering LDL cholesterol on cancer: meta-analysis of individual data from 175,000 people in 27 randomised trials of statin therapy. *PLoS One.* 2012;7:e29849, © National Center for Biotechnology Information.)

and 39,612 participants in 5 trials of more intensive versus less intensive statin therapy (median duration 5.1 years) were obtained. Reducing LDL-C with a statin for about 5 years had no effect on newly diagnosed cancer or on death from such cancers in either the trials of statin versus control (cancer incidence: 3755 [1.4% per year [py]] versus 3738 [1.4% py], RR 1.00 [95% CI 0.96−1.05]; cancer mortality: 1365 [0.5% py] versus 1358 [0.5% py], RR 1.00 [95% CI 0.93−1.08]) or in the trials of more versus less statin (cancer incidence: 1466 [1.6% py] vs 1472 [1.6% py], RR 1.00 [95% CI 0.93−1.07]; cancer mortality: 447 [0.5% py] versus 481 [0.5% py], RR 0.93 [95% CI 0.82−1.06]). Moreover, there was no evidence of any effect of reducing LDL-C with statin therapy on cancer incidence or mortality at any of 23 individual categories of sites, with increasing years of treatment, for any individual statin, or in any given subgroup. In particular, among individuals with low baseline LDL-C (<2 mmol/L), there was no evidence that further LDL-C reduction (from about 1.7 to 1.3 mmol/L) increased cancer risk (381 [1.6% py] versus 408 [1.7% py]; RR 0.92 [99% CI 0.76−1.10]).

Conclusions.—In 27 randomised trials, a median of five years of statin therapy had no effect on the incidence of, or mortality from, any type of cancer (or the aggregate of all cancer) (Figs 1 and 2).

▶ Among the adverse events attributed to statins in the past have been increased incidence of breast and colorectal cancers as shown in the Cholesterol and

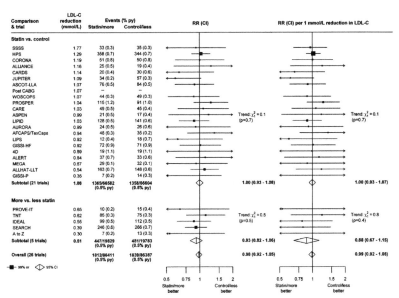

FIGURE 2.—Effects of statin therapy on cancer mortality in each study. Symbols and conventions as in Figure 1. Deaths from cancers known to have been first diagnosed prior to randomization are excluded. (Reprinted from Cholesterol Treatment Trialists' (CTT) Collaboration. Lack of effect of lowering LDL cholesterol on cancer: meta-analysis of individual data from 175,000 people in 27 randomised trials of statin therapy. *PLoS One.* 2012;7:e29849, © National Center for Biotechnology Information.)

Recurrent Events and PROspective Study of Pravastatin in the Elderly at Risk trials, respectively.[1,2] There has been lingering concern over the possibility of increased risk for a variety of malignancies among patients treated with the statins. This concern has been fueled to some degree by observational data that low serum cholesterol levels predispose to the development of malignancy. Confounding such observations is the fact that low serum cholesterol can be a manifestation of the cachexia frequently accompanying malignancy. It is of obvious importance to clarify this issue in a more definitive manner and determine whether the relation between cholesterol lowering with a statin and risk for malignancy is either real or spurious.

In this study, the Cholesterol Treatment Trialists Collaboration (CTTC) performed a patient-level analysis of whether statin therapy is associated with new onset cancer. The CTTC evaluated 175000 patients from 27 prospective randomized clinical trials. No evidence for an increase in malignancy was found (Fig 1), nor was there any signal apparent for an increase in cancer-related mortality (Fig 2). Moreover, there was no increase for risk of cancer depending on length of treatment with a statin, baseline low-density lipoprotein cholesterol, or location-specific organ. There was also no impact of statin therapy on cancer incidence or mortality, irrespective of gender or age.

This is the most definitive evaluation of this issue to date. This meta-analysis is strengthened since these investigators analyzed patient-level data from 27 large clinical trials. One limitation to the data is that the average follow-up was approximately 5 years. These data, however, should be quite reassuring to physicians and patients alike.

P. P. Toth, MD, PhD

References

1. Sacks FM, Pfeffer MA, Moye LA, et al. The effect of pravastatin on coronary events after myocardial infarction in patients with average cholesterol levels. Cholesterol and recurrent events trial investigators. *N Engl J Med.* 1996;335:1001-1009.
2. Shepherd J, Blauw GJ, Murphy MB, et al. Pravastatin in elderly individuals at risk of vascular disease (PROSPER): a randomised controlled trial. *Lancet.* 2002;360:1623-1630.

Risk of Incident Diabetes With Intensive-Dose Compared With Moderate-Dose Statin Therapy: A Meta-analysis

Preiss D, Seshasai SRK, Welsh P, et al (Univ of Glasgow, UK; Univ of Cambridge, UK; et al)
JAMA 305:2556-2564, 2011

Context.—A recent meta-analysis demonstrated that statin therapy is associated with excess risk of developing diabetes mellitus.

Objective.—To investigate whether intensive-dose statin therapy is associated with increased risk of new-onset diabetes compared with moderate-dose statin therapy.

Data Sources.—We identified relevant trials in a literature search of MEDLINE, EMBASE, and the Cochrane Central Register of Controlled Trials (January 1, 1996, through March 31, 2011). Unpublished data were obtained from investigators.

Study Selection.—We included randomized controlled end-point trials that compared intensive-dose statin therapy with moderate-dose statin therapy and included more than 1000 participants who were followed up for more than 1 year.

Data Extraction.—Tabular data provided for each trial described baseline characteristics and numbers of participants developing diabetes and experiencing major cardiovascular events (cardiovascular death, nonfatal myocardial infarction or stroke, coronary revascularization). We calculated trial-specific odds ratios (ORs) for new-onset diabetes and major cardiovascular events and combined these using random-effects model meta analysis. Between-study heterogeneity was assessed using the I^2 statistic.

Results.—In 5 statin trials with 32 752 participants without diabetes at baseline, 2749 developed diabetes (1449 assigned intensive-dose therapy, 1300 assigned moderate-dose therapy, representing 2.0 additional cases in the intensive-dose group per 1000 patient-years) and 6684 experienced cardiovascular events (3134 and 3550, respectively, representing 6.5 fewer cases in the intensive-dose group per 1000 patient-years) over a weighted mean (SD) follow-up of 4.9 (1.9) years. Odds ratios were 1.12 (95% confidence interval [CI], 1.04-1.22; $I^2=0\%$) for new-onset diabetes and 0.84 (95% CI, 0.75-0.94; $I^2=74\%$) for cardiovascular events for participants receiving intensive therapy compared with moderate-dose therapy. As compared with moderate-dose statin therapy, the number needed to harm per year for intensive-dose statin therapy was 498 for new-onset diabetes while the number needed to treat per year for intensive-dose statin therapy was 155 for cardiovascular events.

Conclusion.—In a pooled analysis of data from 5 statin trials, intensive-dose statin therapy was associated with an increased risk of new-onset diabetes compared with moderate-dose statin therapy.

▶ One new concern with stain therapy is an increased risk of new onset diabetes mellitus (DM), which was first identified in the Justification for the Use of Statins in Primary Prevention: An Intervention Trial Evaluating Rosuvastatin trial.[1] Two subsequent meta-analyses confirmed that statin therapy is associated with an increased risk for new onset type 2 DM, with no heterogeneity among the statins.[2,3] In the meta-analysis by Sattar et al, 255 patients would have to be treated for 4 years to observe 1 new case of DM (ie, 1 new case for every 1000 patient years of therapy). It is as yet unclear how statins may affect glucose homeostasis. Despite this risk, it is clear that statins reduce risk for cardiovascular events in both nondiabetic and diabetic patients to an approximately equal degree.[4,5] It is also clear that there is better risk reduction in patients treated with high-dose as opposed to low-dose or moderate-dose statins in the secondary prevention setting.[6] It is not clear, however, if there is a dose dependency to the capacity of statins to increase risk for DM.

This study examined this issue by performing an analysis of pooled data from 5 large statin trials, including the Treating to New Targets trial, the Incremental Decrease in End Points Through Aggressive Lipid Lowering trial, the Aggrastat to Zocor trial, the Pravastatin or Atorvastatin Evaluation and Infection Therapy— Thrombolysis in Myocardial Infarction trial, and the Study of the Effectiveness of Additional Reductions in Cholesterol and Homocysteine, which compared high doses and moderate doses of statins and their effects on cardiovascular outcomes. There were 18.9 cases per 1000 patient years of high-dose statin therapy and 16.9 cases per 1000 patient years, for an absolute difference of 2 cases per 1000 patient years of therapy and a number needed to harm of 498 per year (Fig 1 in the original article). No heterogeneity between study cohorts was detected. There was also no heterogeneity as a function of age, body mass index, high-density lipoprotein cholesterol, or fasting plasma glucose. Curiously, if triglycerides were below the median, this was an independent predictor of increased risk for statin-dependent DM. There is currently no explanation for this, although it may be attributed to play of chance (Fig 2 in the original article). In contrast, there were 6.5 fewer first cardiovascular events per 1000 patient years in patients who received high-dose as opposed to moderate-dose therapy, yielding a number needed to treat to prevent 1 cardiovascular event of 155 per year.

Despite the increased risk for DM, this analysis provides quantitative demonstration of net benefit with statin therapy when comparing moderate doses to high doses of statins. Much work remains to be done in this area. It will be important to elucidate the mechanism(s) by which statin therapy elevates the risk for DM. In the meantime, however, patients should not be discouraged from initiating statin therapy for dyslipidemia, as the benefits of their use still outweigh their risks.

P. P. Toth, MD, PhD

References

1. Ridker PM, Danielson E, Fonseca FA, et al. Rosuvastatin to prevent vascular events in men and women with elevated C-reactive protein. *N Engl J Med.* 2008;359:2195-2207.
2. Rajpathak SN, Kumbhani DJ, Crandall J, Barzilai N, Alderman M, Ridker PM. Statin therapy and risk of developing type 2 diabetes: a meta-analysis. *Diabetes Care.* 2009;32:1924-1929.
3. Sattar N, Preiss D, Murray HM, et al. Statins and risk of incident diabetes: a collaborative meta-analysis of randomised statin trials. *Lancet.* 2010;375: 735-742.
4. Baigent C, Keech A, Kearney PM, et al. Efficacy and safety of cholesterol-lowering treatment: prospective meta-analysis of data from 90,056 participants in 14 randomised trials of statins. *Lancet.* 2005;366:1267-1278.
5. Kearney PM, Blackwell L, Collins R, et al. Efficacy of cholesterol-lowering therapy in 18,686 people with diabetes in 14 randomised trials of statins: a meta-analysis. *Lancet.* 2008;371:117-125.
6. Cannon CP, Steinberg BA, Murphy SA, Mega JL, Braunwald E. Meta-analysis of cardiovascular outcomes trials comparing intensive versus moderate statin therapy. *J Am Coll Cardiol.* 2006;48:438-445.

Effects on 11-year mortality and morbidity of lowering LDL cholesterol with simvastatin for about 5 years in 20 536 high-risk individuals: a randomised controlled trial
Heart Protection Study Collaborative Group (Clinical Trial Service Unit, Oxford, UK)
Lancet 378:2013-2020, 2011

Background.—Findings of large randomised trials have shown that lowering LDL cholesterol with statins reduces vascular morbidity and mortality rapidly, but limited evidence exists about the long-term efficacy and safety of statin treatment. The aim of the extended follow-up of the Heart Protection Study (HPS) is to assess long-term efficacy and safety of lowering LDL cholesterol with statins, and here we report cause-specific mortality and major morbidity in the in-trial and post-trial periods.

Methods.—20 536 patients at high risk of vascular and non-vascular outcomes were allocated either 40 mg simvastatin daily or placebo, using minimised randomisation. Mean in-trial follow-up was 5·3 years (SD 1·2), and post-trial follow-up of surviving patients yielded a mean total duration of 11·0 years (SD 0·6). The primary outcome of the long-term follow-up of HPS was first post-randomisation major vascular event, and analysis was by intention to treat. This trial is registered with ISRCTN, number 48489393.

Findings.—During the in-trial period, allocation to simvastatin yielded an average reduction in LDL cholesterol of 1·0 mmol/L and a proportional decrease in major vascular events of 23% (95% CI 19—28; p<0·0001), with significant divergence each year after the first. During the post-trial period (when statin use and lipid concentrations were similar in both groups), no further significant reductions were noted in either major vascular events (risk ratio [RR] 0·95 [0·89—1·02]) or vascular mortality (0·98 [0·90—1·07]). During the combined in-trial and post-trial periods, no significant differences were recorded in cancer incidence at all sites (0·98 [0·92—1·05]) or any particular site, or in mortality attributed to cancer (1·01 [0·92—1·11]) or to non-vascular causes (0·96 [0·89—1·03]).

Interpretation.—More prolonged LDL-lowering statin treatment produces larger absolute reductions in vascular events. Moreover, even after study treatment stopped in HPS, benefits persisted for at least 5 years without any evidence of emerging hazards. These findings provide further support for the prompt initiation and long-term continuation of statin treatment (Figs 1-3, Table 2).

▶ In the major randomized statin trials, patients have typically been allocated to placebo or statin therapy for approximately 2 to 6 years. The statins have been available for use for just over 20 years. There is great interest in further ascertaining whether benefit and safety persist over the long term. These are extremely important and urgent issues given the fact that many patients initiating statin therapy are likely to require their use for one or more decades to maintain optimal control of their dyslipidemia.

	Simvastatin allocation			Risk ratio (95% CI)	p value
	Simvastatin	Placebo			
In-trial events					
Major coronary event	959/10269 (9·3%)	1287/10267 (12·5%)		0·73 (0·67–0·79)	
Stroke	480/10269 (4·7%)	619/10267 (6·0%)		0·76 (0·68–0·86)	
Revascularisation	981/10269 (9·6%)	1258/10267 (12·3%)		0·76 (0·70–0·83)	
Major vascular event	2153/10269 (21·0%)	2712/10267 (26·4%)		0·77 (0·72–0·81)	p<0·0001
Post-trial events					
Major coronary event	1032/8553 (12·1%)	1021/8172 (12·5%)		0·96 (0·88–1·04)	
Stroke	426/8544 (5·0%)	419/8246 (5·1%)		0·98 (0·86–1·12)	
Revascularisation	671/8015 (8·4%)	672/7572 (8·9%)		0·93 (0·84–1·04)	
Major vascular event	1636/7543 (21·7%)	1566/6967 (22·5%)		0·95 (0·89–1·02)	p=0·17

0·4   0·6   0·8   1·0   1·2   1·4
Favours simvastatin   Favours placebo

FIGURE 1.—First major vascular event during in-trial and post-trial follow-up. Analyses are of numbers of participants having a first post-randomisation event of each type during follow-up, so there is some non-additivity between different types of event. Denominators during the post-trial period are the numbers of randomised patients who had not had the particular outcome or died during the in-trial period. Risk ratios (RRs) are plotted (black squares with area proportional to amount of statistical information in each subdivision) comparing outcome among the participants allocated 40 mg simvastatin daily to that among those allocated placebo, along with their 95% CIs (horizontal lines; ending with arrow head when CI extends beyond scale). For particular subtotals and totals, the result and its 95% CI are represented by a diamond, with the relative risk reduction (and 95% CI) and statistical significance given alongside. A broken vertical line indicates the overall RR. (Reprinted from Heart Protection Study Collaborative Group. Effects on 11-year mortality and morbidity of lowering LDL cholesterol with simvastatin for about 5 years in 20 536 high-risk individuals: a randomised controlled trial. *Lancet*. 2011;378:2013-2020, © 2011, with permission from Elsevier.)

	Simvastatin allocation			Risk ratio (95% CI)	p value
	Simvastatin	Placebo			
In-trial					
Year 1	482/10269 (4·7%)	529/10267 (5·2%)		0·91 (0·80–1·03)	
Year 2	378/9744 (3·9%)	538/9681 (5·6%)		0·69 (0·61–0·79)	
Year 3	361/9286 (3·9%)	507/9053 (5·6%)		0·69 (0·61–0·79)	
Year 4	333/8814 (3·8%)	442/8463 (5·2%)		0·72 (0·62–0·83)	
Year 5+	599/8352 (7·2%)	696/7893 (8·8%)		0·80 (0·72–0·89)	
All in-trial	2153/10269 (21·0%)	2712/10267 (26·4%)		0·77 (0·72–0·81)	p<0·0001
Post-trial					
Year 1	320/7543 (4·2%)	341/6967 (4·9%)		0·86 (0·74–1·00)	
Year 2	343/7099 (4·8%)	333/6487 (5·1%)		0·94 (0·81–1·09)	
Year 3	332/6610 (5·0%)	313/6024 (5·2%)		0·96 (0·83–1·13)	
Year 4	291/6125 (4·8%)	274/5573 (4·9%)		0·96 (0·82–1·14)	
Year 5+	350/5677 (6·2%)	305/5156 (5·9%)		1·05 (0·90–1·22)	
All post-trial	1636/7543 (21·7%)	1566/6967 (22·5%)		0·95 (0·89–1·02)	p=0·17

0·4   0·6   0·8   1·0   1·2   1·4
Favours simvastatin   Favours placebo

FIGURE 2.—First major vascular event by year during in-trial and post-trial follow-up. Conventions as in figure 1. Denominators are the numbers of patients at risk of a first post-randomisation major vascular event at the start of each year. (Reprinted from Heart Protection Study Collaborative Group. Effects on 11-year mortality and morbidity of lowering LDL cholesterol with simvastatin for about 5 years in 20 536 high-risk individuals: a randomised controlled trial. *Lancet*. 2011;378:2013-2020, © 2011, with permission from Elsevier.)

The Heart Protection Study (HPS) investigators evaluated simvastatin therapy in their cohort for an additional 6 years of posttrial follow-up. In the HPS, participants were at increased risk for cardiovascular events. The original trial found significant benefit (23% relative risk reduction) of simvastatin therapy compared with placebo (Fig 1). Six years following the close of the study (for a total of

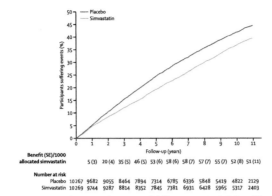

Number at risk

Placebo	10267	9682	9055	8464	7894	7314	6785	6336	5848	5419	4822	2129
Simvastatin	10269	9744	9287	8814	8352	7845	7381	6931	6428	5965	5317	2403

Benefit (SE)/1000 allocated simvastatin: 5 (3) 20 (4) 35 (5) 46 (5) 53 (6) 58 (6) 58 (7) 57 (7) 55 (7) 52 (8) 51 (11)

FIGURE 3.—First major vascular event during total follow-up period. Life-table plot of the effects of simvastatin allocation on percentage of major vascular events during the in-trial and post-trial periods. (Reprinted from Heart Protection Study Collaborative Group. Effects on 11-year mortality and morbidity of lowering LDL cholesterol with simvastatin for about 5 years in 20 536 high-risk individuals: a randomised controlled trial. *Lancet.* 2011;378:2013-2020, © 2011, with permission from Elsevier.)

TABLE 2.—In-Trial and Post-Trial Statin Use (Study and Non-Study), by Year of Follow-up

	Simvastatin-Allocated	Placebo-Allocated
In-trial		
Year 1	8994/10 107 (89%)	389/10 088 (4%)
Year 2	8457/9909 (85%)	889/9826 (9%)
Year 3	8122/9664 (84%)	1608/9563 (17%)
Year 4	7764/9388 (83%)	2262/9241 (24%)
Year 5	6058/7370 (82%)	2345/7225 (32%)
Average	85%	17%
Post-trial		
Year 1	4163/7152 (58%)	4113/6845 (60%)
Year 2	4555/6525 (70%)	4381/6284 (70%)
Year 3	4665/6023 (77%)	4489/5821 (77%)
Year 4	5363/6651 (81%)	5136/6462 (79%)
Year 5	4527/5375 (84%)	4294/5165 (83%)
Average	74%	74%

Data show statin use/alive (in-trial) and statin use/completed forms (post-trial).

11 years of observation), the average percentage of patients in each group taking a statin was 74% (Table 2). During the posttrial period, there was no overall difference in event rates between groups (Figs 1 and 2) although there was a definite persistence of in-trial survival gains (Fig 3). There were no differences detectable in the incidence of nonvascular morbidity or mortality, including cancer, during both the in-trial and posttrial periods.

These data certainly reinforce the growing awareness that long-term statin therapy is safe. Moreover, the data also demonstrate that timely initiation of statin therapy in patients at risk for cardiovascular events incurs benefits that persists and are in no way attenuated over the period evaluated in this posttrial follow-up. This investigation also presents important evidence negating suspicion that long-term statin use is associated with increased risk for malignancy of any particular histologic type or anatomic location.

P. P. Toth, MD, PhD

Stroke and Peripheral Artery Disease

Lipoprotein (a) and Carotid Atherosclerosis in Young Patients With Stroke

Nasr N, Ruidavets JB, Farghali A, et al (Toulouse Univ Hosp, France)
Stroke 42:3616-3618, 2011

Background and Purpose.—Elevated lipoprotein (a) concentration is associated with carotid atherosclerosis in middle-aged and older patients with ischemic stroke. This association has not been explored in young patients with stroke.

Methods.—A retrospective analysis of data from patients aged 16 to 54 years consecutively treated for acute ischemic stroke in a tertiary stroke unit during 4.5 years was performed. We graded carotid atherosclerosis using carotid duplex as: no atherosclerosis (A); plaque without stenosis (B); or stenosis ≥50% (C).

Results.—One hundred ninety-six patients were included (male/female: 119/77; mean age ± SD: 44.3 ± 8.6 years): 115 in Group A; 67 in Group B; and 14 in Group C. Multivariate analysis using polynomial logistic regression showed a graded association of lipoprotein (a) plasma concentration with carotid atherosclerosis ($P<0.001$).

Conclusions.—Our results showed a positive association of lipoprotein (a) plasma concentration with carotid atherosclerosis in young adults with ischemic stroke. This association was strong, graded, and independent of traditional risk factors including cholesterol (Table 3).

▶ In contrast to components of the standard lipid profile (total cholesterol, low-density lipoprotein [LDL]-C, high-density lipoprotein [HDL]-C, triglycerides), lipoprotein(a) (Lp[a]) is an established risk factor for ischemic stroke in older adults. To date, it has not been well established whether Lp(a) is a risk factor for ischemic stroke in young adults. In this study of 196 young adults age 16 to 54 years, Nasr et al evaluated the impact of serum Lp(a) on the risk for ischemic stroke. Carotid atherosclerosis was quantified by duplex ultrasonography, and patients were classified into 3 groups: no atherosclerosis (group

TABLE 3.—Independent Association of Lipoprotein (a) Plasma Concentration with Carotid Atherosclerosis Using Several Cutoff Values*

	Grade B (N = 67)	Grade C (N = 14)	P for Trend
Lipoprotein (a) ≥0.30 g/L	3.11 (1.41−6.84)	7.44 (1.83−27.7)	<0.001
Lipoprotein (a) ≥0.50 g/L	3.38 (1.44−7.91)	10.9 (2.76−42.9)	<0.001

OR indicates odds ratio; CI, confidence interval.
*In each cell, OR (95% CI).

A), plaque without stenosis (group B), and stenosis greater than 50% (group C). Multinomial logistic regression analysis found a graded and highly significant association of Lp(a) with carotid atherosclerosis even after controlling for other established risk factors. For each standard deviation increase in the serum concentration of Lp(a), the odds ratio for carotid atherosclerosis in groups B and C increased to 1.89 and 2.96, respectively. The association remained significant and graded at multiple threshold values for Lp(a) (Table 3).

It is interesting that, although lipids in general correlate poorly with risk for ischemic stroke, Lp(a) correlates quite well, possibly because it is both atherogenic and thrombogenic. Studies are badly needed to better define optimal approaches for reducing risk of ischemic stroke among patients with elevated Lp(a) in both primary and secondary prevention. It remains to be determined if statins or other lipid-modifying medications beneficially impact risk for ischemic stroke in patients with elevated Lp(a).

P. P. Toth, MD, PhD

Statin Use During Ischemic Stroke Hospitalization Is Strongly Associated With Improved Poststroke Survival
Flint AC, Kamel H, Navi BB, et al (Kaiser Permanente, Redwood City, CA; Univ of California, San Francisco, CA; et al)
Stroke 43:147-154, 2012

Background and Purpose.—Statins reduce infarct size in animal models of stroke and have been hypothesized to improve clinical outcomes after ischemic stroke. We examined the relationship between statin use before and during stroke hospitalization and poststroke survival.

Methods.—We analyzed records from 12 689 patients admitted with ischemic stroke to any of 17 hospitals in a large integrated healthcare delivery system between January 2000 and December 2007. We used multivariable survival analysis and grouped-treatment analysis, an instrumental variable method that uses treatment differences between facilities to avoid individual patient-level confounding.

Results.—Statin use before ischemic stroke hospitalization was associated with improved survival (hazard ratio, 0.85; 95% CI, 0.79−0.93; $P<0.001$), and use before and during hospitalization was associated with better rates of survival (hazard ratio, 0.59; 95% CI, 0.53−0.65; $P<0.001$). Patients taking a statin before their stroke who underwent statin withdrawal in the hospital had a substantially greater risk of death (hazard ratio, 2.5; 95% CI, 2.1−2.9; $P<0.001$). The benefit was greater for high-dose (>60 mg/day) statin use (hazard ratio, 0.43; 95% CI, 0.34−0.53; $P<0.001$) than for lower dose (<60 mg/day) statin use (hazard ratio, 0.60; 95% CI, 0.54−0.67; $P<0.001$; test for trend $P<0.001$), and earlier treatment in-hospital further improved survival. Grouped-treatment analysis showed that the association between statin use and survival cannot be explained by patient-level confounding.

Conclusions.—Statin use early in stroke hospitalization is strongly associated with improved poststroke survival, and statin withdrawal in the hospital, even for a brief period, is associated with worsened survival (Figs 1, 3 and Table 2).

▶ Serum lipid levels (including low-density lipoprotein [LDL]-C and high-density lipoprotein [HDL]-C) tend to correlate relatively poorly with risk for ischemic stroke.[1,2] Despite this, statin therapy has been associated with reduced risk for ischemic stroke in both the primary and secondary prevention settings.[3,4] If a stroke occurs, it tends to be smaller, as statins appear to limit infarct size and thereby preserve long-term neurologic functionality. Because the statins appear to exert these benefits independent of their lipid-modifying effects, it is believed that the pleiotropic effects of the statins are neuroprotective by limiting endothelial dysfunction and injury, inflammation, oxidation, and reperfusion injury.

In this fascinating investigation by Flint and coworkers, the impact of statin therapy on poststroke outcomes was quantitated in 12 689 patients in the Kaiser Permanente health care system. Statin therapy reduced mortality of patients with ischemic stroke (Table 2). Taking a statin before hospitalization or before and during hospitalization or initiation of statins during hospitalization reduced

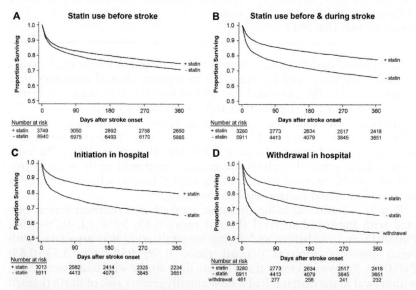

FIGURE 1.—Statin use before and during stroke hospitalization is associated with poststroke survival. **A,** One-year Kaplan-Meier survival curves for statin users before hospitalization (+ statin) and for statin nonusers before hospitalization (− statin). **B,** Survival curves for statin users before and during hospitalization (+ statin) and for statin nonusers before and during hospitalization (− statin). **C,** Survival curves for patients not on a statin before stroke hospitalization but initiated on statin therapy in hospital (+ statin) and for statin nonusers before and during hospitalization (− statin). **D,** Survival curves for statin users before and during hospitalization (+ statin), for statin nonusers before and during hospitalization (− statin), and for patients who were taking a statin before stroke hospitalization but did not receive a statin in hospital (withdrawal). (Reprinted from Flint AC, Kamel H, Navi BB, et al. Statin use during ischemic stroke hospitalization is strongly associated with improved poststroke survival. *Stroke.* 2012;43:147-154, with permission from American Heart Association, Inc.)

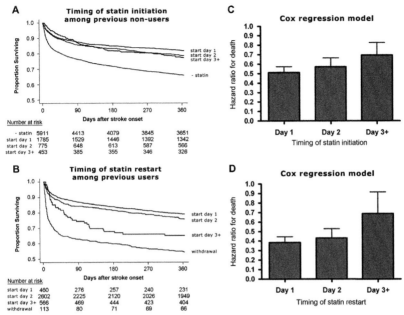

FIGURE 3.—Statin administration early in stroke hospitalization is associated with greater poststroke survival. A, One-year Kaplan-Meier survival curves for patients not taking a statin before stroke hospitalization. Survival curves based on in-hospital statin initiation are as follows: −statin=not treated with a statin; start day 1=statin started Day 1; start day 2=statin started Day 2; and start day 3+=statin started Day 3 or later. B, One-year Kaplan-Meier survival curves for patients who were taking a statin before stroke hospitalization. Survival curves based on in-hospital statin resumption are as follows: withdrawal=not treated with a statin in-hospital; start day 1=statin started Day 1; start day 2=statin started Day 2; and start day 3+=statin started Day 3 or later. C, Increasing hazard of death with delayed in-hospital statin treatment among patients not taking a statin before stroke hospitalization. Hazard ratios from multivariable Cox regression are with reference to the hazard of death among patients treated with a statin (hazard ratio [HR], 1.0). Error bars indicate upper limit of 95% CI (*P*<0.001 for each, *P*<0.001 for log-rank test for trend). D, Increasing hazard of death with delayed in-hospital statin treatment among patients who were taking a statin before stroke hospitalization. HRs from multivariable Cox regression are with reference to the hazard of death among patients not treated with a statin (HR, 1.0; *P*<0.001 for Day 1 and Day 2, *P*=0.019 for Day 3+, *P*<0.001 for log-rank test for trend). (Reprinted from Flint AC, Kamel H, Navi BB, et al. Statin use during ischemic stroke hospitalization is strongly associated with improved poststroke survival. *Stroke.* 2012;43:147-154, with permission from American Heart Association, Inc.)

mortality significantly. Cessation of statin therapy during hospitalization for any reason increased risk of mortality 2.5-fold. In each of these scenarios, Kaplan-Meier survival curves separate relatively quickly and the impact persists (Fig 1). The impact of moderate- versus high-dose statin therapy on mortality following ischemic stroke was also evaluated. Among patients using statins before stroke hospitalization, the cumulative hazard of death over 1 year following stroke was 0.89 (95% confidence interval [CI], 0.82−0.97; *P* < .01) for low to moderate statin dose and 0.65 (95% CI, 0.54−0.79; *P* < .001) for high statin dose compared with no statin. For statin use before and during stroke hospitalization, the hazard ratios were 0.60 (95% CI, 0.54−0.67; *P* < .001) for low- to moderate-dose statin use and 0.43 (95% CI, 0.34−0.53; *P* < .001) for high statin dose compared with

TABLE 2.—Raw Mortality Rates and Adjusted Cox Regression Analysis of Statin Use and Poststroke Survival

Model	1-Y Mortality, No Statin	1-Y Mortality, Statin	P	Hazard Ratio for Death	95% CI	P
Before	28.9%	25.1%	<0.001	0.85	0.79−0.93	<0.001
Before and during	33.8%	22.1%	<0.001	0.59	0.53−0.65	<0.001
Initiation in the hospital	33.8%	19.4%	<0.001	0.55	0.50−0.61	<0.001
Withdrawal in the hospital	46.2%	22.1%	<0.001	2.5	2.1−2.9	<0.001

Before indicates statin use before hospitalization for stroke, irrespective of statin use in the hospital (compared with no statin use before hospitalization, irrespective of statin use in the hospital); Before and during, statin use both before and during hospitalization (compared with no statin use before and during hospitalization); Initiation in the hospital, patients not taking a statin before stroke who began treatment with a statin in the hospital (compared with no statin use before and during hospitalization); Withdrawal in the hospital, patients who were taking a statin before hospitalization but who did not receive a statin in the hospital (compared with statin use both before and during hospitalization).

Percentages for 1 y mortality are unadjusted; P values for unadjusted mortality calculated from Fisher exact test. Hazard ratios represent cumulative 1 y hazard of death from multivariable Cox regression analysis adjusted for age, sex, medical comorbidities, race/ethnicity, year of discharge, and hospital center.

no statin use. There was clear evidence for increasing mortality with delay in initiating statin therapy while patients were hospitalized (Fig 3). The withdrawal of statin therapy was associated with particularly poor outcomes.

This observational study supports a number of conclusions. First, statin therapy should be initiated without delay in patients presenting with ischemic stroke. Second, among patients already on a statin, great care should be taken to avoid discontinuing a statin. Third, high-dose statin therapy outperforms low- to moderate-dose statin therapy in the setting of ischemic stroke. The initiation of statin therapy should be part of any treatment protocol for the acute management of primary or secondary ischemic stroke. Studies such as this are urgently needed to assess the efficacy of statin therapy for managing and preventing transient ischemic attacks.

P. P. Toth, MD, PhD

References

1. Shahar E, Chambless LE, Rosamond WD, et al. Plasma lipid profile and incident ischemic stroke: the Atherosclerosis Risk in Communities (ARIC) study. *Stroke.* 2003;34:623-631.
2. Willey JZ, Xu Q, Boden-Albala B, et al. Lipid profile components and risk of ischemic stroke: the Northern Manhattan Study (NOMAS). *Arch Neurol.* 2009; 66:1400-1406.
3. O'Regan C, Wu P, Arora P, Perri D, Mills EJ. Statin therapy in stroke prevention: a meta-analysis involving 121,000 patients. *Am J Med.* 2008;121:24-33.
4. Amarenco P, Bogousslavsky J, Callahan A 3rd, et al. High-dose atorvastatin after stroke or transient ischemic attack. *N Engl J Med.* 2006;355:549-559.

3 Obesity

Introduction

2012 has been a landmark year for Obesity Medicine, and it is not over yet. The following have occurred and may still occur this year:

1. The American Board of Obesity Medicine (ABOM) was founded and the first certifying exam will be given in November.
2. The first new weight loss drug approved by the FDA in over a decade will hit the market (Belviq or lorcaserin), and the second potentially will be approved as well known as Qnexa or Phentermine/Topiramate.
3. CMS has announced that obesity treatment by primary care providers will be covered by Medicare.

These events are ramifications of the combination efforts of academia, government and the industry to push obesity as a disease to the forefront of health care efforts to improve the well-being of Americans. Since obesity is the most prevalent disease in the United States as well as elsewhere in the world, these events this year will likely change the course of health care in the United States in the next few years and push us toward a better outcome for obesity treatment strategies than we have witnessed in the past 20 years.

All three events above have immediate ramifications for the practitioner, for not only will the subspecialty of Obesity Medicine be recognized, but treatment of the disease will be covered by insurance, and there will be more tools available to help the practitioner care for the obese patient.

The future of obesity treatment is bright, but more needs to be accomplished for health care to finally reverse the epidemic. The epidemic will not be reversed unless PREVENTION is also addressed. Prevention involves altering our environment to ensure that our children do not begin to develop obesity because we know that altering the body set point after it is established is difficult. It involves continued research and continued education of good wellness habits as well as leadership that are supportive and continue to fight for big change on a community and global level.

Prevention must start with research on what the purported causes of obesity really are. Is it the environment of fast food and lack of exercise? Is it ambient temperature and lack of shivering and heat loss through sweating that has slowly increased our BMI? Is it a preservative in our food supply? Is it a change in our body's defended set point due to hypothalamic injury from inflammation due to high fat and calorie ingestion?

The articles presented here address some of the issues regarding causal factors for obesity as well as some of the new drugs that have been used to combat the effects of the environment through satiety. So far, drugs already approved or drugs in the process of being approved for obesity have elicited their effects through two mechanisms:

1. Regulation of appetite and satiety centrally (phentermine, sibutr-amine, lorcaserin, topiramate/phentermine, bupropion/naltrexone)
2. Regulation of absorption of nutrients (orlistat)

The next wave of approvable drugs will hopefully address other pathways such as:

1. Regulation of energy expenditure
2. Regulation of fat oxidation

In addition, new inroads are being formulated with surgical devices that can be inserted without general anesthesia and the incurrent risk of anesthesia as well as the surgical procedure. Surgical procedures will team up with new medications to enhance weight loss and weight maintenance.

Establishing causal factors that are amenable to treatment or prevention will engage the research for an antidote. The field of Obesity Medicine needs more practitioners, advocates, and researchers.

Caroline M. Apovian, MD, FACP, FACN

Diet and Obesity

Long-Term Persistence of Hormonal Adaptations to Weight Loss
Sumithran P, Prendergast LA, Delbridge E, et al (Univ of Melbourne, Victoria, Australia; La Trobe Univ, Melbourne, Victoria, Australia)
N Engl J Med 365:1597-1604, 2011

Background.—After weight loss, changes in the circulating levels of several peripheral hormones involved in the homeostatic regulation of body weight occur. Whether these changes are transient or persist over time may be important for an understanding of the reasons behind the high rate of weight regain after diet-induced weight loss.

Methods.—We enrolled 50 overweight or obese patients without diabetes in a 10-week weight-loss program for which a very-low-energy diet was prescribed. At baseline (before weight loss), at 10 weeks (after program completion), and at 62 weeks, we examined circulating levels of leptin, ghrelin, peptide YY, gastric inhibitory polypeptide, glucagon-like peptide 1, amylin, pancreatic polypeptide, cholecystokinin, and insulin and subjective ratings of appetite.

Results.—Weight loss (mean [$\pm$SE], 13.5 ± 0.5 kg) led to significant reductions in levels of leptin, peptide YY, cholecystokinin, insulin ($P<0.001$ for all comparisons), and amylin ($P = 0.002$) and to increases in levels of ghrelin ($P<0.001$), gastric inhibitory polypeptide ($P = 0.004$), and pancreatic polypeptide ($P = 0.008$). There was also a significant increase in subjective appetite (*P*<0.001). One year after the initial weight loss, there were still significant differences from baseline in the mean levels of leptin (*P*<0.001), peptide YY (*P*<0.001), cholecystokinin (*P* = 0.04), insulin (*P* = 0.01), ghrelin (*P*<0.001), gastric inhibitory polypeptide (*P*<0.001), and pancreatic polypeptide (*P* = 0.002), as well as hunger (*P*<0.001).

Conclusions.—One year after initial weight reduction, levels of the circulating mediators of appetite that encourage weight regain after diet-induced weight loss do not revert to the levels recorded before weight loss. Long-term strategies to counteract this change may be needed to prevent obesity relapse. (Funded by the National Health and Medical Research Council and others; ClinicalTrials.gov number, NCT00870259.)

▶ Lifestyle modifications of diet and exercise are mainstay treatments for weight loss in individuals who are overweight or obese. However, sustained long-term weight loss following caloric restriction and exercise regimens is highly unsuccessful.[1] Multiple factors likely contribute to weight regain after lifestyle interventions; however, 1 plausible mechanism involves aberrations in appetite and satiety hormones. To date, there is little understanding of how appetite regulatory hormones/peptides may contribute to sustained weight loss or weight gain following significant weight loss by lifestyle modification.

In a small (n = 34 completed study), but well-conducted study, Sumithran et al characterized changes in appetite and body weight regulatory hormones after short-term weight loss (10 weeks) and after 1 year of follow-up. A key strength of this study is that the subjects obtained significant short-term weight loss (14%) and sustained weight loss (8%) after 1 year. They present novel findings that key appetite-suppressing hormones, including peptide YY, leptin, cholecystokinin, and insulin were lower after significant weight loss (14%), and these hormones did not return to baseline levels 1 year after weight loss. In addition, ghrelin and gastric inhibitory protein levels were elevated above baseline 1 year after weight loss. This is the first long-term study to demonstrate that appetite-suppressing hormones are lower, and stimulating hormones are elevated 1 year after caloric-induced weight loss, indicating that individuals are predisposed to regain weight after caloric restriction (Fig 2 in the original article). Moreover, in agreement with the biochemical data, subjects' perceived hunger was elevated 1 year following initial weight loss, reinforcing that the propensity to regain weight may be caused by aberrations to regulators of appetite and satiety.

Although this study is suggestive that alterations in satiety hormones contribute to weight regain, we are limited in our interpretations of the findings because of the high attrition rate and small cohort. While the exclusion of premenopausal women from this study is a strong point of the design, we are unable to draw conclusions with regard to the response of these hormones to weight loss in that particular cohort.

Sumithran et al present novel results indicating that alterations in appetite regulator hormones after significant sustained weight loss may predispose moderately obese individuals to regain weight. This reinforces that obesity is a complex multifactorial disease that requires multiple therapeutic strategies to combat this disease. It is postulated that 1 factor that contributes to the success of gastric bypass surgery for profound long-term weight loss is improvements of satiety hormone secretion. Thus, the propensity to regain weight after calorie restriction may be improved by pharmaceutical therapies aimed at improving secretion of satiety hormones. Unfortunately, such agents are lacking in our current arsenal of obesity treatments, and further investigation of the therapeutic potential of satiety hormone modification will enhance our ability to combat this disease.

M. R. Ruth, PhD

Reference

1. Wing RR, Hill JO. Successful weight loss maintenance. *Annu Rev Nutr.* 2001;21: 323-341.

Comparative Effectiveness of Weight-Loss Interventions in Clinical Practice
Appel LJ, Clark JM, Yeh H-C, et al (Johns Hopkins Univ, Baltimore, MD; et al)
N Engl J Med 365:1959-1968, 2011

Background.—Obesity and its cardiovascular complications are extremely common medical problems, but evidence on how to accomplish weight loss in clinical practice is sparse.

Methods.—We conducted a randomized, controlled trial to examine the effects of two behavioral weight-loss interventions in 415 obese patients with at least one cardiovascular risk factor. Participants were recruited from six primary care practices; 63.6% were women, 41.0% were black, and the mean age was 54.0 years. One intervention provided patients with weight-loss support remotely—through the telephone, a study-specific Web site, and e-mail. The other intervention provided in-person support during group and individual sessions, along with the three remote means of support. There was also a control group in which weight loss was self-directed. Outcomes were compared between each intervention group and the control group and between the two intervention groups. For both interventions, primary care providers reinforced participation at routinely scheduled visits. The trial duration was 24 months.

Results.—At baseline, the mean body-mass index (the weight in kilograms divided by the square of the height in meters) for all participants was 36.6, and the mean weight was 103.8 kg. At 24 months, the mean change in weight from baseline was -0.8 kg in the control group, -4.6 kg in the group receiving remote support only ($P<0.001$ for the comparison with the control group), and -5.1 kg in the group receiving in-person support ($P<0.001$ for the comparison with the control group). The percentage of participants who lost 5% or more of their initial weight was 18.8% in the control group, 38.2% in the group receiving remote support only, and 41.4% in the group receiving in-person support. The change in weight from baseline did not differ significantly between the two intervention groups.

Conclusions.—In two behavioral interventions, one delivered with in-person support and the other delivered remotely, without face-to-face contact between participants and weight-loss coaches, obese patients achieved and sustained clinically significant weight loss over a period of 24 months. (Funded by the National Heart, Lung, and Blood Institute and others; ClinicalTrials.gov number, NCT00783315.)

▶ Obesity is known to increase the risk for type 2 diabetes and cardiovascular disease, among many other comorbid conditions. The prevalence of obesity has risen sharply, mainly because of lifestyle changes. It is clear that to halt this epidemic, large-scale, population-based strategies should be implemented. It is also important that weight-loss counseling can be delivered in primary care centers, but there is a paucity of community-based weight-loss trials in which its effectiveness and reproducibility can be evaluated.

The purpose of the trial by Appel et al was to evaluate the long-term (24-month) effectiveness of 2 behavioral weight-loss interventions, differing in personal contact. A total of 415 obese patients were randomized to 3 groups. The control group had in-person individual sessions, the second group had in-person individual sessions plus group sessions, and the third group had in-person support delivered by electronic and telephone contact or a commercial call-center-directed group in which lifestyle interventions were delivered by telephone, Internet, or mail (remote support). The role of the primary care physicians (PCPs) was to support the patients with the weight-loss treatment. The weight loss was similar in the group that received in-person support and remote support, and both were superior to the control group (5.1 kg, 4.6 kg, and 0.8 kg, respectively; Fig 1 in the original article). Patients in both active groups lost more than 5% of initial weight compared with the control group (41% in the in-person group, 38% in the remote group, and 19% in the control group).

This study was one of the longest trials to evaluate remote (telephone, Web-based) interventions. Surprisingly, the effect of in-person and remote counseling yielded similar results. It is not clear if the in-person contact with the PCP influenced the clinical results. Previous studies have shown inferior weight loss in remote counseling compared with frequent in-person sessions.

Unfortunately, neither of the studies (by Wadden and the present study by Appel) were powered to evaluate change in cardiovascular risk factors, and there was no significant change in these parameters in both studies. Nevertheless, when dealing with an epidemic, the use of remote counseling enables providers to offer large-scale, more convenient counseling that can be easily implemented in clinical practice.

R. Ness-Abramof, MD

A Two-Year Randomized Trial of Obesity Treatment in Primary Care Practice
Wadden TA, Volger S, Sarwer DB, et al (Perelman School of Medicine at the Univ of Pennsylvania, Philadelphia; et al)
N Engl J Med 365:1969-1979, 2011

Background.—Calls for primary care providers (PCPs) to offer obese patients behavioral weight-loss counseling have not been accompanied by adequate guidance on how such care could be delivered. This randomized trial compared weight loss during a 2-year period in response to three lifestyle interventions, all delivered by PCPs in collaboration with auxiliary health professionals (lifestyle coaches) in their practices.

Methods.—We randomly assigned 390 obese adults in six primary care practices to one of three types of intervention: usual care, consisting of quarterly PCP visits that included education about weight management; brief lifestyle counseling, consisting of quarterly PCP visits combined with brief monthly sessions with lifestyle coaches who instructed participants about behavioral weight control; or enhanced brief lifestyle counseling, which provided the same care as described for the previous intervention but included meal replacements or weight-loss medication (orlistat or sibutramine), chosen by the participants in consultation with the PCPs, to potentially increase weight loss.

Results.—Of the 390 participants, 86% completed the 2-year trial, at which time, the mean (± SE) weight loss with usual care, brief lifestyle counseling, and enhanced brief lifestyle counseling was 1.7 ± 0.7, 2.9 ± 0.7, and 4.6 ± 0.7 kg, respectively. Initial weight decreased at least 5% in 21.5%, 26.0%, and 34.9% of the participants in the three groups, respectively. Enhanced lifestyle counseling was superior to usual care on both these measures of success ($P = 0.003$ and $P = 0.02$, respectively), with no other significant differences among the groups. The benefits of enhanced lifestyle counseling remained even after participants given sibutramine were excluded from the analyses. There were no significant differences between the intervention groups in the occurrence of serious adverse events.

Conclusions.—Enhanced weight-loss counseling helps about one third of obese patients achieve longterm, clinically meaningful weight loss. (Funded by the National Heart, Lung, and Blood Institute; POWER-UP ClinicalTrials.gov number, NCT00826774.)

▶ The prevalence of obesity has risen sharply during the past 3 decades, reaching epidemic proportions. The causes of obesity are multifactorial, involving genetic, environmental, and psychosocial factors. The obesity epidemic is best explained by a caloric imbalance due to increased caloric intake coupled with decreased physical activity. In order to halt or revert the obesity epidemic, population-based strategies concerning lifestyle changes should be implemented. Modest weight losses of 5% to 10% of initial body weight were shown to improve comorbid conditions and reduce the risk of diabetes.[1] The National Heart, Lung and Blood Institute funded the Practice-based Opportunities for Weight reduction consortium, which conducted a trial of weight loss interventions based on primary care in obese patients with cardiovascular risk factors. The outcomes of 2 studies were published in November 2011 and presented in this article.

In the first study by Wadden et al,[2] usual care (weight loss counseling provided by a primary care physician [PCP] delivered quarterly) was compared to more intensive counseling: quarterly counseling by a PCP in addition to monthly 15-minute, in person counseling by trained assistants or enhanced lifestyle counseling, the same counseling schedule as the intensive counseling but with the added choice of weight loss medications (orlistat or sibutramine) or meal replacements in order to enhance weight loss. The study was designed to evaluate weight loss at 24 months.

A total of 390 obese participants (body mass index 30–50 kg/m^2) were enrolled, and 86% completed the 2-year trial. The mean weight loss with the brief lifestyle counseling group (2.9 kg) and the usual care group (1.7 kg) did not differ significantly; the enhanced lifestyle counseling group lost significantly more weight (4.6 kg) compared to the usual care group (Fig 2 in the original article). Significantly more patients in the enhanced lifestyle group lost at least 5% of initial weight compared to the other groups (35% in the enhanced lifestyle group, 26% in the brief lifestyle group, and 21.5% in the usual care group).

During the study period, sibutramine was withdrawn from the market due to safety issues concerning cardiovascular risk. Even after excluding patients from the analysis who had been given sibutramine, the effect of the enhanced lifestyle group was superior.

It is interesting that a more intensive counseling strategy did not promote superior weight loss compared to the control group. This finding contrasts with previous data in which more intensive counseling yielded better weight loss results.[2]

The strengths of the study are the follow-up of 24 months and the low attrition rate. Since the weight loss medications and meal replacements were provided free to the patients (they are not covered by most health insurance), the reproducibility of this strategy in practice may be problematic. Nevertheless, this study shows that weight loss can be achieved in primary care clinics with minimal staff training.

R. Ness-Abramof, MD

References

1. Knowler WC, Barrett-Connor E, Fowler SE, et al; Diabetes prevention Program Research Group. Reduction in the incidence of type 2 diabetes with lifestyle intervention or metformin. *N Engl J Med.* 2002;346:393-403.
2. Wadden TA, Webb VL, Moran CH, Bailer BA. Lifestyle modification for obesity: new developments in diet, physical activity, and behavior therapy. *Circulation.* 2012;125:1157-1170.

Calcium and vitamin D supplementation is associated with decreased abdominal visceral adipose tissue in overweight and obese adults

Rosenblum JL, Castro VM, Moore CE, et al (Massachusetts General Hosp, Boston; Texas Woman's Univ, Houston)
Am J Clin Nutr 95:101-108, 2012

Background.—Several studies suggest that calcium and vitamin D (CaD) may play a role in the regulation of abdominal fat mass.

Objective.—This study investigated the effect of CaD-supplemented orange juice (OJ) on weight loss and reduction of visceral adipose tissue (VAT) in overweight and obese adults (mean ± SD age: 40.0 ± 12.9 y).

Design.—Two parallel, double-blind, placebo-controlled trials were conducted with either regular or reduced-energy (lite) orange juice. For each 16-wk trial, 171 participants were randomly assigned to 1 of 2 groups. The treatment groups consumed three 240-mL glasses of OJ (regular or lite) fortified with 350 mg Ca and 100 IU vitamin D per serving, and the control groups consumed either unfortified regular or lite OJ. Computed tomography scans of VAT and subcutaneous adipose tissue were performed by imaging a single cut at the lumbar 4 level.

Results.—After 16 wk, the average weight loss ($\sim$2.45 kg) did not differ significantly between groups. In the regular OJ trial, the reduction of VAT was significantly greater ($P = 0.024$) in the CaD group (-12.7 ± 25.0 cm^2) than in the control group (-1.3 ± 13.6 cm^2). In the lite OJ trial, the reduction of VAT was significantly greater ($P = 0.039$) in the CaD group (-13.1 ± 18.4 cm^2) than in the control group (-6.4 ± 17.5 cm^2) after control for baseline VAT. The effect of calcium and vitamin D on VAT remained highly significant when the results of the 2 trials were combined ($P = 0.007$).

Conclusions.—The findings suggest that calcium and/or vitamin D supplementation contributes to a beneficial reduction of VAT. This trial is registered at clinicaltrial.gov as NCT00386672, NCT01363115 (Table 4).

▶ Visceral adipose tissue (VAT) has been associated with insulin resistance and other risk factors for cardiovascular disease. Any intervention that enhances weight loss, particularly loss of VAT, in patients who are participating in a medical weight loss program is desirable.

Findings from this study suggest an effect of calcium and vitamin D supplementation in the form of fortified orange juice on differential VAT loss in overweight and obese individuals who were enrolled in a medical weight loss program without an effect on total weight loss. Vitamin D deficiency is common in the obese, particularly in those with a larger amount of VAT.[1] Vitamin D deficiency is also associated with insulin resistance[2] and cardiovascular disease[3] and may exacerbate these complications associated with obesity. It has been proposed that secondary hyperparathyroidism that occurs as a result of vitamin D deficiency may promote weight gain by impairment in catecholamine-induced lipolysis.[4] Preclinical studies suggested a role of calcium on weight and body fat by means of increased lipolysis and preserved thermogenesis.[5]

This study is one of the few studies available that assesses the effects of calcium and vitamin D on adipose tissue compartments. The strengths of the study include the randomized, double-blind design and the use of a single-slice abdominal CT scan at the level of the lumbar vertebra to assess visceral and subcutaneous fat compartments. The limitation of this study includes the fact that calcium and vitamin D were delivered together in the form of orange juice. The results cannot be generalizable to calcium and vitamin D given separately as pills, and the contribution of effects from calcium and vitamin D cannot be separated. The dose of vitamin D_3 given is relatively small (300 IU/day), consistent with a small rise in serum 25-hydroxy vitamin D levels [25(OH)D] observed in the intervention groups (2–5 ng/mL), and it may be difficult to

TABLE 4.—Changes in Anthropometric and Body-Fat Variables from Baseline to Week 16 in the Control and CaD-Supplemented Groups[1]

Variable	Regular OJ		Lite OJ		Combined	
	Control (n = 34)	CaD (n = 31)	Control (n = 31)	CaD (n = 35)	Control (n = 65)	CaD (n = 66)
Absolute body weight (kg)	−2.4 ± 3.5[2]	−2.2 ± 3.0[2]	−2.3 ± 2.9	−2.9 ± 3.8	−2.4 ± 3.2	−2.5 ± 3.3
Body weight (%)	−3.1 ± 4.4	−2.5 ± 3.2	−3.3 ± 3.8	−3.9 ± 4.7	−3.1 ± 4.0	−3.2 ± 4.1
Absolute BMI (kg/m²)	−0.94 ± 1.37	−0.80 ± 0.99	−1.1 ± 1.1	−1.3 ± 1.5	−1.0 ± 1.0	−1.1 ± 1.3
Absolute waist circumference (cm)	−2.2 ± 4.1	−2.2 ± 3.8	−2.8 ± 2.8	−3.7 ± 4.2	−2.4 ± 3.6	−3.0 ± 4.1
Total abdominal fat (cm²)	−19.5 ± 58.3	−32.3 ± 44.1	−31.6 ± 41.8	−41.9 ± 61.0	−25.3 ± 51.0	−37.6 ± 54.0
SAT (cm²)	−18.3 ± 48.4	−19.6 ± 34.3	−25.3 ± 31.6	−28.8 ± 50.9	−21.6 ± 41.1	−24.8 ± 44.1
VAT (cm²)	−1.3 ± 13.6	−12.7 ± 25.0*,[2]	−6.4 ± 17.5	−13.1 ± 18.4[3]	−3.7 ± 15.7	−12.9 ± 21.8**
VAT (%)	−4 ± 19	−9 ± 13	−5 ± 20	−16 ± 18*	−5 ± 19	−13 ± 16*

*,**Significantly different from the control value.

*P < 0.05.

**P < 0.01. CaD, calcium and vitamin D; lite, reduced energy; OJ, orange juice; SAT, subcutaneous adipose tissue; VAT, visceral adipose tissue.

[1] All values are means ± SDs. Changes in the anthropometric and body-fat variables between the control and experimental groups over time were made by using unadjusted, independent-sample, 2-sided t tests.

[2] ANCOVA was used to adjust for baseline total abdominal fat in the regular OJ trial. Differences in change in body weight were not significant (adjusted P = 0.755), and differences in the change in VAT remained significant (adjusted P = 0.02).

[3] ANCOVA was used to adjust for baseline VAT in the Lite OJ trial. Differences in the change in VAT were significant (P = 0.039).

attribute the biological effects observed to such small changes in serum 25(OH) D alone (Table 4). The larger decline in VAT in the intervention group reached statistical significance but was not associated with an improvement in fasting glucose, insulin, or lipid profile, thus the clinical significance of these results needs to be confirmed.

Future studies to assess the effects of calcium and vitamin D separately and using a higher vitamin D dose is warranted before calcium and vitamin D supplementation could be recommended routinely for patients in medical weight loss programs.

P. Pramyothin, MD

References

1. Cheng S, Massaro JM, Fox CS, et al. Adiposity, cardiometabolic risk, and vitamin D status: the Framingham Heart Study. *Diabetes.* 2010;59:242-248.
2. Liu E, Meigs JB, Pittas AG, et al. Plasma 25-hydroxyvitamin d is associated with markers of the insulin resistant phenotype in nondiabetic adults. *J Nutr.* 2009;139: 329-334.
3. Wang TJ, Pencina MJ, Booth SL, et al. Vitamin D deficiency and risk of cardiovascular disease. *Circulation.* 2008;117:503-511.
4. McCarty MF, Thomas CA. PTH excess may promote weight gain by impeding catecholamine-induced lipolysis-implications for the impact of calcium, vitamin D, and alcohol on body weight. *Med Hypotheses.* 2003;61:535-542.
5. Zemel MB. Mechanisms of dairy modulation of adiposity. *J Nutr.* 2003;133: 252S-256S.

Replacing caloric beverages with water or diet beverages for weight loss in adults: main results of the Choose Healthy Options Consciously Everyday (CHOICE) randomized clinical trial

Tate DF, Turner-McGrievy G, Lyons E, et al (The Univ of North Carolina at Chapel Hill)
Am J Clin Nutr 95:555-563, 2012

Background.—Replacement of caloric beverages with noncaloric beverages may be a simple strategy for promoting modest weight reduction; however, the effectiveness of this strategy is not known.

Objective.—We compared the replacement of caloric beverages with water or diet beverages (DBs) as a method of weight loss over 6 mo in adults and attention controls (ACs).

Design.—Overweight and obese adults [$n = 318$; BMI (in kg/m^2): 36.3 ± 5.9; 84% female; age (mean ± SD): 42 ± 10.7 y; 54% black] substituted noncaloric beverages (water or DBs) for caloric beverages ($\geq$200 kcal/d) or made dietary changes of their choosing (AC) for 6 mo.

Results.—In an intent-to-treat analysis, a significant reduction in weight and waist circumference and an improvement in systolic blood pressure were observed from 0 to 6 mo. Mean (±SEM) weight losses at 6 mo were −2.5 ± 0.45% in the DB group, −2.03 ± 0.40% in the Water group, and −1.76 ± 0.35% in the AC group; there were no significant differences between groups. The chance of achieving a 5% weight loss at 6 mo was greater in the DB group than in the AC group (OR: 2.29; 95% CI: 1.05, 5.01; $P = 0.04$). A significant reduction in fasting glucose at 6 mo ($P = 0.019$) and improved hydration at 3 ($P = 0.0017$) and 6 ($P = 0.049$) mo was observed in the Water group relative to the AC group. In a combined analysis, participants assigned to beverage replacement were 2 times as likely to have achieved a 5% weight loss (OR: 2.07; 95% CI: 1.02, 4.22; $P = 0.04$) than were the AC participants.

Conclusions.—Replacement of caloric beverages with noncaloric beverages as a weight-loss strategy resulted in average weight losses of 2% to 2.5%. This strategy could have public health significance and is a simple, straightforward message. This trial was registered at clinicaltrials.gov as NCT01017783.

▶ Obesity is a major global health problem and an important risk factor for type 2 diabetes mellitus (T2DM), cardiovascular disease, and cancer, among many other comorbidities. The American Heart Association released a scientific statement recommending reductions in added-sugar intake to no more than 100 to 150 kcal/day for most Americans, since it identifies sugar-sweetened beverages as the primary source of added sugar, contributing to the obesity and T2DM epidemic. It is believed that sugar-sweetened beverages cause weight gain because of their high caloric content and low satiety, and coupled with incomplete compensation for the calories ingested, this leads to an increased total caloric intake. Due to its rapid absorption and its high glycemic load, sweetened beverages may, independent of obesity, promote insulin resistance and inflammation, while high-fructose corn syrup, a widely used sweetener, may increase visceral adiposity and cause dyslipidemia and ectopic fat deposition.[1]

This study evaluated the effect of promoting weight loss at 6 months by replacing caloric beverages with noncaloric beverages (water or diet beverages) versus a control group who received instruction about healthy choices but included no changes in drinking habits. This study was unique because although participants were instructed concerning healthy choices, just the change in drinking pattern was randomized and reinforced with monthly meetings. At the end of the study all groups lost weight, without a significant difference between groups. The diet beverage group lost 2.5% of initial body weight, the water group lost −2%, and the healthy choices group lost 1.76% of initial body weight (Fig 3 in the original article). Combining the 2 beverage replacement groups, twice as many achieved more than 5% weight loss compared to the healthy choices group.

Although the weight loss effect of this study is modest, as mentioned in the article, the potential for population-based changes is important. A simple and straight statement can be made: Changes in the choice of beverages can make a substantial change in weight and possibly in other health-related outcomes.

R. Ness-Abramof, MD

Reference

1. Malik VS, Popkin BM, Bray GA, Després J-P, Hu FB. Contemporary reviews in cardiovascular medicine: sugar-sweetened beverages, obesity, type 2 diabetes mellitus, and cardiovascular disease risk. *Circulation.* 2010;121:1356-1364.

Epidemiology and Complications of Obesity

Hypertriglyceridemic waist: a simple clinical phenotype associated with coronary artery disease in women
Blackburn P, Lemieux I, Lamarche B, et al (Université du Québec à Chicoutimi, Saguenay, Canada; Centre de recherche de l'Institut universitaire de cardiologie et de pneumologie de Québec, Canada; Université Laval, Québec, Canada; et al)
Metabolism 61:56-64, 2012

The aim of the present study was to compare the ability of the hypertriglyceridemic waist phenotype and the National Cholesterol Education Program—Adult Treatment Panel III (NCEP-ATP III) clinical criteria to predict coronary artery disease (CAD) risk in a sample of women. We studied 254 women among whom the presence/absence of CAD was assessed by angiography. The *hypertriglyceridemic waist phenotype* was defined as having both a high waist circumference (≥85 cm) and increased fasting triglyceride levels (≥1.5 mmol/L), whereas the presence of at least 3 of the 5 NCEP-ATP III criteria was used as the "reference" screening approach to identify women with the features of the metabolic syndrome. Women with hypertriglyceridemic waist were characterized by higher adiposity indices as well as by a more disturbed fasting metabolic risk profile compared with women without this phenotype. Similar differences were observed when comparing the metabolic profile of women with vs without at least 3 of the NCEP-ATP III clinical criteria. Moreover, differences in the Framingham risk score were essentially similar when women were considered at low or high risk by either hypertriglyceridemic waist or by NCEP-ATP III clinical criteria ($P < .0001$). Finally, both clinical phenotypes were predictive of CAD (hypertriglyceridemic waist: relative odds ratio, 2.1; 95% confidence interval, 1.1-3.8; $P = .02$; NCEP-ATP III clinical criteria: relative odds ratio, 2.5; 95% confidence interval, 1.4-4.6; $P < .003$). These results suggest that hypertriglyceridemic waist is a simple screening tool to identify women with clustering metabolic abnormalities and at increased CAD risk.

▶ The metabolic syndrome comprises a cluster of risk factors that increase the risk for type 2 diabetes mellitus (type 2 DM) and cardiovascular disease. The risk factors include increased glucose levels, high blood pressure, elevated triglycerides, low high-density lipoprotein cholesterol, and a high waist circumference as a marker of obesity. Meeting 3 of 5 of the diagnostic criteria fulfills the diagnosis of the syndrome. The prevalence of the syndrome has been increasing worldwide due to the increasing prevalence of obesity.

The cutoff for waist circumference differs among ethnical groups and recommendations of different health organizations. The initial threshold for waist circumference by the American Heart Association/National Heart, Lung, and Blood Institute (AHA/NHLBI) was a waist circumference of 88 cm or more for women and 102 cm or more for men.[1] This cutoff was changed according to ethnic specific cutoffs; for whites a cutoff of 80 cm or more for women and 94 cm or more for men has been recommended.[2] When using the AHA/NHLBI definition for the United States, the higher or lower waist circumference thresholds do not significantly change the diagnosis of the metabolic syndrome because of the high prevalence of the other components of the syndrome in the population and because of the high prevalence of obesity.

The metabolic syndrome criteria are not the only criteria proposed to identify high-risk patients. The hypertriglyceridemic waist, a combination of increased waist circumference and high fasting triglyceride level, has also been shown to identify high-risk patients for cardiovascular disease and type 2 DM and may be an easier way to screen in clinical practice.

This study compared the diagnostic ability of the hypertriglyceridemic waist phenotype and the National Cholesterol Education Program—Adult Treatment Panel III (NCEP-ATP III) to predict coronary artery disease (CAD) risk in women referred for coronary angiography. The study enrolled 254 women, in which the diagnosis of the hypertriglyceridemic waist was a waist circumference of 85 cm or more and increased fasting triglyceride of 1.5 mmol/L or more (133 mg/dL). As expected, women with the hypertriglyceridemic waist had higher adiposity and increased metabolic abnormalities. There was no significant difference for the diagnosis of high-risk or low-risk women when comparing the hypertriglyceridemic waist and the NCEP-ATP III criteria, with both criteria encompassing a higher risk for CAD (hypertriglyceridemic waist: relative odds ratio, 2.1; 95% confidence interval, 1.1–3.8; $P = .02$; NCEP-ATP III clinical criteria: relative odds ratio, 2.5; 95% confidence interval, 1.4–4.6; $P < .003$). The hypertriglyceridemic waist and NCEP diagnosed different subgroups of high-risk patients, a result that is concordant with previous studies.

This study reinforces the hypertriglyceridemic waist as a way to identify high-risk patients using a relatively easy and accessible clinical tool.

R. Ness-Abramof, MD

References

1. Grundy SM, Brewer HB Jr, Cleeman JI, Smith SC Jr, Lenfant C, for the Conference Participants. NHLBI/AHA Conference Proceedings: definition of metabolic syndrome: report of the National Heart, Lung, and Blood Institute/American Heart Association conference on scientific issues related to definition. *Circulation.* 2004; 109:433-438.
2. Alberti KG, Eckel RH, Grundy SM, et al. Harmonizing the metabolic syndrome: a joint interim statement of the International Diabetes Federation Task Force on Epidemiology and Prevention; National Heart, Lung, and Blood Institute; American Heart Association; World Heart Federation; International Atherosclerosis Society; and International Association for the Study of Obesity. *Circulation.* 2009;120: 1640-1645.

The effect of increasing obesity on the response to and outcome of assisted reproductive technology: a national study

Luke B, a Society for Assisted Reproductive Technology writing group (Michigan State Univ, East Lansing; et al)
Fertil Steril 96:820-825, 2011

Objective.—To evaluate the effect of increasing female obesity on response to and outcome of assisted reproductive technology (ART) treatment.

Design.—Historical cohort study.

Setting.—Clinic-based data.

Patient(s).—A total of 152,500 ART cycle starts from the Society for Assisted Reproductive Technology Clinical Outcomes Reporting System for 2007–2008, limited to women with documented height and grouped by body mass index (BMI, [weight/height^2]).

Intervention(s).—None.

Main Outcome Measure(s).—Cycle cancellation overall, cycle cancellation due to low response, treatment failure (not pregnant vs. pregnant), and pregnancy failure (fetal loss or stillbirth vs. live birth), as adjusted odds ratios and 95% confidence intervals, with cycles among normal-weight women as the reference group.

Result(s).—Cycle cancellation overall and cancellation due to low response using autologous oocytes significantly paralleled increasing BMI. The odds of treatment failure rose significantly with autologous-fresh cycles, from 1.03 for cycles among overweight women (BMI 25.0–29.9) to 1.53 for cycles among women with BMIs $\geq$50.0 kg/m^2. Likewise, the odds of pregnancy failure were most significant with increasing BMI among women with autologous-fresh cycles, increasing from 1.10 for cycles to overweight women to 2.29 for cycles to women with BMI $\geq$50.0 kg/m^2.

Conclusion(s).—These results indicate significantly higher odds of cycle cancellation. In addition, treatment and pregnancy failures with increasing obesity significantly increased starting with overweight women.

▶ The prevalence of overweight and obesity in women of childbearing age has increased markedly during the past 30 years. Approximately 25% of women in the United States who become pregnant are obese. Obese pregnant women are at high risk of maternal and fetal complications. Maternal complications include increased risk of gestational diabetes, hypertension, and pre-eclampsia and eclampsia as well as an increased need for cesarean section. Obese women are often insulin resistant. In women with polycystic ovary syndrome, insulin-mediated overstimulation of ovarian steroidogenesis and decreased sex hormone–binding globulin cause oligomenorrhea and infertility. Furthermore, obese women require higher doses of gonadotropins to achieve a proper ovarian response, have lower pregnancy rates after in vitro fertilization, and have higher spontaneous abortion rates.[1]

The authors evaluated the effect of female obesity on response and outcome of assisted reproductive technology treatment (ART). The database included 152 500 ART cycles. Only cycles in women with documented height and weight were included in the study. The study population was stratified based on body mass index (BMI) from underweight to BMI greater than 50 kg/m^2. The high number of cycles and the inclusion of women with very high BMIs were unique to this database. Women with higher BMIs had a higher incidence of ovulating disorder (eg, polycystic ovarian syndrome) and tubal factors compared to women with lower BMIs in which there was a higher prevalence of endometriosis. With increasing BMI, the chances of cycle cancellation were higher, particularly in autologous fresh cycles, and the chances of achieving an intrauterine pregnancy and a live birth were lower. This trend began in the over-weight range. One of the main limitations of the study is that the data are not presented in a per-women basis, but rather on a per-cycle basis, meaning that women with cycle failures were overrepresented. This study emphasizes another poor obstetric outcome related to obesity.

R. Ness-Abramof, MD

Reference

1. Pasquali R, Pelusi C, Genghini S, Cacciari M, Gambineri A. Obesity and reproductive disorders in women. *Hum Reprod Update.* 2003;9:359-372.

Obesity Is Not Protective against Fracture in Postmenopausal Women: GLOW
Compston JE, for the Glow Investigators (Cambridge Univ Hosps NHS Foundation Trust, UK; et al)
Am J Med 124:1043-1050, 2011

Objective.—To investigate the prevalence and incidence of clinical fractures in obese, postmenopausal women enrolled in the Global Longitudinal study of Osteoporosis in Women (GLOW).

Methods.—This was a multinational, prospective, observational, population-based study carried out by 723 physician practices at 17 sites in 10 countries. A total of 60,393 women aged ≥55 years were included. Data were collected using self-administered questionnaires that covered domains that included patient characteristics, fracture history, risk factors for fracture, and anti-osteoporosis medications.

Results.—Body mass index (BMI) and fracture history were available at baseline and at 1 and 2 years in 44,534 women, 23.4% of whom were obese (BMI ≥30 kg/m^2). Fracture prevalence in obese women at baseline was 222 per 1000 and incidence at 2 years was 61.7 per 1000, similar to rates in nonobese women (227 and 66.0 per 1000, respectively). Fractures in obese women accounted for 23% and 22% of all previous and incident fractures, respectively. The risk of incident ankle and upper leg fractures was significantly higher in obese than in nonobese women, while the risk of wrist fracture was significantly lower. Obese women with fracture were more likely to have experienced early menopause and to report 2 or

TABLE 2.—Frequency of Fractures by Skeletal Location in Obese, Nonobese, and Underweight Women (Rates per 1000 Women)

	Previous Fracture				Incident Fracture (Within 2 Years of Baseline)			
Fracture Site	Group 1: Obese (n = 10,441)	Group 2: Nonobese (n = 33,349)	Group 3: Underweight (n = 744)	P Value*	Group 1: Obese (n = 10,441)	Group 2: Nonobese (n = 33,349)	Group 3: Underweight (n = 744)	P Value*
Clavicle	11.0	12.5	21.6		2.0	2.3	1.4	
Upper arm	28.9	26.3	39.2		6.1	6.0	6.8	
Wrist	67.0	85.7	108	1 vs 2, 1 vs 3	12.1	15.4	17.6	1 vs 2
Spine	18.6	20.9	33.9	1 vs 3	5.6	7.0	8.1	
Rib	35.6	41.2	58.0	1 vs 2, 1 vs 3	8.1	9.3	1.4	2 vs 3
Hip	11.2	15.9	43.3	1 vs 2, 1 vs 3, 2 vs 3	3.8	4.6	11.0	1 vs 3
Pelvis	6.0	10.6	23.0	1 vs 2, 1 vs 3, 2 vs 3	1.9	2.7	8.1	1 vs 3
Ankle	75.3	55.2	50.0	1 vs 2, 1 vs 3	13.3	8.5	6.9	1 vs 3
Upper leg	9.7	7.5	13.5		3.7	2.5	5.4	
Lower leg	28.9	23.0	27.0	1 vs 2	5.3	3.6	2.7	1 vs 2

*We performed pairwise comparisons among the 3 groups, and report any results where Fisher's exact test $P \leq .017$ (for example, 1 vs 2 means the difference between group 1 [obese] and group 2 [nonobese] is statistically significant at alpha = .017 level).

more falls in the past year. Self-reported asthma, emphysema, and type 1 diabetes were all significantly more common in obese than nonobese women with incident fracture. At 2 years, 27% of obese women with incident fracture were receiving bone protective therapy, compared with 41% of nonobese and 57% of underweight women.

Conclusions.—Our results demonstrate that obesity is not protective against fracture in postmenopausal women and is associated with increased risk of ankle and upper leg fractures (Table 2).

▶ Low body weight is a known risk factor for fractures, particularly hip fractures. Obesity has been known to be protective against fractures. This protective effect is possibly mediated through a higher bone density in obese individuals and the padding effect of fat during falls. On the other hand, obese individuals have lower vitamin D levels, with a compensatory secondary hyperparathyroidism and its deleterious effect on bone, and they may be more prone to falls, increasing fracture risk.[1]

Because of the increasing prevalence of overweight and obesity in the population, it is important to redefine the risk of fractures in obese individuals. A meta-analysis that evaluated body mass index (BMI) as a risk factor for fractures showed a nonlinear relationship between fracture and BMI, with a marked increase in the risk of fractures from normal to low BMI, but just a modest decrease in risk from normal to high BMI.[2]

The Global Longitudinal Study of Osteoporosis in Women is a multinational, prospective, observational study in 10 countries that recruited more than 60 000 postmenopausal women. The present study evaluated the prevalence and incidence of clinical fractures (self-reported) in obese postmenopausal women. Data on BMI and fractures were available for 44 534 women, of which 23.4% were obese (BMI $\geq$ 30 kg/m^2). Obese women had a higher risk of incident ankle and upper leg fractures and a lower risk of wrist fractures. Underweight women had a higher relative and absolute risk of hip and pelvic fractures compared to normal weight and obese women (Table 2). The risk of spinal fractures in this study could not be accurately assessed since most of these fractures were not clinically apparent but were diagnosed by radiographic studies. Obese women who fractured had a higher incidence of asthma, emphysema, and type 1 diabetes, but comorbidities were self-reported.

Another important finding in this study is that obese women were less likely to be given antifracture therapy compared with normal weight and underweight women, meaning that fractures in this population were not perceived to be fragility fractures. Because obese women have higher BMI, they were not included in most studies for fracture prevention, and the effect of therapy in obese women still needs to be investigated. Nevertheless, because of the increasing prevalence of obesity and the additional comorbidities associated with fractures in this population, studies are needed to better understand risks and appropriate antifracture therapy for obese individuals.

R. N. Abramof, MD

References

1. Nielson CM, Srikanth P, Orwoll ES. Obesity and fracture in men and women: an epidemiologic perspective. *J Bone Miner Res.* 2012;27:1-10.
2. Johnell O, Kanis JA, Oden A, et al. Predictive value of BMD for hip and other fractures. *J Bone Miner Res.* 2005;20:1185-1194.

New Developments in Obesity

A PGC1—α—dependent myokine that drives brown—fat—like development of white fat and thermogenesis

Boström P, Wu J, Jedrychowski MP, et al (Dana-Farber Cancer Inst and Harvard Med School, Boston, MA; Harvard Med School, Boston, MA; et al)
Nature 481:463-468, 2012

Exercise benefits a variety of organ systems in mammals, and some of the best—recognized effects of exercise on muscle are mediated by the transcriptional co—activator PPAR—γ co—activator—1 α (PGC1—α). Here we show in mouse that PGC1—α expression in muscle stimulates an increase in expression of FNDC5, a membrane protein that is cleaved and secreted as a newly identified hormone, irisin. Irisin acts on white adipose cells in culture and *in vivo* to stimulate UCP1 expression and a broad program of brown—fat—like development. Irisin is induced with exercise in mice and humans, and mildly increased irisin levels in the blood cause an increase in energy expenditure in mice with no changes in movement or food intake. This results in improvements in obesity and glucose homeostasis. Irisin could be therapeutic for human metabolic disease and other disorders that are improved with exercise (Fig 6).

▶ Research investigating the potential to increase energy expenditure as a treatment modality for obesity has flourished in recent years. The identification of brown adipose tissue (BAT) in adults[1] has catalyzed this research, and particular attention has been invested in understanding its contribution to whole-body metabolism. Previous studies have found that PPAR-γ co-activator-1 α (PGC1-α) is a transcriptional coactivator that has a fundamental role in energy metabolism, including modulation of uncoupling protein 1 and BAT thermogenesis. Upregulation of PGC1-α in skeletal muscle of mice has been found to be protective against obesity and diabetes development,[2] suggesting that it may induce systemic effects on energy metabolism by regulating the secretion of factors from skeletal muscle. Identification of such mediators would make great advances in the treatment of obesity.

In a superbly conducted study, Bostrom and colleagues identified a novel blood-secreted hormone they coined *irisin*, a cleaved fragment of FNDC5 that is regulated by PGC1-α. Through a series of experiments utilizing cell culture and mouse models, this study demonstrates that irisin induces browning of white adipose tissue through upregulation of UCP-1 and Cidea mRNA expression (Fig 6). Moreover, mice fed a high-fat diet were protected against obesity and diabetes with exogenous administration of irisin (Fig 6). This study also

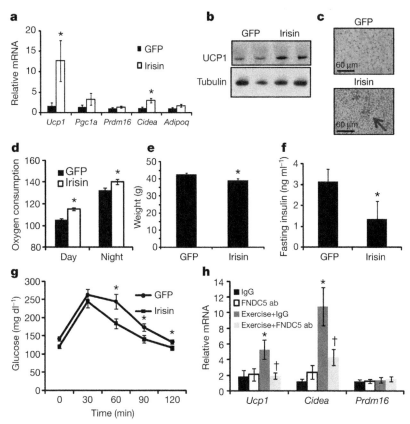

FIGURE 6.—Irisin induces browning of white adipose tissues *in vivo* and protects against diet-induced obesity and diabetes. a—c, Wild-type BALB/c mice were injected with 10^{10} GFP- or FNDC5-expressing adenoviral particles intravenously ($n = 7$ for each group). a, b, Animals were killed after 10 days and inguinal/subcutaneous fat pads were collected and analysed using qPCR analysis of indicated mRNAs (a) and western blot against UCP1 (b). c, Representative images from immunohistochemistry against UCP1 in these mice. All results in a—c were repeated two times with similar results. d—g, C57BL/6 mice fed a 60% kcal high-fat diet for 20 weeks were intravenously injected with GFP- or FNDC5-expressing adenovirus and all analyses were done 10 days thereafter ($n = 7$ for both groups). d, Oxygen consumption at day and night. e, Body weights of mice 10 days after injection with indicated adenovirus. f, Fasting plasma insulin measured using enzyme-linked immunosorbent assay (ELISA). g, Intraperitoneal glucose tolerance test. h, Mice were injected intraperitoneally with 50 μg of rabbit IgG or a rabbit anti-FNDC5 antibody (ab) and were either subjected to swimming for 7 days or kept sedentary ($n = 10$ for all groups). Data show mRNA expression levels from inguinal white adipose tissue. All data in d—j were performed at least twice in a separate mouse cohort with similar results. $\dagger P < 0.05$ compared to exercise and IgG. One-way ANOVA was used for statistics in h. All other statistics were performed using Student's *t*-test, and bar graphs are mean ± s.e.m. (Reprinted by permission from Macmillan Publishers Ltd: Nature. Boström P, Wu J, Jedrychowski MP, et al. A PGC1–α–dependent myokine that drives brown—fat—like development of white fat and thermogenesis. *Nature*. 2012;481:463-468, Copyright 2012.)

demonstrated that by blocking the actions of irisin, the benefits of exercise on browning BAT were not observed.

While this study offers novel insight into the potential therapeutic potential of irisin, the interpretation of the results is limited to mouse models, and caution must be taken when considering the potential application in humans. However, the authors did demonstrate that human and mouse irisin is identical and, thus, irisin likely has a highly conserved function in mammals. Therefore, it is plausible that irisin may have similar positive effects on energy expenditure in humans.

Boström et al have identified and characterized a novel polypeptide secreted by skeletal muscle that increases the thermogenic activity of adipose tissue and whole-body energy expenditure. Thus, irisin offers great potential as a therapeutic agent in the treatment of obesity. Future research should be directed at characterizing the function of irisin in humans to aid in the development of new pharmaceutical treatments of obesity.

M. Ruth, PhD

References

1. Cypess AM, Lehman S, Williams G, et al. Identification and importance of brown adipose tissue in adult humans. *N Engl J Med.* 2009;360:1509-1517.
2. Wenz T, Rossi SG, Rotundo RL, Spiegelman BM, Moraes CT. Increased muscle PGC-1alpha expression protects from sarcopenia and metabolic disease during aging. *Proc Natl Acad Sci U S A.* 2009;106:20405-20410.

Impact of weight change, secular trends and ageing on cardiovascular risk factors: 10-year experiences from the SOS study
Sjöström CD, Lystig T, Lindroos AK (Sahlgrenska Univ Hosp, Göteborg, Sweden)
Int J Obes 35:1413-1420, 2011

Objective.—Many short-term studies indicate that 5% weight loss in the obese is enough to induce significant improvements of cardiovascular risk factors. However, it is not known what degree of weight loss is required to improve risk factors over a more extended period of time or how ageing and secular trends *per se* are influencing risk factors during long-term follow-up.

Methods.—Patients examined after 10 years in the intervention study Swedish Obese Subjects were used for the current analysis. Surgically treated subjects ($n = 959$) and conventionally treated obese controls ($n = 842$) were pooled to obtain a study group with a large range of weight changes. The patients were divided in 11 groups based on the amount of weight change. Analysis of covariance was used to determine the necessary weight change over 10 years for a significant alteration of a risk factor. In a linear regression of risk factor change by weight change, the y intercept was interpreted as the effect of 10 years ageing and secular trends on a given risk factor in the absence of weight change.

Results.—The necessary weight loss for significant improvement of risk factors ranged from 10 to 44 kg. At zero weight change, 10 years of ageing was associated with significant increases in systolic blood pressure, pulse pressure, high-density lipoprotein cholesterol and glucose, and with significant decreases in diastolic blood pressure, total cholesterol, triglycerides and insulin.

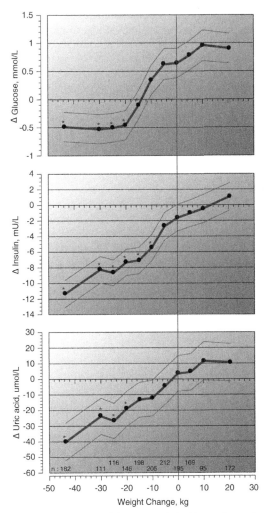

FIGURE 3.—Adjusted means (± 95% confidence interval) for 10-year changes in glucose, insulin and uric acid in 1801 obese patients. Study population divided into 11 delta weight classes. *Denotes a significant ($P < 0.05$) difference in the level of risk factor change as compared with reference (red vertical line). For interpretation of the references to color in this figure legend, the reader is referred to web version of this article. (Reprinted by permission from Macmillan Publishers Ltd: International Journal of Obesity. Sjöström CD, Lystig T, Lindroos AK. Impact of weight change, secular trends and ageing on cardiovascular risk factors: 10-year experiences from the SOS study. *Int J Obes.* 2011;35:1413-1420, Copyright 2011.)

Conclusions.—The necessary weight loss to maintain a favourable effect on risk factors in an obese population is larger than previously indicated by short-term studies. Treatment effects are influenced by non-weight change-dependant shifts in risk factor levels (Fig 3).

▶ Numerous previous studies have established that modest weight loss (∼5%) improves blood pressure, blood lipid profiles, and glucose metabolism and thus lowers the risk of developing cardiometabolic disease.[1,2] However, much of our current knowledge on the beneficial effects of weight loss is based on shorter-term follow-up periods (≤ 2 years), and few long-term studies have investigated the effects of modest body weight loss on risk factors for cardiometabolic disease. In order to establish treatment guidelines, it is critical to understand the degree of weight loss that will provide long-term benefit to obese patients for risk factors of cardiometabolic disease.

In the article under review, the authors challenge the notion that modest weight loss ($\sim 4\%$) appreciably improves long-term cardiovascular disease and type 2 diabetes risk factors in severely obese adults (body mass index [BMI] $> 34 \text{ kg/m}^2$). The current study examined a cohort of patients (n $= 1801$) from the Swedish Obesity Study (SOS) with at least 10 years of follow-up. The SOS is a large (N $= 4047$) prospective long-term intervention study that examined the effects of surgical versus conventional weight loss interventions on various outcomes. The authors demonstrated that 5 kg or 4% body weight reduction in severely obese adults did not affect systolic or diastolic blood pressure, blood glucose and insulin, uric acid, triglycerides, and total and high-density lipoprotein cholesterol over 10 years of follow-up. On the other hand, the authors noted that at least 10 to 45 kg, or 9% to 38%, weight loss was required to induce significant improvements in cardiometabolic risk factors after 10 years (Fig 3).

Some of the key limitations of this study include inclusion of both surgical and lifestyle weight loss subjects. It is widely accepted that surgical weight loss induces changes in physiology that are not observed when weight loss is achieved through nonsurgical methods. For example, gastric bypass surgery modifies the secretion of glucagon-like peptide-1 (GLP-1), a factor critical to glucose metabolism.[3] In addition, the cohort of subjects included in this study was limited to subjects with a BMI greater than 34 kg/m^2. As such, the findings of this study are not generalizable to individuals who are overweight or who have moderate obesity.

Overall, this study provides evidence that significant long-term benefit of weight loss on metabolic disease is only achieved with 10 kg ($> 9\%$) or greater weight loss. No long-term benefits were attributed to 5 kg of body weight loss ($\sim 4\%$), suggesting that individuals with severe to morbid obesity must achieve at least 10 kg or 9% body weight loss to have significant benefits on cardiometabolic risk factors 10 years after initial weight loss. Future studies should be directed at examining the long-term benefits of the degree of weight loss on cardiometabolic risk and disease outcome for overweight and obese populations in order to establish weight loss guidelines. This study challenges the current notion that modest weight loss can improve long-term cardiometabolic risk and suggests that weight loss expectations may need to be revised to ensure that more beneficial long-term outcomes are achieved.

M. Ruth, PhD

References

1. Goldstein DJ. Beneficial health effects of modest weight loss. *Int J Obes Relat Metab Disord.* 1992;16:397-415.
2. Blackburn G. Effect of degree of weight loss on health benefits. *Obes Res.* 1995;3: 211s-216s.

3. Pournaras DJ, Osborne A, Hawkins SC, et al. Remission of type 2 diabetes after gastric bypass and banding: mechanisms and 2 year outcomes. *Ann Surg.* 2010; 252:966-971.

Obesity is associated with hypothalamic injury in rodents and humans
Thaler JP, Yi C-X, Schur EA, et al (Univ of Washington, Seattle; Univ of Cincinnati, OH; et al)
J Clin Invest 122:153-162, 2012

Rodent models of obesity induced by consuming high-fat diet (HFD) are characterized by inflammation both in peripheral tissues and in hypothalamic areas critical for energy homeostasis. Here we report that unlike inflammation in peripheral tissues, which develops as a consequence of obesity, hypothalamic inflammatory signaling was evident in both rats and mice within 1 to 3 days of HFD onset, prior to substantial weight gain. Furthermore, both reactive gliosis and markers suggestive of neuron injury were evident in the hypothalamic arcuate nucleus of rats and mice within the first week of HFD feeding. Although these responses temporarily subsided, suggesting that neuroprotective mechanisms may initially limit the damage, with continued HFD feeding, inflammation and gliosis returned permanently to the mediobasal hypothalamus. Consistent with these data in rodents, we found evidence of increased gliosis in the mediobasal hypothalamus of obese humans, as assessed by MRI. These findings collectively suggest that, in both humans and rodent models, obesity is associated with neuronal injury in a brain area crucial for body weight control.

▶ Previous experimental evidence suggests that similar to systemic and tissue-specific inflammation, diet-induced rodent models of obesity also display inflammation of the hypothalamus. High-fat feeding in rodents induces an inflammatory response of the hypothalamus that results in increased food intake and weight gain.[1] As such, inflammatory damage to the central appetite and metabolic regulatory center appears to be an integral part of the pathogenesis of obesity; however, the underlying mechanisms have not been established, and little is known regarding this phenomenon in humans. Further understanding of this process would greatly benefit the advancement of obesity treatment.

Thaler et al present novel findings detailing the time course of hypothalamic inflammation during high-fat feeding in rodents. Intriguingly, hypothalamic inflammation was detected very early in the course of high-fat feeding (within 24 hours), much earlier than other key metabolic tissues, including skeletal muscle and adipose tissue. Patterns characteristic of neuronal injury, such as reactive gliosis, were apparent at early stages of high-fat feeding (Fig 3 in the original article). These findings show that the area of the brain vital to metabolic and appetite regulation is injured and inflamed in response to a high-fat diet, suggesting that early injury to the hypothalamus plays a pathogenic role in the development of diet-induced obesity. Their experiments were extensive and included measures of several markers of inflammation and brain injury at numerous time points during the progression of obesity. The thoroughness of their experimental design lends considerable weight to the interpretation of their findings and provides a strong foundation for implementing human studies.

The authors also reported that there was a positive correlation between body mass index and gliosis in a set of retrospectively analyzed magnetic resonance imaging patient scans. Although this is suggestive of a role for hypothalamic injury and inflammation in the pathogenesis of human obesity, we are limited in our interpretation of these findings due to the retrospective analyses and cannot infer causation. Future studies in controlled settings of overfeeding in carefully selected subjects should be conducted to better delineate hypothalamic injury and inflammation in human obesity.

Overall, Thaler et al present novel findings from a well-conducted rodent study demonstrating that inflammation and injury of the hypothalamus occur early in the course of obesity development. These findings are suggestive of an integral and potentially causal role of the hypothalamus in obesity development and present an area that clearly requires attention as we continue to devise treatment strategies for obesity.

M. R. Ruth, PhD

Reference

1. Lumeng CN, Saltiel AR. Inflammatory links between obesity and metabolic disease. *J Clin Invest.* 2011;121:2111-2117.

Pharmacological Treatment of Obesity

Two-year sustained weight loss and metabolic benefits with controlled-release Phentermine/Topiramate in obese and overweight adults (SEQUEL): a randomized, placebo-controlled, phase 3 extension study
Garvey WT, Ryan DH, Look M, et al (Univ of Alabama at Birmingham; Pennington Biomedical Res Ctr, Baton Rouge, LA; San Diego Sports Medicine, CA; et al)
Am J Clin Nutr 95:297-308, 2012

Background.—Obesity is a serious chronic disease. Controlled-release phentermine/topiramate (PHEN/TPM CR), as an adjunct to lifestyle modification, has previously shown significant weight loss compared with placebo in a 56-wk study in overweight and obese subjects with ≥2 weight-related comorbidities.

Objective.—This study evaluated the long-term efficacy and safety of PHEN/TPM CR in overweight and obese subjects with cardiometabolic disease.

Design.—This was a placebo-controlled, double-blind, 52-wk extension study; volunteers at selected sites continued with original randomly assigned treatment [placebo, 7.5 mg phentermine/46 mg controlled-release topiramate (7.5/46), or 15 mg phentermine/92 mg controlled-release topiramate (15/92)] to complete a total of 108 wk. All subjects participated in a lifestyle-modification program.

Results.—Of 866 eligible subjects, 676 (78%) elected to continue in the extension. Overall, 84.0% of subjects completed the study, with similar completion rates between treatment groups. At week 108, PHEN/TPM CR was associated with significant, sustained weight loss (intent-to-treat with last observation carried forward; $P < 0.0001$ compared with placebo); least-squares mean percentage changes from baseline in body weight were −1.8%, −9.3%, and −10.5% for placebo, 7.5/46, and 15/92, respectively. Significantly more PHEN/TPM CR—treated subjects at each dose achieved ≥5%, ≥10%, ≥15%, and ≥20% weight loss compared with placebo ($P < 0.001$). PHEN/TPM CR improved cardiovascular and metabolic variables and decreased rates of incident diabetes in comparison with placebo. PHEN/TPM CR was well tolerated over 108 wk, with reduced rates of adverse events occurring between weeks 56 and 108 compared with rates between weeks 0 and 56.

Conclusion.—PHEN/TPM CR in conjunction with lifestyle modification may provide a well-tolerated and effective option for the sustained treatment of obesity complicated by cardiometabolic disease. This trial was registered at clinicaltrials.gov as NCT00796367.

▶ The prevalence of obesity in the United States has reached 35% and is associated with multiple adverse effects, including hypertension, hyperlipidemia, and diabetes.[1] A modest weight reduction of only 10% leads to improvement in obesity related comorbidities; however, achieving and maintaining this degree of weight loss remains challenging. Currently, there are no definitive pharmacologic treatment options for obesity. Existing pharmacotherapy includes phentermine and orlistat. Phentermine, a sympathomimetic amine, achieves a weight loss of less than 10% and is only approved for short-term use. Orlistat, a gastric lipase inhibitor, shows a maximal weight loss of 7% and is often not tolerated because of its gastrointestinal side effects.[2] Thus, long-term, effective treatment options are needed to treat obesity.

The SEQUEL trial was a 2-year study that evaluated the efficacy and safety of a novel combination drug that combines phentermine plus topiramate for the treatment of obesity. Phentermine is a sympathomimetic amine that suppresses appetite and has been approved for short-term treatment of obesity (< 3 months). Topiramate was initially marketed as an anti-epileptic drug and was later approved for the prophylaxis of migraine headaches. In clinical trials, subjects using topiramate were noted to have dose-related weight loss. Subsequently, clinical trials evaluated topiramate for weight loss confirmed this effect. The rationale for combining topiramate with phentermine is 2-fold. First, the combination targets more than 1 pathway to satiety in the hopes of maximizing the weight loss effect. Second, lower doses of each drug are used to minimize the potential adverse effects.[3]

Initial data on the combination of phentermine plus topiramate was published in the CONQUER trial, which was a 52-week double-blind randomized controlled trial that assigned 2487 obese subjects with a body mass index of 27 to 45 kg/m^2 and 2 or more weight-related comorbidities to receive placebo, mid-dose (phentermine 7.5 mg plus topiramate 46 mg), or full-dose (phentermine 15 mg plus topiramate 92 mg) treatment for 52 weeks. Mean weight loss at 1 year was 7.8%, 9.8%, and 1.2% for mid-dose, full-dose, and placebo, respectively.[4] The SEQUEL trial was a 52-week extension of the CONQUER trial, with 78% of subjects electing to continue in the extension. Results from the SEQUEL show sustained weight loss at 2 years, with mean weight loss of 9.3%, 10.5%, and 1.8% for mid-dose, full-dose, and placebo, respectively. In addition to weight loss, treatment showed significant improvement in weight related comorbidities, including lower fasting glucose and insulin values (compared with placebo) and improvement in both systolic and diastolic blood pressure as well as lipid parameters. Side effects of treatment include paresthesia, dry mouth, constipation, and headache. Serious adverse events were rare and occurred at similar rates for treatment versus placebo groups.

The SEQUEL trial demonstrates the effectiveness of long-term treatment with the novel combination of phentermine and topiramate. The magnitude of weight loss achieved may have a meaningful impact on treating or preventing obesity-related comorbidities. Although longer-term studies are needed to fully elucidate potential risks, this unique combination treatment may fill the current void in the pharmacologic treatment of obesity.

A. Powell, MD

References

1. Flegal KM, Carroll MD, Kit BK, Ogden CL. Prevalence of obesity and trends in the distribution of body mass index among US adults, 1999-2010. *JAMA.* 2012; 307:491-497.
2. Foxcroft DR, Milne R. Orlistat for the treatment of obesity: rapid review and cost-effectiveness model. *Obes Rev.* 2000;1:121-126.
3. Bray GA, Hollander P, Klein S, et al. A 6-month randomized, placebo-controlled, dose-ranging trial of topiramate for weight loss in obesity. *Obes Res.* 2003;11: 722-733.
4. Gadde KM, Allison DB, Ryan DH, et al. Effects of low-dose, controlled-release, phentermine plus topiramate combination on weight and associated comorbidities in overweight and obese adults (CONQUER): a randomized, placebo-controlled, phase 3 trial. *Lancet.* 2011;377:1341-1352.

Surgical Treatment of Obesity

Bariatric Surgery versus Intensive Medical Therapy in Obese Patients with Diabetes
Schauer PR, Kashyap SR, Wolski K, et al (Cleveland Clinic, OH; et al)
N Engl J Med 366:1567-1576, 2012

Background.—Observational studies have shown improvement in patients with type 2 diabetes mellitus after bariatric surgery.

Methods.—In this randomized, nonblinded, single-center trial, we evaluated the efficacy of intensive medical therapy alone versus medical therapy plus Roux-en-Y gastric bypass or sleeve gastrectomy in 150 obese patients with uncontrolled type 2 diabetes. The mean (±SD) age of the patients was 49 ± 8 years, and 66% were women. The average glycated hemoglobin level was $9.2 \pm 1.5\%$. The primary end point was the proportion of patients with a glycated hemoglobin level of 6.0% or less 12 months after treatment.

Results.—Of the 150 patients, 93% completed 12 months of follow-up. The proportion of patients with the primary end point was 12% (5 of 41 patients) in the medical therapy group versus 42% (21 of 50 patients) in the gastric-bypass group ($P = 0.002$) and 37% (18 of 49 patients) in the sleeve-gastrectomy group ($P = 0.008$). Glycemic control improved in all three groups, with a mean glycated hemoglobin level of $7.5 \pm 1.8\%$ in the medical-therapy group, $6.4 \pm 0.9\%$ in the gastric-bypass group ($P<0.001$), and $6.6 \pm 1.0\%$ in the sleeve-gastrectomy group ($P = 0.003$). Weight loss was greater in the gastric-bypass group and sleeve-gastrectomy group (-29.4 ± 9.0 kg and -25.1 ± 8.5 kg, respectively) than in the medical-therapy group (-5.4 ± 8.0 kg) ($P<0.001$ for both comparisons). The use of drugs to lower glucose, lipid, and blood-pressure levels decreased significantly after both surgical procedures but increased in patients receiving medical therapy only. The index for homeostasis model assessment of insulin resistance (HOMA-IR) improved significantly after bariatric surgery. Four patients underwent reoperation. There were no deaths or life-threatening complications.

Conclusions.—In obese patients with uncontrolled type 2 diabetes, 12 months of medical therapy plus bariatric surgery achieved glycemic control in significantly more patients than medical therapy alone. Further study will be necessary to assess the durability of these results. (Funded by Ethicon Endo-Surgery and others; ClinicalTrials.gov number, NCT00432809.)

▶ The prevalence of type 2 diabetes mellitus (type 2 DM) has been increasing rapidly during the last 3 decades due to the increasing prevalence of obesity. More than 30% of the US population is obese with a body mass index (BMI) ≥ 30 kg/m^2. Currently, bariatric surgery is the most efficacious treatment yielding substantial and sustained weight loss. A recent meta-analysis by Buchwald et al, in which patients had a mean BMI of 47.9 kg/m^2, mean weight loss was 38.5 kg or 55.9% of excess body weight with 78% of the patients having complete resolution of diabetes and 86.6% having resolution or improvement in control of type 2 diabetes. Diabetes resolution and weight loss were greater for patients undergoing biliopancreatic diversion/duodenal switch, followed by gastric bypass and less in patients having banding procedures.[1]

There is an increasing interest in the effect of bariatric surgery in improving or even curing type 2 DM. Bariatric surgery is also referred to as *metabolic surgery*, with a trend in performing this surgery in diabetic patients with lower BMIs.

Recently, 2 prospective studies evaluating the effect of bariatric surgery versus intensive lifestyle changes in the control and resolution of type 2 diabetes were published.

The first study, by Schauer et al, included 150 patients with uncontrolled diabetes with a BMI range of 27 to 40 kg/m^2. The patients were randomly assigned to medical therapy, Roux-en-Y gastric bypass, or sleeve gastrectomy. The primary endpoint of the study was glycemic control at 1 year (proportion of patients achieving an A1c of 6% or less with or without diabetic medications); secondary endpoints included other parameters associated with cardiovascular risk factors, weight loss, and changes in medications. At the end of the first year, substantially more patients who had bariatric surgery had an A1c of 6% or less, had a greater decrease in A1c, and were taking fewer medications for glucose control (Fig 1 in the original article). Patients on the gastric bypass group who achieved an A1c of 6% or less did so without the need for medications, while 28% of the sleeve gastrectomy patients still required diabetic medications. There was no mortality during the study, with 4 patients requiring reoperation during this year.

It is known that longstanding diabetes and need for multiple glucose-lowering therapies, including insulin, will lower the rate of remission of type 2 diabetes after bariatric surgery. In this study, the mean duration of diabetes was 8 years, with an average use of 3 glucose-lowering medications and a high use of insulin therapy (44%). The strength of the study is the randomization of the patients with uncontrolled, longstanding diabetes to 3 treatment arms and the evaluation of 2 bariatric surgery techniques: gastric bypass and sleeve gastrectomy. The outcome between the 2 bariatric arms did not differ significantly concerning glucose control, although the study was not powered to compare between the 2 bariatric arms.

The improvement in glucose control was observed already 3 months after surgery, as has been reported in a previous study, probably due to changes in gut hormones in addition to weight loss.

As mentioned by the authors, the limitation of the study is that it was conducted in a bariatric surgery center in highly selected patients with a relatively low incidence of complications and, therefore, it is not clear if these results can be generalized. The long-term durability of the glycemic effect of surgery will be evaluated in a follow-up study. It is worth mentioning that aiming for normoglycemia (A1c < 6%) in high-risk patients with the use of hypoglycemic medications cannot be advocated after the results of the Action to Control Cardiovascular Risk in Diabetes study in which patients in the intensive therapy had a greater mortality risk, possibly due to hypoglycemia.[2]

We are just starting the era of metabolic surgery. Further studies should address the long-term effect of surgery in controlling or curing type 2 diabetes and specific patient characteristics for the choice of the right candidate for the appropriate surgical procedure.

R. N. Abramof, MD

References

1. Buchwald H, Estok R, Fahrbach K, et al. Weight and type 2 diabetes after bariatric surgery: systematic review and meta-analysis. *Am J Med.* 2009;122:248-256.e5.
2. Action to Control Cardiovascular Risk in Diabetes Study Group, Gerstein HC, Miller ME, Byington RP, et al. Effects of intensive glucose lowering in type 2 diabetes. *N Engl J Med.* 2008;358:2545-2559.

Bariatric Surgery versus Conventional Medical Therapy for Type 2 Diabetes
Mingrone G, Panunzi S, De Gaetano A, et al (Università Cattolica S. Cuore, Rome, Italy; Inst of Systems Analysis and Computer Science (IASI), Rome, Italy; et al)
N Engl J Med 366:1577-1585, 2012

Background.—Roux-en-Y gastric bypass and biliopancreatic diversion can markedly ameliorate diabetes in morbidly obese patients, often resulting in disease remission. Prospective, randomized trials comparing these procedures with medical therapy for the treatment of diabetes are needed.

Methods.—In this single-center, nonblinded, randomized, controlled trial, 60 patients between the ages of 30 and 60 years with a body-mass index (BMI, the weight in kilograms divided by the square of the height in meters) of 35 or more, a history of at least 5 years of diabetes, and a glycated hemoglobin level of 7.0% or more were randomly assigned to receive conventional medical therapy or undergo either gastric bypass or biliopancreatic diversion. The primary end point was the rate of diabetes remission at 2 years (defined as a fasting glucose level of <100 mg per deciliter [5.6 mmol per liter] and a glycated hemoglobin level of <6.5% in the absence of pharmacologic therapy).

Results.—At 2 years, diabetes remission had occurred in no patients in the medical-therapy group versus 75% in the gastric-bypass group and 95% in the biliopancreatic-diversion group ($P<0.001$ for both comparisons). Age, sex, baseline BMI, duration of diabetes, and weight changes were not significant predictors of diabetes remission at 2 years or of improvement in glycemia at 1 and 3 months. At 2 years, the average baseline glycated hemoglobin level ($8.65 \pm 1.45\%$) had decreased in all groups, but patients in the two surgical groups had the greatest degree of improvement (average glycated hemoglobin levels, $7.69 \pm 0.57\%$ in the medical-therapy group, $6.35 \pm 1.42\%$ in the gastric-bypass group, and $4.95 \pm 0.49\%$ in the biliopancreatic-diversion group).

Conclusions.—In severely obese patients with type 2 diabetes, bariatric surgery resulted in better glucose control than did medical therapy. Preoperative BMI and weight loss did not predict the improvement in hyperglycemia after these procedures. (Funded by Catholic University of Rome; ClinicalTrials.gov number, NCT00888836.)

▶ Obesity is a known risk factor for many comorbidities including type 2 diabetes mellitus (type 2 DM), cardiovascular disease, and hypertension. A weight loss of 5% to 10% of initial body weight was shown to improve risk factors including glucose control. Bariatric surgery is one of the most effective procedures to promote substantial and sustained weight loss. Bariatric surgery also markedly improves diabetes control or even may promote remission of diabetes.[1] The effect of bariatric surgery on diabetes depends on several factors including the duration of diabetes, need for multiple medications, and type of bariatric surgery. Remission from diabetes is greatest with the biliopancreatic surgery followed by Roux-en-Y bypass surgery, with the restrictive procedures (gastric banding) reporting lower rates of remission of type 2 DM and of weight loss. It is clear that weight loss alone is not the only factor affecting glucose control. Incretins are hormones that augment insulin postprandial insulin response and reduce appetite, among other metabolic effects. Glucagonlike peptide 1 (GLP-1) is secreted by the distal ileum in response to nutrients. One of the mechanisms by which there is an immediate improvement in glucose control following Roux-en-Y gastric bypass is an increase in GLP-1 concentrations. The change in gut-derived hormones is eminent following bypass surgeries such as the Roux-en-Y procedure and biliopancreatic diversion but not on the restrictive procedures such as gastric banding or sleeve gastrectomy.[2]

In the study by Mingrone, 60 obese patients (with a body mass index [BMI] $\geq$ 35 kg/m^2) with type 2 DM for at least 5 years, and an A1C of $\geq$ 7% were randomly assigned to conventional medical therapy or to either gastric bypass surgery or biliopancreatic diversion. The primary endpoint was remission of type 2 DM at 2 years defined as a fasting glucose of less than 100 mg/dL or a glycated hemoglobin level of less than 6.5% without hypoglycemic therapy. At the end of 2 years, 75% of patients who had the bypass surgery and 95% of the patients who had biliopancreatic diversion reached the primary endpoint and were on remission from diabetes, whereas none of the patients on the conventional therapy was on remission. Interestingly, age, sex, baseline BMI or duration of diabetes or weight change did not predict the change in glucose at 1 and 3 months or remission of type 2 DM. It is important to emphasize that the rate of weight loss did not correlate with remission of type 2 DM, possibly because of additional factors known to improve glucose homeostasis. In this study, the effect of the biliopancreatic diversion surgery was similar to the Roux-en-Y bypass surgery, unlike reports of superior metabolic effect with the biliopancreatic surgery.

This study was not powered to evaluate cardiovascular disease outcome or the long-term effects of surgery, such as nutritional and metabolic complications such as bone loss. This study was done in a single center by experienced surgeons with a relatively low rate of complications; therefore, it will be difficult to replicate in worldwide practices. Furthermore, diabetes is known to be a progressive disease, and the long-term efficacy of bariatric surgery in promoting remission of type 2 DM still needs to be assessed. Nevertheless, this study confirms the superiority of malabsorptive bariatric surgery in improving glucose control and inducing remission of type 2 DM. Surgery may be appropriate for obese patients with type 2 DM not controlled by medical therapy alone.

R. Ness-Abramof, MD

References

1. Meijer RI, van Wagensweld BA, Siegert CE, Eringa EC, Serné EH, Smulders YM. Bariatric surgery as a novel treatment for type 2 diabetes mellitus: a systematic review. *Arch Surg.* 2011;146:744-750.
2. Schernthaner G, Brix JM, Kopp HP, Scherthaner GH. Cure of type 2 diabetes by metabolic surgery? A critical analysis of the evidence in 2010. *Diabetes Care.* 2011;34:S355-S360.

4 Thyroid

Introduction

I have selected many different studies for the 2012 YEAR BOOK. These papers have an important impact for the practice in Endocrinology. I would like to introduce two of them:

In 2011 Marcocci et al published a work in the *New England Journal of Medicine*. The authors performed a randomized, double-blind, placebo-controlled trial to determine the effect of selenium (an antioxidant agent). Altogether, 159 patients with mild Graves' orbitopathy were enrolled. The patients were given sodium selenite (100 μg twice daily), or placebo (twice daily) orally for 6 months and were then followed for 6 months after treatment was withdrawn. At the 6-month evaluation, treatment with selenium was associated with an improved quality of life and less eye involvement and slowed the progression of Graves' orbitopathy, as compared with placebo. The Clinical Activity Score (CAS) decreased in all groups, but the change was significantly greater in the selenium-treated patients. This prospective trial showed for the first time that selenium has a positive effect of the outcome of mild GO. These data have a direct clinical consequence for many patients with active GO.[1]

Another important publication was that of Wells and coworkers investigating the role of vandetanib for the treatment of metastasized medullary thyroid cancer (MTC). Vandetanib is a once-daily oral agent that selectively targets RET, VEGFR, and EGFR signaling. The aim of this study was to investigate the effectiveness of vandetanib in an international, randomized, placebo-controlled, double-blind, phase III trial (ZETA) to evaluate vandetanib 300 mg/d in patients with locally advanced or metastatic MTC. Between December 2006 and November 2007, 331 patients were randomly assigned to receive vandetanib or placebo. Of those patients, 37% had progressed and 15% had died. The study met its primary objective of PFS prolongation with vandetanib versus placebo. Statistically significant advantages for vandetanib were also seen for objective response rate, disease control rate, and biochemical response. The benefit that was demonstrated in PFS for patients receiving vandetanib compared with placebo was observed in patients with the hereditary or the sporadic form of MTC. Because of the small number of patients with sporadic MTC who were *RET* negative and the large number of patients who were *RET* unknown, the subgroup analyses of PFS and objective response rate by *RET* mutation status are inconclusive. Nonetheless, vandetanib is a promising agent for the treatment of patients with progressive MTC.[2]

These are just a two examples of brilliant studies published in 2011. I hope you enjoy reading these and the other articles.

Matthias Schott, MD, PhD

References

1. Marcocci C, Kahaly GJ, Krassas GE, et al. Selenium and the course of mild Graves' orbitopathy. *N Engl J Med.* 2011;364:1920-1931.
2. Wells SA Jr, Robinson BG, Gagel RF, et al. Vandetanib in patients with locally advanced or metastatic medullary thyroid cancer: a randomized, double-blind phase III trial. *J Clin Oncol.* 2012;30:134-141.

Autoimmunity

Selenium and the Course of Mild Graves' Orbitopathy

Marcocci C, for the European Group on Graves' Orbitopathy (Univ of Pisa, Italy; et al)

N Engl J Med 364:1920-1931, 2011

Background.—Oxygen free radicals and cytokines play a pathogenic role in Graves' orbitopathy.

Methods.—We carried out a randomized, double-blind, placebo-controlled trial to determine the effect of selenium (an antioxidant agent) or pentoxifylline (an antiinflammatory agent) in 159 patients with mild Graves' orbitopathy. The patients were given sodium selenite (100 μg twice daily), pentoxifylline (600 mg twice daily), or placebo (twice daily) orally for 6 months and were then followed for 6 months after treatment was withdrawn. Primary outcomes at 6 months were evaluated by means of an overall ophthalmic assessment, conducted by an ophthalmologist who was unaware of the treatment assignments, and a Graves' orbitopathy–specific quality-of-life questionnaire, completed by the patient. Secondary outcomes were evaluated with the use of a Clinical Activity Score and a diplopia score.

Results.—At the 6-month evaluation, treatment with selenium, but not with pentoxifylline, was associated with an improved quality of life ($P<0.001$) and less eye involvement ($P = 0.01$) and slowed the progression of Graves' orbitopathy ($P = 0.01$), as compared with placebo. The Clinical Activity Score decreased in all groups, but the change was significantly greater in the selenium-treated patients. Exploratory evaluations at 12 months confirmed the results seen at 6 months. Two patients assigned to placebo and one assigned to pentoxifylline required immunosuppressive therapy for deterioration in their condition. No adverse events were evident with selenium, whereas pentoxifylline was associated with frequent gastrointestinal problems.

Conclusions.—Selenium administration significantly improved quality of life, reduced ocular involvement, and slowed progression of the disease in patients with mild Graves' orbitopathy. (Funded by the University of

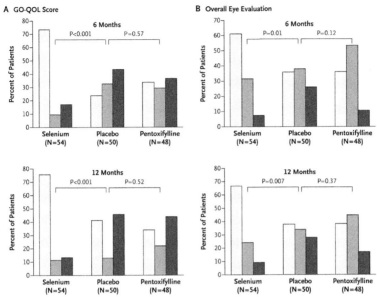

FIGURE 2.—Primary End Points. Panel A shows the changes reflected in the score on the Graves' orbitopathy—specific quality-of-life questionnaire (GO-QOL) at 6 months and 12 months. This questionnaire measures limitations in visual functioning (as a consequence of diplopia, decreased visual acuity, or both) and in psychosocial functioning (as a consequence of a changed appearance). Panel B shows the changes at 6 months and 12 months in overall results of the eye evaluation performed by an ophthalmologist who was unaware of the treatment assignments. The quality of life and overall eye evaluations were considered to be improved, unchanged, or worsened according to predefined criteria. Differences in proportions were tested with the use of the contingency 3×2 chi-square test. (Reprinted from Marcocci C, for the European Group on Graves' Orbitopathy, Selenium and the course of mild graves' orbitopathy. *N Engl J Med.* 2011;364:1920-1931. Copyright 2011, Massachusetts Medical Society. All rights reserved.)

Pisa and the Italian Ministry for Education, University and Research; EUGOGO Netherlands Trial Register number, NTR524) (Fig 2).

▶ Approximately half the patients with Graves disease have ocular involvement (Graves orbitopathy [GO]). Moderately severe and active forms of GO can be effectively treated with glucocorticoids, orbital irradiation, or both, whereas milder forms may improve spontaneously and generally require only local measures to control symptoms. The aim of the present study was to investigate the role of selenium for the treatment of GO. Selenium is a trace mineral and an essential nutrient for selenocysteine synthesis. Selenocysteine is incorporated into several selenoproteins, mostly enzymes, in which selenium acts as a reduction-oxidation center and functions as an antioxidant. A number of in vitro studies have suggested that increased generation of oxygen free radicals plays a pathogenic role in GO. Selenium also has an important effect on the immune system and might be beneficial in patients with Hashimoto thyroiditis or Graves disease.

The authors performed a randomized, double-blind, placebo-controlled trial to determine the effect of selenium (an antioxidant agent). In comparison, pentoxifylline (an anti-inflammatory agent) was also investigated. Altogether, 159 patients with mild GO were enrolled. The patients were given sodium selenite (100 µg twice daily), pentoxifylline (600 mg twice daily), or placebo (twice daily) orally for 6 months and were then followed up for 6 months after treatment was withdrawn. At the 6-month evaluation, treatment with selenium, but not with pentoxifylline, was associated with an improved quality of life ($P < .001$) and less eye involvement ($P = .01$) and slowed the progression of GO ($P = .01$), as compared with placebo (Fig 2). The Clinical Activity Score (CAS) decreased in all groups, but the change was significantly greater in the selenium-treated patients. Exploratory evaluations at 12 months confirmed the results seen at 6 months. No adverse events were evident with selenium, whereas pentoxifylline was associated with frequent gastrointestinal problems.

This prospective trial showed for the first time that selenium has a positive effect of the outcome of mild GO. Positive effects were also seen for the quality of life. It has to be mentioned that an improvement of the CAS was also seen in the placebo group as well as in the pentoxifylline group. However, this study has 2 major limitations: (1) the authors did not quantify the serum selenium levels and (2) patients living in selenium-deficient areas were enrolled. This may also explain the positive effect of a selenium treatment.

M. Schott, MD, PhD

Evidence of a Combined Cytotoxic Thyroglobulin and Thyroperoxidase Epitope-Specific Cellular Immunity in Hashimoto's Thyroiditis

Ehlers M, Thiel A, Bernecker C, et al (Univ Hosp Duesseldorf, Germany)
J Clin Endocrinol Metab 2012 [Epub ahead of print]

Context.—Hashimoto's thyroiditis (HT) is a common autoimmune disease leading to thyroid destruction due to lymphocytic infiltration. Only rare data are available regarding the recognition of specific cellular antigens, *e.g.* of thyroperoxidase (TPO) and thyroglobulin (Tg).

Objective.—The aim of this study was to quantify and characterize TPO- and Tg-epitope-specific CD8-positive T cells of HT patients.

Design.—Six different human leukocyte antigen (HLA)-A2 restricted, TPO- or Tg-specific tetramers were synthesized and used for measuring CD8-positive T cells in HT patients and controls.

Results.—The frequency of peripheral TPO- and Tg-specific CD8-positive T cells was significantly higher in HLA-A2-positive HT patients (2.8 ± 9.5%) compared with HLA-A2-negative HT patients (0.5 ± 0.7%), HLA-A2-positive nonautoimmune goiter patients (0.2 ± 0.4%), and HLA-A2-positive healthy controls (0.1 ± 0.2%). The frequency of Tg-specific T cells (3.0%) was very similar to those of TPO-specific CD8-positive T cells (2.9%). Subgroup analyses revealed a steady increase of the number of epitope-specific CD8-positive T cells from 0.6 ± 1.0% at initial diagnosis up to 9.4 ± 18.3% in patients with long-lasting disease. Analyses of the number of thyroid-infiltrating cells as well as the cytotoxic capacity revealed a similar picture for TPO- and Tg-specific T cells.

Conclusion.—We here report for the first time that both antigens, TPO and Tg, are recognized by CD8-positive T cells and are involved in the thyroid destruction process leading to clinical disease manifestation.

▶ Hashimoto's thyroiditis (HT) is among the most common human autoimmune diseases. HT is characterized by infiltration of the thyroid gland by autoreactive T and B cells causing thyroid cell death and production of anti—thyroid peroxidase (anti-TPO) and antithyroglobulin (anti-Tg) antibodies. It is still under major debate whether TPO or Tg (or possibly another antigen) represents the major target of the cellular immune process. The aim of this study was to quantify and characterize TPO- and Tg-epitope-specific CD8-positive T cells of HT patients. In this study, the authors found that the frequency of Tg-specific T cells (3.0%) was very similar to those of TPO-specific CD8-positive T cells (2.9%) (Fig 1 in the original article). Importantly, subgroup analyses found a steady increase of the number of epitope-specific CD8-positive T cells from 0.61% ± 1.01% at initial diagnosis up to 9.43% ± 18.27% in patients with long-lasting disease (Fig 2 in the original article). Analyses of the number of thyroid infiltrating cells as well as the cytotoxic capacity showed a similar picture for TPO- and Tg-specific T cells. This is crucial, as the opposite development of antigen-specific cell numbers was thought to be correct. In addition, this study shows a clear correlation between epitope-specific thyroid-infiltrating T cells and the magnitude of hypothyroidism.

Remarkably, the Tg-specific T cells were clearly elevated in the peripheral blood at the time of clinical disease manifestation whereas a reverse distribution was observed in the thyroid aspirates. This phenomenon may suggest an ostensible role for Tg-specific T cells at disease initiation, besides an incremental role for the TPO-specific T cells during disease progress due to epitope-spreading. These data, therefore, support the idea of a combined TPO- and Tg-specific cytotoxic immune response in HT patients. Irrespectively, the authors are still unable to definitely answer the question, which of both antigens is initially recognized by the immune system, including the possibility of a different—antigen recognized by T cells resulting in an antigen spreading? Nonetheless, this study gives a more precise insight into the pathophysiology of HT.

T. Baehring, PhD

A prospective study of lymphocyte subpopulations and regulatory T cells in patients with chronic hepatitis C virus infection developing interferon-induced thyroiditis
Soldevila B, Alonso N, Martínez-Arconada MJ, et al (Universitat Autónoma de Barcelona, Badalona, Spain; Hospital Universitari Germans Trias i Pujol, Badalona, Spain)
Clin Endocrinol 75:535-543, 2011

Objective.—One of the side effects of interferon-alpha (IFN-α) therapy is interferon-induced thyroiditis (IIT). The role of lymphocyte subpopulations in IIT remains to be defined. The aim of this study was to assess different peripheral blood lymphocyte subpopulations, mainly CD4$^+$CD25 $^+$CD127low/-FoxP3$^+$ regulatory T cells (Tregs), in patients with chronic hepatitis C virus (HCV) infection who developed IIT.

Design, Patients and Methods.—From 120 patients with chronic HCV who started antiviral treatment, those who developed IIT (IIT patients) were selected and compared with patients who did not develop IIT (Co-HCV). Peripheral blood mononuclear cells were obtained before treatment (BT), mid-treatment (MT), end of treatment (ET), 24 weeks post-treatment (PT) and at appearance of IIT (TT).

Results.—Eleven patients developed IIT: three Hashimoto's thyroiditis, one Graves'disease, one positive antithyroidal antibodies, one nonautoimmune hypothyroidism and five destructive thyroiditis. During antiviral treatment, an increase in CD8$^+$ and in Tregs was observed in both groups. A decrease in CD3$^+$, CD19$^+$ and NKT lymphocyte subpopulations was also observed (all $P < 0.05$). However, no changes were observed in the percentage of CD4$^+$, CD3$^+\gamma\delta^+$ and iNKT lymphocytes, Th1/Th2 balance and Bcl2 expression on B cells when BT was compared with ET. At the appearance of IIT (TT), IIT patients had a higher Th1 response (CCR5$^+$CCR7$^-$) ($P < 0.01$) and a higher Tregs percentage ($P < 0.05$) than Co-HCV.

Conclusions.—Our results point to the immunomodulatory effects of IFN-α on different lymphocyte subpopulations and a possible role of Th1 response and Tregs in patients with HCV who developed IIT.

▶ The standard therapy for chronic hepatitis C virus (HCV) infection currently consists of pegylated interferon-alfa (pegIFN-a) and ribavirin (RBV). Several studies have demonstrated a high incidence of thyroid disease, a frequent side effect of interferon-alfa, occurring in up to 40% of patients during treatment. With the exception of direct toxic effects on the thyroid combined with genetic predisposition, interferon-alfa-induced pathophysiological mechanisms that lead to thyroiditis have not been well defined. Since interferon-alfa has been linked to a T-helper-1 shift, in addition to induction of enhanced activity of different immune cells, the authors intended to investigate peripheral blood lymphocyte subpopulations in affected patients, thereby particularly focusing on regulatory T cells, which are phenotypically characterized by CD4$^+$CD25$^+$CD127 low-FoxP3$^+$ and play a fundamental role in the maintenance of self-tolerance. A total of 120 patients with HCV received antiviral treatment and 11 developed interferon-induced thyroiditis. Hashimoto thyroiditis, Graves disease, and destructive thyroiditis were represented by the affected population. No correlation was found between thyroiditis and the duration of treatment, nor between thyroiditis and the response to antiviral treatment. The authors observed a significant difference concerning the dynamics of different lymphocyte populations when comparing HCV patients without treatment with those who received antiviral treatment. There were no significant differences in the patient population suffering from thyroiditis. However, at the appearance of interferon-induced thyroiditis, patients showed an elevated Th1 response and interestingly an increased amount of regulatory T cells when compared to the control group. At first sight, these findings seem paradoxical; however, an increased regulatory T cell population has been previously observed in autoimmune thyroiditis[1] and could be attributed to a malfunction in this population. Consequently, further studies are needed to analyze the functional capacity of regulatory T cells in HCV patients who suffer from interferon-alfa—induced thyroiditis. Until malfunction can be ruled out, it must be concluded that an increase of regulatory T cells cannot predict the onset of thyroiditis. It would be reasonable to unravel the pathophysiological mechanisms in order to develop immune therapies that prevent the onset of thyroiditis under antiviral therapy. This article also provides interesting documentation concerning the immunological monitoring of HCV patients under antiviral treatment.

M. Schott, MD, PhD

A. Thiel, MD

Reference

1. Marazuela M, García-López MA, Figueroa-Vega N, et al. Regulatory T cells in human autoimmune thyroid disease. *J Clin Endocrinol Metab*. 2006;91:3639-3646.

Induction of Autoimmune Thyroiditis by Depletion of CD4+CD25+ Regulatory T cells in Thyroiditis-Resistant IL-17, But Not Interferon-γ Receptor, Knockout Nonobese Diabetic-H2h4 Mice

Horie I, Abiru N, Sakamoto H, et al (Nagasaki Univ Graduate School of Biomedical Sciences, Japan; et al)
Endocrinology 152:4448-4454, 2011

Iodine-induced experimental autoimmune thyroiditis in the nonobese diabetic (NOD)-H2h4 mouse is a prototype of animal models of Hashimoto's thyroiditis in humans. Recent studies have shown the resistance to thyroiditis of NOD-H2h4 mice genetically deficient for either IL-17 or interferon (IFN)-γ, implicating both of T helper type 1 (Th1) and Th17 immune responses in disease pathogenesis. However, we hypothesized that robust induction of a single arm of effector T cells (either Th1 or Th17) might be sufficient for inducing thyroiditis in NOD-H2h4 mice. To address this hypothesis, enhanced immune responses consisting of either Th1 or Th17 were induced by anti-CD25 antibody-mediated depletion of regulatory T cells (Treg) in thyroiditis-resistant IL-17 knockout (KO) or IFN-γ receptor (IFN-γR) KO, respectively, NOD-H2h4 mice. Depletion of Treg in IL-17 KO mice (*i.e.* Th1 enhancement) elicited antithyroglobulin autoantibodies and thyroiditis. Immunohistochemical analysis of the thyroid glands revealed the similar intrathyroidal lymphocyte infiltration patterns, with CD4+T and CD19+ B cells being dominant between the wild-type and Treg-depleted IL-17 KO mice. In contrast, Treg-depleted IFN-γR KO mice remained thyroiditis resistant. Intracellular cytokine staining assays showed differentiation of Th1 cells in IL-17 KO mice but not of Th17 cells in IFN-γR KO mice. Our findings demonstrate that a robust Th1 immune response can by itself induce thyroiditis in otherwise thyroiditis-resistant IL-17 KO mice.

Thus, unlike Th17 cells in IFN-γR KO mice, Th1 cells enhanced by Treg depletion can be sustained and induce thyroiditis.

▶ Mimicking human Hashimoto thyroiditis, nonobese diabetic H2^{h4} mice develop anti-Tg autoantibodies and intrathyroidal lymphocyte infiltration when given iodine in their drinking water. The cellular pathomechanisms—T helper type 1 and T helper type (Th) 17—have been shown to play a crucial role in the initiation of autoimmune thyroiditis in knockout models, as knocking out 1 of each effector T cell subgroup resulted in a resistance toward developing thyroiditis.[1,2] However, considering a variety of other autoimmune diseases, Th1 and Th17 partly exhibited converse influences on the development and course of disease in vivo. Furthermore, although protective effects were shown either for Th1 or Th17 in different autoimmune diseases in vivo, a variety of antigen-specific effector T cells induced artificially in vitro appeared to be pathogenic. On the basis of these findings, the authors hypothesized and consequently demonstrated in this study that subsequent to depletion of regulatory T cells (Treg), autoimmune thyroiditis and anti-Tg antibodies were induced in otherwise thyroiditis-resistant interleukin-17 knockout mice. However, interferon-γ knockout mice maintained their resistance against thyroiditis subsequent to depletion of Tregs (Fig 4 in the original article). Thus, in contrast to previous studies, the authors propose that a Th1 immune response is sufficient for the initiation of an autoimmune thyroiditis in predisposed animals. This may be attributed to an enhanced Th1 immune response, compensating for Th17 deficiency. Another explanation may be revealed by in vitro experiments. It has been proposed that Th17 cells exhibit a high plasticity and thereby low stability, and indeed they may not be pathogenic in their original condition but actually convert into Th1 cells prior to biological actions in autoimmune diseases. This study seems to suggest a major role for Th1 in autoimmune thyroiditis; however, this may be limited to the basic conditions in this specific mouse model, with iodine being the main trigger. Further studies in humans and other mouse models are needed to clarify the role and plasticity of Th17 cells and other effector T cells in autoimmune thyroiditis.

A. Thiel, MD

M. Schott, MD, PhD

References

1. Horie I, Abiru N, Nagayama Y, et al. T helper type 17 immune response plays an indispensable role for development of iodine-induced autoimmune thyroiditis in nonobese diabetic-H2h4 mice. *Endocrinology.* 2009;150:5135-5142.
2. Yu S, Sharp GC, Braley-Mullen H. Dual roles for IFN-γ, but not for IL-4, in spontaneous autoimmune thyroiditis in NOD.H-2h4 mice. *J Immunol.* 2002;169: 3999-4007.

Protein Kinase Cε Regulates Proliferation and Cell Sensitivity to TGF-1β of CD4⁺ T Lymphocytes: Implications for Hashimoto Thyroiditis
Mirandola P, Gobbi G, Masselli E, et al (Univ of Parma, Italy)
J Immunol 187:4721-4732, 2011

We have studied the functional role of protein kinase Cε (PKCε) in the control of human CD4⁺ T cell proliferation and in their response to TGF-1β. We demonstrate that PKCε sustains CD4⁺ T cell proliferation triggered in vitro by CD3 stimulation. Transient knockdown of PKCε expression decreases IL-2R chain transcription, and consequently cell surface expression levels of CD25. PKCε silencing in CD4 T cells potentiates the inhibitory effects of TGF-1β, whereas in contrast, the forced expression of PKCε virtually abrogates the inhibitory effects of TGF-1β. Being that PKCε is therefore implicated in the response of CD4 T cells to both CD3-mediated proliferative stimuli and TGF-1β antiproliferative signals, we studied it in Hashimoto thyroiditis (HT), a pathology characterized by abnormal lymphocyte proliferation and activation. When we analyzed CD4 T cells from HT patients, we found a significant increase of PKCε expression, accounting for their enhanced survival, proliferation, and decreased sensitivity to TGF-1β. The increased expression of PKCε in CD4⁺ T cells of HT patients, which is described for the first time, to our knowledge, in this article, viewed in the perspective of the physiological role of PKCε in normal Th lymphocytes, adds knowledge to the molecular pathophysiology of HT and creates potentially new pharmacological targets for the therapy of this disease.

▶ The protein kinase Cs (PKCs), in particular PKCε, have a critical role in the activation and proliferation of lymphocytes, which express several PKC isoforms that are upregulated and activated on T cell stimulation. In vivo experiments demonstrated that PKCε plays a key role in inflammation and immunity.

The present data demonstrate that PKCε sustains human CD4⁺ T cell duplication in vitro. Suppression of PKCε expression impaired CD3-mediated activation and proliferation: cell cultures transfected with small interfacing RNA (siRNA) PKCε showed more cells that did not duplicate at all and an overall decrease of the proliferating fraction of the cell culture, without affecting cell viability. In contrast, upregulation of PKCε expression in CD4⁺ cells transfected with wild type PKCε promoted cell proliferation. This effect was specific to PKCε because it could not be observed in cells transfected with a mutated, kinase-inactive PKCε isoform (PKCεm) and was rescued by siRNA-resistant PKCε (PKC1234R) expression. Searching for a mechanistic explanation for these observations, the authors found that, although the cell surface expression of activation markers like CD71 and CD95 was not affected, the expected upregulation of CD25 expression was prevented in stimulated CD4⁺ T cells by the suppression of PKCε expression. Using multiple TCR-independent T cell activators (PHA, PMA, and ionomycin), the authors observed that PKCε expression and activation were upregulated in stimulated CD4⁺ cells. Ionomycin, an activator of classical PKCs, activated PKCε as well and promoted its late upregulation, in agreement with recent data reported from another group showing that PKCε can be downstream of PKCa.[1]

The increased expression of PKCε in CD4$^+$ T cells of Hashimoto thyroiditis (HT) patients (Fig 8 in the original article), described in this article for the first time viewed in the perspective of the physiological role of PKCε in normal Th lymphocytes, adds knowledge to the molecular pathophysiology of HT and creates potentially new pharmacological targets for the therapy of this disease.

A. Thiel, MD

M. Schott, MD, PhD

Reference

1. Durgan J, Cameron AJ, Saurin AT, et al. The identification and characterization of novel PKCepsilon phosphorylation sites provide evidence for functional cross-talk within the PKC superfamily. *Biochem J.* 2008;411:319-331.

Simultaneous Occurrence of Subacute Thyroiditis and Graves' Disease

Hoang TD, Mai VQ, Clyde PW, et al (Natl Naval Med Ctr, Wisconsin, Bethesda, MD)

Thyroid 21:1397-1400, 2011

Background.—Rare cases of Graves' disease occurring years after subacute thyroiditis (SAT) have been reported. Here, we present the first known case of simultaneous occurrence of Graves' disease and SAT.

Patient Findings.—A 41-year-old woman presented with 10 days of neck pain, dysphagia, and hyperthyroid symptoms. Neck pain had initially started at the base of the right anterior neck and gradually spread to her upper chest, the left side of her neck, and bilateral ears. Physical examination revealed a heart rate of 110 beats/minute and a diffusely enlarged tender thyroid gland without evidence of orbitopathy. There was a resting tremor of the fingers and brisk deep tendon reflexes. Laboratory values: thyrotropin <0.01 mcIU/mL (nL 0.39−5.33), free thyroxine 2.0 ng/dL (nL 0.59−1.60), free T3 6.6 pg/mL (nL 2.3−4.2), thyroglobulin 20.1 ng/mL (nL 2.0−35.0), thyroglobulin antibody 843 IU/mL (nL 0−80), thyroperoxidase antibody 130 IU/mL (nL 0−29), thyroid stimulating hormone receptor antibody 22.90 IU/L (nL < 1.22), thyroid stimulating immunoglobulins 299 units (nL < 140), erythrocyte sedimentation rate 120 mm/h (nL 0−20), and C-reactive protein 1.117 mg/dL (nL 0−0.5). Human leukocyte antigen (HLA) typing revealed DRB1, DR8, B35, B39, DQB1, DQ4, and DQ5. A thyroid ultrasound showed an enlarged heterogeneous gland with mild hypervascularity. Fine-needle aspiration (FNA) biopsies of both thyroid lobes revealed granulomatous thyroiditis. The thyroid scan showed a diffusely enlarged gland and heterogeneous trapping. There was a focal area of relatively increased radiotracer accumulation in the right upper pole. The 5-hour uptake (^{123}I) was 6.6% (nL 4−15). The patient was symptomatically treated. Over the next several weeks, she developed hypothyroidism requiring levothyroxine treatment.

Summary.—This case illustrates a rare simultaneous occurrence of Graves' disease and SAT. Previous case studies have shown that Graves' disease may develop months to years after an episode of SAT. A strong family history of autoimmune thyroid disorders was noted in this patient. Genetic predilection was also shown by HLA typing.

Conclusion.—Although the occurrence of SAT with Graves' disease may be coincidental, SAT-induced autoimmune alteration may promote the development of Graves' disease in susceptible patients. Genetically mediated mechanisms, as seen in this patient by HLA typing and a strong family history, may also be involved.

▶ Autoimmune alterations induced by subacute thyroiditis have been proposed to be causative in the development of Graves disease. The deferred occurrence of Graves disease in patients who suffered from subacute thyroiditis within an interval of 4 months to 8 years has been reported previously. In this case report, the authors introduce the simultaneous incidence of both diseases, thereby underlining the recently proposed pathophysiologic correlations.[1] The authors present a 41-year-old white woman with typical signs of hyperthyroidism combined with symptoms induced by subacute thyroiditis. Graves ophthalmopathy was clinically ruled out. Laboratory results, ultrasonography, and fine-needle aspiration confirmed the clinical diagnosis. During the course of disease, she eventually developed hypothyroidism, which was quite unusual, as only less than 1% of affected patients become hypothyroid subsequent to subacute thyroiditis. The incidence of Graves disease following subacute thyroiditis has been linked to stress on the immune system in predisposed patients, release or expression of autoantigens in susceptible patients, and, last but not least, to genetic susceptibility toward the disease. Risk factors leading to the induction of an acute thyroiditis were ruled out in this patient. However, interestingly, human leukocyte antigen typing revealed a genetic predilection for both Graves disease (HLADRB1, DQB1) and subacute thyroiditis (HLA-B35) supporting the theory of genetic susceptibility. Additionally, the authors propose autoimmunity induced by viral infection. Apart from the fact that the simultaneous appearance of both disorders might be coincidental, this case report reveals strong evidence for pathophysiologic interactions between subacute thyroiditis and Graves disease. Consequently, a regular monitoring for Graves disease seems reasonable in patients subsequent to recovery from subacute thyroiditis. Furthermore, the exact pathophysiologic process leading to these clinical findings is still nebulous and demands further clarification.

A. Thiel, MD

M. Schott, MD, PhD

Reference

1. Nakano Y, Kurihara H, Sasaki J. Graves' disease following subacute thyroiditis. *Tohoku J Exp Med.* 2011;225:301-309.

Fibroblasts Expressing the Thyrotropin Receptor Overarch Thyroid and Orbit in Graves' Disease

Smith TJ, Padovani-Claudio DA, Lu Y, et al (Univ of Michigan Med School, Ann Arbor; et al)
J Clin Endocrinol Metab 96:3827-3837, 2011

Context.—Graves' disease (GD) is a systemic autoimmune syndrome comprising manifestations in thyroid and orbital connective tissue. The link between these two tissues in GD eludes our understanding. Patients with GD have increased frequency of circulating monocyte lineage cells known as fibrocytes. These fibrocytes infiltrate orbital connective tissues in thyroid-associated ophthalmopathy and express functional TSH receptor (TSHR).

Objective.—The aim of the study was to identify and characterize CD34+ fibrocytes in thyroid tissue.

Design/Setting/Participants.—Patients undergoing surgical thyroidectomy at two academic medical centers were recruited to the study.

Main Outcome Measures.—We performed immunohistochemistry, flow cytometry, real-time PCR, cytokine-specific ELISA, and cell differentiation.

Results.—CD34+ColI+CXCR4+TSHR+ cells can be identified *in situ* in thyroid tissue from donors with GD, Hashimoto's thyroiditis, or in normal-appearing tissue. Thyroid fibroblasts cultivated from these glands express a CD34−ColI+CXCR4+TSHR+ phenotype. TSHR levels are higher than those in orbital fibroblasts. When treated with TSH, thyroid fibroblasts generate IL-6 and IL-8. The induction of IL-6 can be blocked by dexamethasone, a chemical inhibitor of Akt/Pkb, and by knocking down Akt with a specific small interfering RNA. When treated with TGF-β or rosiglitazone, thyroid fibroblasts differentiate into myofibrocytes or adipocytes, respectively.

Conclusions.—ColI+CXCR4+TSHR+ thyroid fibroblasts resemble orbital fibroblasts and circulating fibrocytes. CD34+ fibrocytes appear to infiltrate both tissues in GD. Thyroid fibroblasts lose CD34 display in culture, unlike orbital fibroblasts and circulating fibrocytes. Fibrocytes and their fibroblast derivatives may participate in the pathogenesis of thyroid autoimmunity after TSHR activation. They could represent a therapeutic target for these diseases.

▶ Graves disease (GD) remains a poorly understood autoimmune syndrome, impacting several tissues, including the thyroid and orbit. The aim of this study was to identify and characterize CD34 fibrocytes in thyroid tissue. The authors of this study found that thyroid fibroblasts not only display thyrotropin receptor (TSHR), but when ligated with TSH and the monoclonal antibody M22, they can also produce the proinflammatory cytokines, interleukin-6 (IL-6) and IL-8 (Figs 4-6 in the original article). TSHR display was detected by flow cytometry in all strains of cells, regardless of whether donors presented with autoimmune thyroid disease or had an isolated malignancy but were otherwise healthy. Thus, thyroid fibroblasts join an ever-lengthening list of tissues and fibroblast types that display functional TSHR, as described in the past. The finding that TSHR can initiate signaling in fibroblasts and provoke cytokine production could open several potential avenues for therapy development. It is possible that aspects of tissue remodeling occurring in GD and other thyroid autoimmune processes such as hormone therapy might be mediated through fibroblast-displayed TSHR. It is notable that the levels of the receptor exceed those found previously on orbital fibroblasts. Several laboratory groups have demonstrated that TSHR levels in orbital fibroblasts can be upregulated after adipogenic differentiation. Thyroid fibroblasts do not appear to require further cell differentiation to display TSHR or respond to TSH. Unlike orbital fibroblasts cultivated from patients with GD and thromboangiitis obliterans, thyroid fibroblasts fail to display CD34 in culture (Fig 4 in the original article). This finding is not surprising considering the previous observations that fibrocytes subjected to prolonged culture can also lose CD34 expression.[1] Thus, the expression of CD34 appears to represent a labile and nondurable surface marker of fibrocytes and the fibroblasts differentiated from them.

Further studies are required to more fully elucidate the roles of these cells in autoimmune thyroid disease. From the current findings, it seems possible that thyroid fibroblasts, by virtue of their display of functional TSHR, might be targeted directly by anti-TSHR antibodies in GD and by the elevated serum levels of TSH frequently encountered in hormone therapy. It is thus possible that fibrocytes could mediate intrathyroidal events associated with both diseases and could represent attractive therapeutic targets.

A. Thiel, MD

M. Schott, MD, PhD

Reference

1. Keeley EC, Mehrad B, Strieter RM. The role of fibrocytes in fibrotic diseases of the lungs and heart. *Fibrogenesis Tissue Repair.* 2011;4:2.

Outcome of Graves' Orbitopathy after Total Thyroid Ablation and Glucocorticoid Treatment: Follow-Up of a Randomized Clinical Trial

Leo M, Marcocci C, Pinchera A, et al (Univ of Pisa, Italy)
J Clin Endocrinol Metab 97:E44-E48, 2012

Context.—In a previous study, we found that total thyroid ablation (thyroidectomy plus ^{131}I) is associated with a better outcome of Graves' orbitopathy (GO) compared with thyroidectomy alone, as observed shortly (9 months) after glucocorticoid (GC) treatment.

Objective.—The objective of the study was to evaluate the outcome of GO in the same patients of the previous study over a longer period of time.

Design.—This was a follow-up of a randomized study.

Setting.—The study was conducted at a referral center.

Patients.—Fifty-two of 60 original patients with mild to moderate GO participated in the study.

Interventions.—Patients randomized into thyroidectomy (TX) or total thyroid ablation and treated with GC were reevaluated in 2010, namely 88.0 ± 17.7 months after GC, having undergone an ophthalmological follow-up in the intermediate period.

Main Outcome Measures.—The main outcome measures included the following: 1) GO outcome; 2) time to GO best possible outcome and to GO improvement; and 3) additional treatments.

Results.—GO outcome at the end of the follow-up was similar in the two groups. However, the time required for the best possible outcome to be achieved was longer in the TX group (24 *vs.* 3 months, $P = 0.0436$), as was the time required for GO to improve (60 *vs.* 3 months, $P = 0.0344$). Additional treatments were given to a similar proportion of patients in each group (TX, 28%, total thyroid ablation, 25.9%), but they affected GO beneficially more often in the TX group (28 *vs.* 3.7%, *P*: 0.0412).

Conclusions.—Compared with thyroidectomy alone, total thyroid ablation allows the achievement of the best possible outcome and an improvement of GO within a shorter period of time (Fig 1).

▶ Treatment of hyperthyroidism in patients with Graves' orbitopathy (GO) is controversial. A conservative strategy based on antithyroid drugs is favored by some, whereas others, based on a proposed pathogenetic link between thyroid and orbital tissues, advocate an ablative strategy because removal of thyroid antigens could be beneficial for GO. In this study, the authors investigated the same patients that have already been studied over a longer period of time. Patients underwent a new evaluation on average approximately 7 years after glucocorticoid (GC) treatment, when GO outcome was similar, regardless of thyroid treatment. Nevertheless, this study shows that ablation may still have some advantages. Thus, the periods required to the best GO outcome and to GO improvement were shorter in total thyroid ablation (TTA). Whereas near-total thyroidectomy (TX) patients needed approximately 2 years to the best GO outcome and approximately 5 years to GO improvement, TTA patients needed only 3 months for both. The overlap concerning time to best outcome (Fig 1) should explain the relatively high, yet significant, *P* values. TSH receptor antibody (TRAb) reflect GO severity and activity. Thus, a shorter period would have been expected in TTA for TRAb to decrease or disappear. However, there was no difference with TX. In addition, approximately 25% of the patients still had detectable TRAb at the end of the follow-up, regardless of thyroid treatment, although the levels decreased over time. It may therefore be argued that the TTA advantages may not reflect a greater/faster attenuation of autoimmunity but rather other, unknown phenomena. Whatever the case, this study still shows some apparent advantages of ablation on the GO outcome, which may have clinical implications. To some extent, results in the long term reflected additional treatments, which were given to a similar proportion of patients in each group and affected favorably GO more often in TX. Nevertheless, additional treatments did not influence our conclusions, because GO outcome and time to improvement were not affected when the authors considered only patients who had not received these treatments.

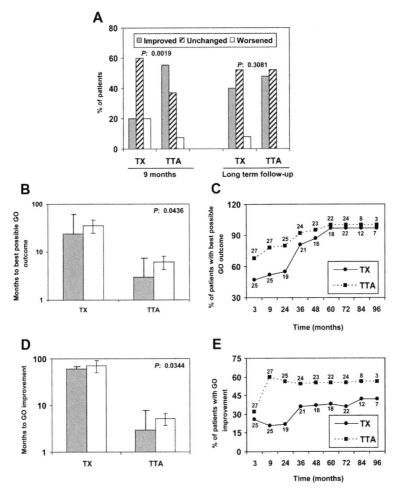

FIGURE 1.—A, Overall outcome of GO 9 months after the completion of glucocorticoid treatment and then in 2010 (long term follow-up), after a mean period of 88.0 ± 17.7 months (range 19–129). B, Median ± IQR (*gray columns*) and mean ± SD (*white columns*) time required to achieve the best possible outcome (the outcome observed at the end of the follow-up) of GO. C, Percent of patients reaching the best possible GO outcome over time. Number of patients available at each time point is indicated. D, Median ± IQR (*gray columns*) and mean ± SD (*white columns*) time required to reach an improvement of GO. E, Percent of patients with GO improvement over time. Number of patients available at each time point is indicated. (Reprinted from Leo M, Marcocci C, Pinchera A, et al. Outcome of Graves' orbitopathy after total thyroid ablation and glucocorticoid treatment: follow-up of a randomized clinical trial. *J Clin Endocrinol Metab.* 2012;97:E44-E48, Copyright 2012, with permission from The Endocrine Society.)

Some issues and possible weaknesses of this study should be considered. First, the study cannot answer the question whether an ablative strategy is preferable to a conservative one. Second, patients were given GC, which certainly affected GO. Thus, it is not known whether ablation is beneficial in patients not given GC. Third, there was a 45-day difference between TX and TTA in terms of timing of GC administration. Whether this affected GO is unknown. Fourth, this evaluation was not part of the original protocol, and the frequency of visits might have been affected by GO severity.

M. Schott, MD, PhD
A. Thiel, MD

Euthyroid Goiter

High-Intensity Focused Ultrasound Ablation of Thyroid Nodules: First Human Feasibility Study

Esnault O, Franc B, Ménégaux F, et al (ENT & Cervicofacial Surgery (Private Practice), Paris, France; Ambroise Paré Hosp, Boulogne Billancourt, France; Pitié Salpêtrière Hosp, Paris, France; et al)
Thyroid 21:965-973, 2011

Background.—Thyroid surgery is common, but complications may occur. High-intensity focused ultrasound (HIFU) is a minimally invasive alternative to surgery. We hypothesized that an optimized HIFU device could be safe and effective for ablating benign thyroid nodules without affecting neighboring structures.

Methods.—In this open, single-center feasibility study, 25 patients were treated with HIFU with real-time ultrasound imaging 2 weeks before a scheduled thyroidectomy for multinodular goiter. Thyroid ultrasonography imaging, thyroid function, were evaluated before and after treatment. Adverse events were carefully recorded. Each patient received HIFU for one thyroid nodule, solid or mixed, with mean diameter ≥8 mm, and no suspicion of malignancy. The HIFU device was progressively adjusted with stepwise testing. The energy level for ablation ranged from 35 to 94 J/pulse for different groups of patients. One pathologist examined all removed thyroids.

Results.—Three patients discontinued treatment due to pain or skin microblister. Among the remaining 22 patients, 16 showed significant changes by ultrasound. Macroscopic and histological examinations showed that all lesions were confined to the targeted nodule without affecting neighboring structures. At pathological analysis, the extent of nodule destruction ranged from 2% to 80%. Five out of 22 patients had over 20% pathological lesions unmistakably attributed to HIFU. Seventeen cases had putative lesions including nonspecific necrosis, hemorrhage, nodule detachment, cavitations, and cysts. Among these 17 cases, 12 had both ultrasound changes and cavitation at histology that may be expected for an HIFU effect. In the last three patients ablated at the highest energy level, significant ultrasound changes and complete coagulative necrosis were observed in 80%, 78%, and 58% of the targeted area, respectively. There were no major complications of ablation.

Conclusion.—This study showed the potential efficacy of HIFU for human thyroid nodule ablation. Lesions were clearly visible by histology and ultrasound after high energy treatments, and safety and tolerability were good. We identified a power threshold for optimal necrosis of the target thyroid tissue. Further studies are ongoing to assess nodule changes at longer follow-up times.

▶ Adults show a high prevalence of thyroid nodules; up to 40% are affected when identified by ultrasonography. Even if malignancy is ruled out efficiently, disease progress often necessitates surgical therapy. However, consideration of the risk—benefit evaluation concerning long-term follow-up of thyroid nodules versus the risks of thyroid surgery is commonly challenging in many individual cases. Therefore, therapeutic alternatives to surgery would be of significant value. This study introduces high-intensity focused ultrasound scan as being a minimally invasive alternative to surgery. Importantly, the authors emphasize the tissue-conserving properties of this method when compared with other minimally invasive therapies that have been focused on recently. Being less invasive and also having minimal side effects, the therapeutic value of high-intensity, focused ultrasound scan is currently also being assessed for gynecologic tumors, hepatocellular or renal-cell carcinomas, and hyperparathyroidism. Localized prostate cancer is actually routinely treated in several centers worldwide by high-intensity, focused ultrasound scan. In this study, 25 patients with benign thyroid nodules were treated previous to thyroidectomy. The primary goals of the study were first to assess safety and side effects and second to determine technical treatment parameters. Mild side effects, including local pain, mild skin burns, cough and skin microblisters, were minimized due to modification of the device and appropriate analgesia. Dysphonia or vocal cord palsy was not observed in this study. Furthermore, improvement of the pulse-energy for optimal clinical results combined with few adverse effects was a central objective of this study. However, the success of treatment could not be clearly assessed because of the small population size. Additionally, lacking an exact definition of the hallmarks of a high-intensity, focused, ultrasound-induced lesion and also because of permanent improvement of the technical parameters, the extent of nodule destruction varied from 2% to 80%. Promisingly, after treatment optimization, nodule destruction ranged from 58% to 80% ($n = 3$). Further studies on a larger scale will be needed for optimization according to the size and consistency of the nodules, for identification of ultrasonographic factors predictive of successful high-intensity, focused ultrasound effects, for assessment of the relevance of laboratory parameters, and also to improve the targeting and mapping. Altogether, this study introduces an interesting alternative therapeutic approach for benign thyroid nodules, especially because high-intensity, focused ultrasound, when compared with radiofrequency and laser ablation, required smaller safety margins and was less operator dependent.

A. Thiel, MD
M. Schott, MD, PhD

The Prevalence and Features of Thyroid Pyramidal Lobes as Assessed by Computed Tomography

Park JY, Kim DW, Park JS, et al (Inje Univ College of Medicine, Busan, South Korea; et al)
Thyroid 22:173-177, 2012

Background.—The pyramidal lobe is an accessory lobe of the thyroid gland. The prevalence of the pyramidal lobe in thyroid glands and its features have been studied in autopsy series but there is little information regarding its parameters in patients or normal subjects. The purpose of the current study was to assess the frequency, location, and size of the pyramidal lobe using computed tomography (CT) of the neck.

Methods.—From January to December 2010, 327 patients who underwent neck CT for trauma, thyroid cancer, pharyngolaryngeal malignancy, a palpable neck mass, cervical lymphadenopathy, and vocal cord paralysis were enrolled in the study. Their neck CTs were retrospectively analyzed by a single radiologist. Small pyramidal lobes (< 9 mm) were not included in the study.

Results.—A pyramidal lobe was present in 41.3% (135/327) of the patients; some pyramidal lobes showed complete separation from the thyroid gland (12.6%, 17/135). There was no difference in the frequency of pyramidal lobe detection by gender ($p > 0.05$, Fisher's exact test). The pyramidal lobe predominantly originated from the left thyroid gland in 54.1% (73/135) of patients. There were two patients in whom the pyramidal lobe was located bilaterally (one case from both the right and left sides of the thyroid gland and one case from the left side and midline of the thyroid gland). The average length and volume of the pyramidal lobes were 25.0 mm and 129.4 mm^3, respectively. The upper margin of the pyramidal lobe was most commonly located at the level of the thyroid cartilage.

Conclusion.—The prevalence of the pyramidal lobe in the left lobe of the thyroid gland is somewhat greater than 50% using the criteria employed in this study. Neck CT is useful for detecting the presence, size, configuration, and location of the pyramidal lobe.

▶ Because the pyramidal lobe in living patients is an accessory anatomical part of the thyroid, insufficient knowledge regarding it is available. As yet, studies referring to the prevalence and features of the pyramidal lobe were restricted to autopsy series. This study analyzed the prevalence, size, and anatomic location of the accessory lobe via computed tomography in a population of 327 patients characterized by a broad spectrum of diseases. Independent of gender and age, pyramidal lobes were found in 41.3% of the patients and most frequently originated from the left thyroid gland. The prevalence of the pyramidal lobe was not associated with distinct diseases. Furthermore, the continuity with the main thyroid gland and the average length and volume were assessed, revealing significantly larger pyramidal lobes in women. The upper part of the pyramidal lobes was most commonly abreast with the thyroid cartilage. Altogether, this study might be very valuable in clinical practice, as an exact mapping of the glandular landmarks and anatomic measurements of the thyroid will hopefully be helpful for the surgeon to avoid postoperative complications subsequent to thyroidectomy and neck dissection.[1] Importantly, in thyroid cancer, remnant thyroid tissue is most likely to be the focus of recurrence, and the amount of remnant thyroid tissue after thyroid surgery can significantly influence the outcome of radioactive iodine ablation because radioactive iodine preferentially targets healthy thyroid tissue when compared with malignant thyroid cells. Further studies are required to approve the clinical relevance of these facts. To give but one example, a negative correlation between the augmented knowledge regarding the pyramidal lobe and the recurrence rate in thyroid cancer could possibly emerge and would be eligible. If a significant benefit is indeed affirmed in future studies, a standardized preoperative neck computed tomography scan would be warrantable.

M. Schott, MD, PhD

A. Thiel, MD

Reference

1. Ozgur Z, Celik S, Govsa F, Ozgur T. Anatomical and surgical aspects of the lobes of the thyroid glands. *Eur Arch Otorhinolaryngol.* 2011;268:1357-1363.

Hypothyroidism

Increased Risk for Non-Autoimmune Hypothyroidism in Young Patients with Congenital Heart Defects

Passeri E, Frigerio M, De Filippis T, et al (Università degli Studi di Milano, San Donato Milanese, Italy; Istituto di Ricovero e Cura A Carattere Scientifico (IRCCS) Policlinico San Donato, Italy; IRCCS Istituto Auxologico Italiano, Milan, Italy; et al)

J Clin Endocrinol Metab 96:E1115-E1119, 2011

Context.—Newborns with congenital hypothyroidism (CH) have an increased risk for congenital heart defects (CHD) due to a common embryonic developmental program between thyroid gland and heart and great vessels.

Objective.—Our objective was to investigate the prevalence and origin of thyroid disorders in young patients with CHD.

Design and Setting.—We conducted a prospective observational study between January 2007 and January 2009 in academic Pediatric Cardiosurgery and Endocrinology.

Patients.—Patients included 324 children (164 males, 160 females, aged 0.2−15.4 yrs) with CHD.

Intervention.—Subjects underwent hormonal and genetic screening.

Main Outcome Measures.—Serum TSH and thyroid hormone levels were assessed.

Results.—Two CHD patients were diagnosed with CH at the neonatal screening (1:162). Mild hypothyroidism (serum TSH >4.0 μU/ml) was diagnosed and confirmed 6 months later [TSH = 5.4 ± 1.5 μU/ml; free

$T_4 = 1.3 \pm 0.2$ ng/dl (normal values 0.8–1.9)] in 37 children (11.5%) who were negative at neonatal screening. Hypothyroidism was not related to type of CHD, whereas TSH levels positively correlated with serum N-terminal pro-type B natriuretic peptide levels. Biochemical and ultrasound findings consistent with thyroid autoimmunity were present in three of 37 hypothyroid children (8.1%). One patient had hemiagenesis (2.7%). Variations in candidate genes were screened in CHD patients. *NKX2.5* coding sequence was normal in all samples. A 3-Mb microdeletion in 22q11.2 was detected in three patients (8.3%), whereas only known polymorphisms were identified in *TBX1* coding sequence.

Conclusions.—CHD patients have an increased risk for both CH (10-fold higher) and acquired mild hypothyroidism (3-fold higher). Unrecognized mild hypothyroidism may negatively affect the outcome of CHD children, suggesting that thyroid function should be repeatedly checked. Thyroid autoimmunity and 22q11.2 microdeletions account for small percentages of these cases, and still unknown mechanisms underline such a strong association.

▶ Different studies have found a significantly increased risk for congenital heart defects in children with congenital hypothyroidism. Consequently, common pathways in thyroid and cardiovascular development seem to be inevitable. As congenital heart defects are recognized as the most common congenital malformation, and hypothyroidism may very well have a negative impact on the course of disease in affected children, especially as they increasingly survive until adulthood, the authors investigated the prevalence and origin of thyroid disorders in patients suffering from congenital heart defects. Furthermore, transcription factors, which have been found to be associated with the embryonic development of both thyroid and heart, were analyzed in all participants. Three hundred twenty-four patients were enrolled into the study. Hypothyroidism was diagnosed in 12% of the patients, consequently resulting in a significantly higher risk for hypothyroidism in children with congenital heart defects. Serum thyroid-stimulating hormone (TSH) levels correlated with serum N-terminal pro-type B natriuretic peptide (NT-proBNP) levels; however, no association with disease severity could be observed in this study. Nevertheless, NT-proBNP levels are related to ventricular dysfunction and volume overload, therefore, implicating a relevant association between the extent of hypothyroidism and cardial dysfunction. Interestingly, only 8% of the affected children presented with thyroid autoimmunity, although autoimmune thyroid disease is the most frequent cause of acquired hypothyroidism in children. Besides 3 patients with DiGeorge syndrome, analysis of the known transcription factors involved in embryonic development did not evoke any path-breaking insights. Further studies are obligatory to estimate the clinical relevance of an early treatment for mild and severe hypothyroidism in children with congenital heart defects. Furthermore, the causal connection between hypothyroidism and congenital heart defects is still nebulous, as known pathways do not elucidate the findings in this study.

A. Thiel, MD
M. Schott, MD, PhD

Serum TSH within the Reference Range as a Predictor of Future Hypothyroidism and Hyperthyroidism: 11-Year Follow-Up of the HUNT Study in Norway

Åsvold BO, Vatten LJ, Midthjell K, et al (Norwegian Univ of Science and Technology, Trondheim, Norway; Norwegian Univ of Science and Technology, Levanger, Norway; et al)
J Clin Endocrinol Metab 97:93-99, 2012

Context.—Serum TSH in the upper part of the reference range may sometimes be a response to autoimmune thyroiditis in early stage and may therefore predict future hypothyroidism. Conversely, relatively low serum TSH could predict future hyperthyroidism.

Objective.—The objective of the study was to assess TSH within the reference range and subsequent risk of hypothyroidism and hyperthyroidism.

Design and Setting.—This was a prospective population-based study with linkage to the Norwegian Prescription Database.

Subjects.—A total of 10,083 women and 5,023 men without previous thyroid disease who had a baseline TSH of 0.20–4.5 mU/liter and who participated at a follow-up examination 11 yr later.

Main Outcome Measures.—Predicted probabilities of developing hypothyroidism or hyperthyroidism during follow-up, by categories of baseline TSH, were estimated.

Results.—During 11 yr of follow-up, 3.5% of women and 1.3% of men developed hypothyroidism, and 1.1% of women and 0.6% of men developed hyperthyroidism. In both sexes, the baseline TSH was positively associated with the risk of subsequent hypothyroidism. The risk increased gradually from TSH of 0.50–1.4 mU/liter [women, 1.1%, 95% confidence interval (CI) 0.8–1.4; men, 0.3%, 95% CI 0.1–0.6] to a TSH of 4.0–4.5 mU/liter (women, 31.5%, 95% CI 24.6–39.3; men, 14.7%, 95% CI 7.7–26.2). The risk of hyperthyroidism was higher in women with a baseline TSH of 0.20–0.49 mU/liter (3.9%, 95% CI 1.8–8.4) than in women with a TSH of 0.50–0.99 mU/liter (1.4%, 95% CI 0.9–2.1) or higher (∼1.0%).

Conclusion.—TSH within the reference range is positively and strongly associated with the risk of future hypothyroidism. TSH at the lower limit of the reference range may be associated with an increased risk of hyperthyroidism (Table 3).

▶ In this longitudinal population-based study, serum thyroid-stimulating hormone (TSH) within the reference range was positively and strongly associated with the risk of future hypothyroidism. The risk increased gradually from TSH of 0.50 to 1.4 mU/L to TSH of 4.0 to 4.5 mU/L (Fig 1 in the original article). The association of TSH with future hypothyroidism was essentially similar in women and men, but at any given TSH level, the absolute risk of hypothyroidism was higher in women than in men (Table 3). The risk of hyperthyroidism was higher in women with TSH of 0.20 to 0.49 mU/L than in women with higher TSH levels.

TABLE 3.—Age-Adjusted Predicted Probabilities (with 95% CI) of Hypothyroidism[a] at Follow-Up According to Categories of Baseline TSH in Women, by Age, Smoking, and BMI at Baseline[b]

TSH (mU/liter)	Hypothyroid, n/Total	Probability (%)	(95% CI)	Hypothyroid, n/Total	Probability (%)	(95% CI)
		20–49 yr of age			50–69 yr of age	
0.20–0.49	0/74	—		1/103	—	
0.50–1.4	28/2160	1.3	(0.9–1.9)	20/2371	0.8	(0.5–1.3)
1.5–1.9	25/1020	2.4	(1.7–3.6)	32/1398	2.3	(1.6–3.2)
2.0–2.4	23/575	4.0	(2.7–5.9)	26/821	3.2	(2.2–4.6)
2.5–2.9	24/305	7.8	(5.3–11.4)	38/454	8.3	(6.1–11.3)
3.0–3.4	23/164	13.9	(9.4–20.1)	26/231	11.2	(7.7–15.9)
3.5–3.9	13/83	15.7	(9.3–25.1)	28/171	16.4	(11.6–22.7)
4.0–4.5	21/56	37.3	(25.7–50.6)	27/97	27.8	(19.8–37.5)
		Nonsmokers			Smokers	
0.20–0.49	1/104	—		0/72	—	
0.50–1.4	31/2812	1.1	(0.8–1.6)	17/1704	1.0	(0.6–1.6)
1.5–1.9	32/1758	1.8	(1.3–2.6)	25/654	3.8	(2.5–5.5)
2.0–2.4	34/1113	3.0	(2.2–4.2)	15/279	5.3	(3.2–8.7)
2.5–2.9	41/609	6.7	(5.0–9.0)	21/146	14.5	(9.6–21.2)
3.0–3.4	33/322	10.2	(7.4–14.0)	16/73	21.8	(13.7–32.7)
3.5–3.9	34/222	15.4	(11.2–20.8)	7/32	21.7	(10.7–39.2)
4.0–4.5	35/121	28.9	(21.5–37.7)	13/31	40.5	(24.8–58.3)
		BMI <25.0 kg/m^2			BMI ≥25.0 kg/m^2	
0.20–0.49	0/77	—		1/100	—	
0.50–1.4	21/2067	1.0	(0.6–1.5)	27/2456	1.1	(0.7–1.6)
1.5–1.9	17/967	1.7	(1.1–2.7)	40/1446	2.7	(2.0–3.7)
2.0–2.4	22/546	3.9	(2.5–5.8)	27/849	3.2	(2.2–4.6)
2.5–2.9	24/263	8.7	(5.8–12.7)	38/495	7.7	(5.7–10.5)
3.0–3.4	19/148	12.3	(8.0–18.6)	30/247	12.3	(8.7–17.0)
3.5–3.9	15/82	18.2	(11.2–28.1)	26/172	15.3	(10.6–21.5)
4.0–4.5	19/52	35.4	(23.6–49.3)	29/101	29.2	(21.1–38.9)

Editor's Note: Please refer to original journal article for full references.

[a]Defined as prescription of levothyroxine, or TSH above 4.50 mU/liter combined with free T$_4$ below 9.0 pmol/liter, in people without a history of hyperthyroidism.

[b]Due to missing information on smoking or BMI, 31 and 15 women were excluded from the analyses by smoking and BMI, respectively.

These results are of special importance. It has been suggested that the upper limit of the reference range for TSH should be lowered, in part based on the observation that people with TSH in the upper part of the reference range are at increased risk of hypothyroidism.[1] This study's results indicate, however, that most people with TSH between 2.5 and 4.5 mU/L do not develop hypothyroidism during 11 years of follow-up. Furthermore, the association of TSH with the risk of hypothyroidism appears to be gradual across the reference range, with no cutoff point that distinctly separates TSH levels that are associated with increased risk of hypothyroidism from TSH levels that are not. Nonetheless, a substantial proportion of people with TSH in the uppermost part of the reference range developed hypothyroidism, which gives support to the suggestion that follow-up of thyroid function in these individuals may be appropriate. In summary, this longitudinal population-based study shows that serum TSH concentrations within the reference range are positively and strongly associated with the risk of developing hypothyroidism during 11 years of follow-up in both women and men. Conversely,

TSH at the lower limit of the reference range may be associated with an increased risk of hyperthyroidism.

A. Thiel, MD

M. Schott, MD, PhD

Reference

1. Wartofsky L, Dickey RA. The evidence for a narrower thyrotropin reference range is compelling. *J Clin Endocrinol Metab.* 2005;90:5483-5488.

Miscellaneous

A Mutation in the Thyroid Hormone Receptor Alpha Gene

Bochukova E, Schoenmakers N, Agostini M, et al (Univ of Cambridge Metabolic Res Laboratories and Natl Inst for Health Res Cambridge Biomedical Res Centre, UK; et al)

N Engl J Med 366:243-249, 2012

Thyroid hormones exert their effects through alpha (TRα1) and beta (TRβ1 and TRβ2) receptors. Here we describe a child with classic features of hypothyroidism (growth retardation, developmental retardation, skeletal dysplasia, and severe constipation) but only borderline-abnormal thyroid hormone levels. Using whole-exome sequencing, we identified a de novo heterozygous nonsense mutation in a gene encoding thyroid hormone receptor alpha (*THRA*) and generating a mutant protein that inhibits wild-type receptor action in a dominant negative manner. Our observations are consistent with defective human TRα-mediated thyroid hormone resistance and substantiate the concept of hormone action through distinct receptor subtypes in different target tissues (Table 1).

▶ It has been proposed that thyroid hormones mediate diverse actions in humans via distinct receptor subtypes in different target tissues. In this study, the authors affirm this concept by analyzing a novel mutation in the thyroid-hormone receptor alpha gene. Thyroid hormones act through nuclear receptor proteins, which are ligand-inducible transcription factors mediating the expression of target genes in different tissues. The receptor proteins are subclassified according to their genetic origin. The genes *THRA* and *THRB* encode the receptor subtypes TRα1, TRβ1, and TRβ2. Contrary to TRα1, which seems to be most abundant in bone, the gastrointestinal tract, cardiac and skeletal muscle, and the central nervous system, TRβ1 is predominantly found in the liver and kidney along with TRβ2, showing a predominant distribution in the hypothalamus, pituitary, cochlea, and retina. In this study the authors present the case of a child with clinical features of hypothyroidism (growth retardation, developmental retardation, skeletal dysplasia, and severe constipation), with almost normal thyroid hormone levels. They reveal a de novo causative mutation in the *THRA* gene, impairing the wild-type receptor function in a dominant negative manner and consequently leading to resistance of the target tissues toward thyroid hormone. Presenting an abnormally low blood pressure and heart rate, a reduced basal metabolic

TABLE 1.—Biochemical and Metabolic Measurements in the Patient*

Variable	Baseline	After Thyroxine Treatment	Reference Values
Thyroxine (μg/dl)			
Total	3.3	10.6	7.4–12.1[†]
Free	0.5	1.5	0.8–1.7[‡]
Triiodothyronine			
Total (ng/dl)	155	260	130–221[†]
Free (ng/dl)	0.4	0.7	0.3–0.5[‡]
Reverse (ng/ml)	0.07	0.2	0.21–0.37[†]
Thyroid-stimulating hormone (mU/liter)	1.04	<0.03	0.8–6.2[‡]
Sex hormone–binding globulin (nmol/liter)	146	131	20–81[†]
Insulin-like growth factor 1 (ng/ml)	59	96	67–257[†]
Pulse (bpm)[§]	71	69	
Blood pressure (mm Hg)[§]	82/51	77/43	
Basal metabolic rate (MJ/day)[¶]	3.49	4.08	4.06

Editor's Note: Please refer to original journal article for full references.

*To convert the values for total thyroxine to nanomoles per liter or free thyroxine to picomoles per liter, multiply by 12.87. To convert the values for total triiodothyronine to nanomoles per liter, multiply by 0.01536. To convert the values for free triiodothyronine to picomoles per liter, multiply by 15.36. To convert the values for insulin-like growth factor 1 to nanomoles per liter, divide by 7.7.

[†]Values are from 23 healthy control subjects who were matched with the patient according to age, sex, and body-mass index.

[‡]Reference ranges in children from 1 to 5 years of age are from Kapelari et al.[3]

[§]Detailed reference values are shown in Figure 4 in the Supplementary Appendix.

[¶]The basal metabolic rate was measured by means of indirect calorimetry with the use of a ventilated hood. The reference value is the predicted basal metabolic rate of the patient on the basis of her age, sex, and body composition.

rate, subnormal insulin-like growth factor-1 (IGF-1) levels, subnormal levels of serum free T3 and free T4, normal thyrotropin levels with elevated sex-hormone binding globulin levels, only the thyroid hormones and IGF-1 levels were restored appropriately or superphysiologically in the child after thyroxine treatment. However, the level of sex hormone–binding globulin remained high, the pulse rate and blood pressure remained abnormally low, and the clinical features of hypothyroidism persisted, underlining the concept of distinct thyroid-hormone receptor actions in different tissues (Table 1). Whole-exome sequencing of a DNA sample from the patient uncovered one heterozygous de novo mutation (c1207 G→T, p.E403X) in *THRA*. The abnormal receptor failed to activate a thyroid-hormone–responsive reporter gene and mediated substantial repression of basal promoter activity in a dominant negative manner due to structural modeling, thus leading to the facilitation of corepressor-binding and failure of free T3 recruitment. In summary, this article focuses on tissue-specific responsiveness (tissues predominant for TRβ) versus tissue-specific resistance (tissues predominant for TRα1) toward thyroid hormones. This study adds to our insight into tissue-specific functions of thyroid hormones and may contribute to future receptor-specific therapeutic possibilities.

A. Thiel, MD
M. Schott, MD, PhD

Treatment of Amiodarone-Induced Thyrotoxicosis Type 2: A Randomized Clinical Trial

Eskes SA, Endert E, Fliers E, et al (Univ of Amsterdam, The Netherlands; et al)
J Clin Endocrinol Metab 97:499-506, 2012

Context.—Amiodarone-induced thyrotoxicosis (AIT) type 2 is self-limiting in nature, but most physicians are reluctant to continue amiodarone. When prednisone fails to restore euthyroidism, possibly due to mixed cases of AIT type 1 and 2, perchlorate (ClO_4) might be useful because ClO_4 reduces the cytotoxic effect of amiodarone on thyrocytes.

Objectives.—Our objectives were to demonstrate the feasibility of continuation of amiodarone in AIT type 2 and to evaluate the usefulness of ClO_4 (given alone or in combination with prednisone) in AIT type 2.

Design and Setting.—A randomized multicenter study was conducted in 10 Dutch hospitals.

Methods.—Patients with AIT type 2 were randomized to receive prednisone 30 mg/d (group A, n = 12), sodium perchlorate 500 mg twice daily (group B, n = 14), or prednisone plus perchlorate (group C, n = 10); all patients continued amiodarone and were also treated with methimazole 30 mg/d. Follow-up was 2 yr.

Main Outcome Measures.—Treatment efficacy (defined as TSH values ≥ 0.4 mU/liter under continuation of amiodarone) and recurrent thyrotoxicosis were evaluated.

Results.—Initial therapy was efficacious in 100, 71, and 100% of groups A, B, and C, respectively ($P = 0.03$). The 29% failures in group B became euthyroid after addition of prednisone. Neither the time to reach TSH of 0.4 mU/liter or higher [8 wk (4—20), 14 wk (4—32), and 12 wk (4—28) in groups A, B, and C respectively] nor the time to reach free T_4 of 25 pmol/liter or below [4 wk (4—20), 12 wk (4—20), and 8 wk (4—20) in groups A, B, and C) were significantly different between groups (values as median with range). Recurrent thyrotoxicosis occurred in 8.3%.

Conclusion.—Euthyroidism was reached despite continuation of amiodarone in all patients. Prednisone remains the preferred treatment modality of AIT type 2, because perchlorate given alone or in combination with prednisone had no better outcomes (Table 2).

▶ Amiodarone-induced thyrotoxicosis (AIT) type 2 is caused by a destructive thyroiditis due to direct cytotoxic effects of the drug on thyrocytes. The nature of destructive thyroiditis is that of a self-limiting disease. The aim of this study was to demonstrate the feasibility of continuation of amiodarone in AIT type 2 and to evaluate the usefulness of perchlorate (given alone or in combination with prednisone) in AIT type 2. The authors could demonstrate that euthyroidism was reached despite continuation of amiodarone in all patients. Details are given in Table 2. The authors showed that prednisone remains the preferred treatment modality of AIT type 2, because perchlorate given alone or in combination with prednisone had no better outcomes.

TABLE 2.—Treatment Outcomes in Patients with AIT Type 2

	Group A (n = 12) Prednisone + Methimazole	Group B (n = 14) Perchlorate + Methimazole	Group C (n = 10) Prednisone + Perchlorate + Methimazole
Efficacy of treatment[a]			
TSH ≥ 0.4 mU/liter on initial therapy	12 (100%)	10 (71%)	10 (100%)
TSH ≥ 0.4 mU/liter on additional therapy	NA	4 (29%)	NA
Time to FT_4 ≤ 25 pmol/liter (wk)[b]	4 (4–20)	12 (4 –20)	8 (4–20)
Time to TSH ≤ 0.4 mU/liter (wk)[b]	8 (4–20)	14 (4 –32)	12 (4 –28)
Amiodarone continued	12 (100%)	14 (100%)	10 (100%)
Recurrent thyrotoxicosis	1	0	2
Time of recurrence (wk)	24	NA	12 and 76
Time to TSH ≥ 0.4 mU/liter (wk)	8	NA	4
Follow-up			
Amiodarone continued until end of follow-up	12 (100%)	14 (100%)	10 (100%)
Follow-up < 2 yr	0	2[c]	1[d]
Follow-up 2 yr	12	12	9
TSH 0.4 –5.0 mU/liter at 2 yr	10	11	6
TSH > 5.0 mU/liter at 2 yr	2	1	3
On levothyroxine at 2 yr	3	1	1

NA, Not applicable.
[a]Defined as TSH of 0.4 mU/liter or higher while amiodarone is continued.
[b]Median (range).
[c]Sudden cardiac death and cardiac transplant.
[d]Agranulocytosis upon methimazole treatment of recurrent thyrotoxicosis.

This study is the first prospective, controlled trial indicating that discontinuation of amiodarone in AIT type 2 is not necessary for restoration of euthyroidism. One may argue that the time to normalize free thyroxine (T_4) and thyroid-stimulating hormone (TSH) is longer when amiodarone is continued. A recent retrospective study identified 8 patients with AIT type 2 assembled in the period 2003 through 2008 who were treated with prednisone under continuation of amiodarone. When compared with 32 matched controls with AIT type 2 treated with prednisone after discontinuation of amiodarone, median time to first normalization of thyroid hormone levels did not significantly differ between both groups (24 and 31 days, respectively).[1] Because of a higher rate of recurrences in patients continuing amiodarone, the median time for stably restoring euthyroidism was much longer in this group. To establish whether continuation of amiodarone in prednisone-treated AIT type 2 patients really affects cure time will require a randomized clinical trial comparing continuation of amiodarone with stopping amiodarone. Continuation of amiodarone carries a risk of recurrent thyrotoxicosis. The authors observed an incidence of 8.3% at 2-year follow-up. An open Japanese study reported 6% recurrences of AIT type 2 occurring 5 to 8 years after the first episode.[2] In agreement with that study, the recurrences in this study were also mild and responded quickly to therapy. In this study, there was a high incidence of hypothyroidism, which, although frequently transient in nature, persisted in many cases until the end of follow-up. One could argue that continuation of amiodarone would result in more cases of hypothyroidism.

However, this appears unlikely because 17% of AIT type 2 patients in whom amiodarone was discontinued developed permanent hypothyroidism within 2 years after successful treatment with steroids.[3] This study had some limitations. As indicated, the authors did not apply color flow Doppler sonography to discriminate AIT types, because this method was not available in all centers. The number of patients in each treatment modality is rather small in the study. In view of this limited sample size, the results may not be generalized to all cases of AIT type 2, and, as indicated by the authors, they authors cannot exclude the possibility that in specific circumstances, discontinuation of amiodarone might be necessary.

A. Thiel, MD

M. Schott, MD, PhD

References

1. Bogazzi F, Bartalena L, Tomisti L, Rossi G, Brogioni S, Martino E. Continuation of amiodarone delays restoration of euthyroidism in patients with type 2 amiodarone-induced thyrotoxicosis treated with prednisone: a pilot study. *J Clin Endocrinol Metab.* 2011;96:3374-3380.
2. Sato K, Shiga T, Matsuda N, et al. Mild and short recurrence of type II amiodarone-induced thyrotoxicosis in three patients receiving amiodarone continuously for more than 10 years. *Endocr J.* 2006;53:531-538.
3. Bogazzi F, Dell'Unto E, Tanda ML, et al. Long-term outcome of thyroid function after amiodarone-induced thyrotoxicosis, as compared to subacute thyroiditis. *J Endocrinol Invest.* 2006;29:694-699.

Thyroid Cancer

Vandetanib in Patients With Locally Advanced or Metastatic Medullary Thyroid Cancer: A Randomized, Double-Blind Phase III Trial

Wells SA Jr, Robinson BG, Gagel RF, et al (Natl Insts of Health, Bethesda, MD; Univ of Sydney, Australia; Univ of Texas MD Anderson Cancer Ctr, Houston; et al)

J Clin Oncol 30:134-141, 2012

Purpose.—There is no effective therapy for patients with advanced medullary thyroid carcinoma (MTC). Vandetanib, a once-daily oral inhibitor of RET kinase, vascular endothelial growth factor receptor, and epidermal growth factor receptor signaling, has previously shown antitumor activity in a phase II study of patients with advanced hereditary MTC.

Patients and Methods.—Patients with advanced MTC were randomly assigned in a 2:1 ratio to receive vandetanib 300 mg/d or placebo. On objective disease progression, patients could elect to receive open-label vandetanib. The primary end point was progression-free survival (PFS), determined by independent central Response Evaluation Criteria in Solid Tumors (RECIST) assessments.

Results.—Between December 2006 and November 2007, 331 patients (mean age, 52 years; 90% sporadic; 95% metastatic) were randomly assigned to receive vandetanib (231) or placebo (100). At data cutoff (July 2009; median follow-up, 24 months), 37% of patients had progressed and

15% had died. The study met its primary objective of PFS prolongation with vandetanib versus placebo (hazard ratio [HR], 0.46; 95% CI, 0.31 to 0.69; *P* < .001). Statistically significant advantages for vandetanib were also seen for objective response rate (*P* < .001), disease control rate (*P* = .001), and biochemical response (*P* < .001). Overall survival data were immature at data cutoff (HR, 0.89; 95% CI, 0.48 to 1.65). A final survival analysis will take place when 50% of the patients have died. Common adverse events

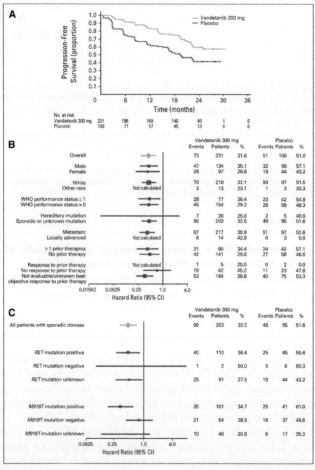

FIGURE 2.—(A) Kaplan-Meier curve of progression-free survival (PFS; intention-to-treat population; all randomly assigned patients); derived from all available centralized Response Evaluation Criteria in Solid Tumors (RECIST) assessments. (B) Forest plot of hazard ratios for PFS according to baseline characteristics and disease status. (C) Forest plot of hazard ratios for PFS according to rearranged during transfection (*RET*) mutation status and *M918T* mutation status in patients with sporadic medullary thyroid carcinoma. (B, C) A hazard ratio < 1 favors vandetanib. The analyses were performed using a log-rank test with treatment as the only factor. (Reprinted from Wells SA Jr, Robinson BG, Gagel RF, et al, Vandetanib in patients with locally advanced or metastatic medullary thyroid cancer: a randomized, double-blind phase III trial. *J Clin Oncol.* 2012;30:134-141, Copyright 2012, with permission from American Society of Clinical Oncology. All rights reserved.)

(any grade) occurred more frequently with vandetanib compared with placebo, including diarrhea (56% *v* 26%), rash (45% *v* 11%), nausea (33% *v* 16%), hypertension (32% *v* 5%), and headache (26% *v* 9%).

Conclusion.—Vandetanib demonstrated therapeutic efficacy in a phase III trial of patients with advanced MTC (ClinicalTrials.gov NCT00410761) (Fig 2).

▶ Medullary thyroid carcinoma (MTC), a malignancy of the parafollicular C cells of the thyroid gland, accounts for approximately 5% of all thyroid cancers and presents either sporadically (75% of patients) or in a hereditary pattern. Neither radiotherapy nor chemotherapy has demonstrated durable objective responses in patients with advanced MTC. Germline mutations in the RET (rearranged during transfection) proto-oncogene occur in virtually all patients with hereditary MTC. Approximately 50% of patients with sporadic MTC have somatic RET mutations, and 85% of them have the M918 T mutation. Evidence from preclinical studies of molecular-targeted therapeutics with activity against RET demonstrate that RET kinase is a potential therapeutic target in MTC 1. Other signaling pathways likely to contribute to the growth and invasiveness of MTC include vascular endothelial growth factor receptor (VEGFR)-dependent tumor angiogenesis and epidermal growth factor receptor (EGFR)-dependent tumor cell proliferation. Vandetanib is a once-daily oral agent that selectively targets RET, VEGFR, and EGFR signaling.[1] The aim of the present study was to investigate the effectiveness of vandetanib in an international, randomized, placebo-controlled, double-blind, phase III trial (ZETA) to evaluate vandetanib 300 mg/d in patients with locally advanced or metastatic MTC. Between December 2006 and November 2007, 331 patients were randomly assigned to receive vandetanib or placebo. Thirty-seven percent of patients had progressed, and 15% had died. The study met its primary objective of progression-free survival (PFS) prolongation with vandetanib versus placebo. This is beautifully shown in Fig 2. Statistically significant advantages for vandetanib were also seen for objective response rate, disease control rate, and biochemical response. The benefit that was demonstrated in PFS for patients receiving vandetanib compared with placebo was observed in patients with the hereditary or the sporadic form of MTC. Because of the small number of patients with sporadic MTC who were RET negative and the large number of patients who were RET unknown, the subgroup analyses of PFS and objective response rate by RET mutation status are inconclusive. Unfortunately, the overall survival of both groups looks very similar. However, this might be because of the crossover design of this study. Even though side effects are also seen, the drug has major implications for the treatment of metastatic (growing) MTC for which no other effective therapies are available.

M. Schott, MD, PhD

Reference

1. Carlomagno F, Vitagliano D, Guida T, et al. ZD6474, an orally available inhibitor of KDR tyrosine kinase activity, efficiently blocks oncogenic RET kinases. *Cancer Res.* 2002;62:7284-7290.

CXCR4 expression correlates with the degree of tumor infiltration and *BRAF* status in papillary thyroid carcinomas

Torregrossa L, Giannini R, Borrelli N, et al (Université di Pisa, Italy; et al)
Mod Pathol 25:46-55, 2012

Emerging evidence indicates that interactions between chemokine receptors and their ligands may have a critical role in several steps of tumor development, including tumor growth, progression, and metastasis. In this report, we retrospectively evaluated CXCR4 expression in a consecutive series of 200 papillary thyroid carcinomas. We investigated the relationship between the clinicopathological features of the tumors and mutations in the *BRAF* gene to verify whether overexpression of CXCR4 is linked to more aggressive behavior in thyroid tumors. CXCR4 protein expression was evaluated by immunohistochemical staining. A final staining score was calculated by adding the score representing the percentage of positive cells to the intensity score. The CXCR4 expression of each papillary thyroid carcinoma sample was normalized by calculating the z score for each final staining score. Univariate analysis was used to correlate CXCR4 expression with the papillary thyroid carcinoma variant, the degree of neoplastic infiltration, the American Joint Commission on Cancer stage, the presence of lymphocytic thyroiditis and the mutation status of the *BRAF* gene. Multiple regression analysis confirmed a strong association between CXCR4, *BRAF* mutation and the degree of neoplastic infiltration. These data clearly indicate that the chemokine receptor expression induced by oncogenic activation could be the major determinant of the local aggressiveness of neoplastic cells. In conclusion, our data indicate that CXCR4 expression and *BRAF* mutation status could cooperatively induce and promote a more aggressive phenotype in papillary thyroid carcinoma through several pathways and specifically increase the tumors spread outside of the thyroid gland (Table 1).

▶ Papillary thyroid carcinomas account for more than 80% of all thyroid cancers. Because thyroid cancer is the most common endocrine malignancy and because of the development of local and distant metastases or tumor recurrence in many patients during the course of the disease, novel therapeutic approaches are indeed warrantable. Different chemokines and their receptors have been proposed to be involved in tumor growth, progression, and metastasis.[1] In this study, the authors focus on the expression of the chemokine receptor CXCR4, which has been demonstrated to play an important role in a variety of human cancers regarding migration and metastatic processes in the context with its ligand CXCL12. Interestingly, the receptor expression inversely correlated with tumor size and no significant association was observed among age at diagnosis, gender, multifocality, and CXCR4 protein expression. However, a significant correlation was revealed between CXCR4 expression and papillary thyroid carcinoma subgroups, degree of neoplastic infiltration, lymphocytic thyroiditis, besides *BRAF* V600E-mutated tumors (Table 1). Concordant with other studies,[2] the authors revealed high CXCR4 levels in the tall cell and classic subgroups, whereas low levels

TABLE 1.—Correlation Between CXCR4 Immunohistochemical Expression and Clinicopathological Features

Clinical–Pathological Features	CXCR4 FSS Mean FSS	P	CXCR4 z Score High n (%)	Low n (%)	P	OR (95% CI)
Age at diagnosis						
Patients <45 years (n = 110)	3.36 ± 2.3	0.5	33 (30.0)	77 (70.0)	0.072	0.59 (0.33–1.05)
Patients ≥45 years (n = 90)	3.53 ± 2.5		38 (42.2)	52 (57.8)		
Gender						
Male (n = 45)	3.73 ± 2.5	0.38	17 (37.8)	28 (62.2)	0.72	1.14 (0.57–2.26)
Female (n = 155)	3.35 ± 2.4		54 (34.8)	101 (65.2)		
PTC variants						
MicroPTC (n = 68)	3.79 ± 2.6	0.00005	29 (42.6)	39 (57.4)		
FV (n = 39)	1.74 ± 1.6		2 (5.0)	37 (95.0)	<0.00005	b
CV (n = 83)	3.66 ± 2.2		32 (38.5)	51 (61.5)		
TCV (n = 10)	5.80 ± 1.6		8 (80.0)	2 (20.0)		
Multifocality[a]						
No (n = 153)	3.50 ± 2.4	0.62	53 (34.6)	100 (65.4)	0.64	1.17 (0.60–2.30)
Yes (n = 47)	3.23 ± 2.4		18 (38.3)	29 (61.7)		
Lymph node metastasis						
No (n = 145)	3.18 ± 2.5	0.019	46 (31.7)	99 (68.3)	0.07	1.79 (0.95v3.39)
Yes (n = 55)	4.10 ± 2.1		25 (45.5)	30 (54.5)		
Degree of neoplastic infiltration						
A (n = 55)	2.18 ± 2.0	0.00005	8 (14.5)	47 (85.5)		
B (n = 45)	2.93 ± 2.7		11 (24.4)	34 (75.6)	<0.00005	b
C (n = 30)	4.16 ± 2.3		15 (50.0)	15 (50.0)		
D (n = 70)	4.44 ± 2.0		37 (52.8)	33 (47.2)		
AJCC stages						
I (n = 169)	3.31 ± 2.4	0.04	53 (31.4)	116 (68.6)		
II (n = 5)	1.80 ± 2.6		1 (20.0)	4 (80.0)	0.063	b
III (n = 18)	4.55 ± 2.2		12 (66.7)	6 (33.3)		
IVa (n = 8)	4.50 ± 2.4		5 (62.5)	3 (37.5)		
Lymphocytic thyroiditis						
No (n = 128)	3.13 ± 2.5	0.022	38 (29.7)	90 (70.3)	0.022	2.00 (1.10–3.65)
Yes (n = 72)	3.98 ± 2.2		33 (45.8)	39 (54.2)		
BRAF status						
Wild type (n = 110)	2.40 ± 2.2	0.00005	21 (19.1)	89 (80.9)	<0.00005	5.30 (2.82–9.96)
V600E mutated (n = 90)	4.70 ± 2.0		50 (55.5)	40 (44.5)		

Abbreviations: AJCC, American Joint Commission on Cancer; CI, confidence interval; CV, classical variant of PTC; FV, follicular variant of PTC;
FSS, final staining score; OR, odds ratio; PTC, papillary thyroid carcinoma; TCV, tall cell variant of PTC.
[a]The neoplasm with the greatest size or the highest pT status has always been analyzed in the presence of multifocality.
[b]Not done.

were detected in the follicular variants. The inverse correlation of CXCR4 expression and tumor size indicates that the subgroups play a superior role in the distribution and incidence of the chemokine receptor. However, other groups have recently revealed converse results.[3] Converse results were also obtained in comparison to other groups regarding the association between CXCR4 and extrathyroidal extension of the tumor besides CXCR4 expression by malignant epithelial cells and inflammation. Possibly the number of cases or the study population may explain the divergent findings. Thus, further studies are needed to unravel these contradictions. However, since a strong association between the *BRAF* mutation and tumor invasiveness has been demonstrated previously[4] and a significant association between CXCR4, *BRAF*, and the degree of neoplastic infiltration was confirmed in this study, it is likely that CXCR4 plays an important role in tumor progress. Therefore, further studies are needed and CXCR4 may potentially be applied for the differential diagnosis of malignant versus benign thyroid nodules.

A. Thiel, MD

M. Schott, MD, PhD

References

1. Müller A, Homey B, Soto H, et al. Involvement of chemokine receptors in breast cancer metastasis. *Nature.* 2001;410:50-56.
2. Torregrossa L, Faviana P, Filice ME, et al. CXC chemokine receptor 4 immunodetection in the follicular variant of papillary thyroid carcinoma: comparison to galectin-3 and hector battifora mesothelial cell-1. *Thyroid.* 2010;20:495-504.
3. Wagner PL, Moo TA, Arora N, et al. The chemokine receptors CXCR4 and CCR7 are associated with tumor size and pathologic indicators of tumor aggressiveness in papillary thyroid carcinoma. *Ann Surg Oncol.* 2008;15:2833-2841.
4. Basolo F, Torregrossa L, Giannini R, et al. Correlation between the BRAF V600E mutation and tumor invasiveness in papillary thyroid carcinomas smaller than 20 millimeters: analysis of 1060 cases. *J Clin Endocrinol Metab.* 2010;95:4197-4205.

Immunoglobulin G expression and its colocalization with complement proteins in papillary thyroid cancer

Qiu Y, Korteweg C, Chen Z, et al (Shantou Univ Med College, China)
Mod Pathol 25:36-45, 2012

Except for the well-known immunoglobulin G (IgG) producing cell types, ie, mature B lymphocytes and plasma cells, various non-lymphoid cell types, including human cancer cells, neurons, and some specified epithelial cells, have been found to express IgG. In this study, we detected the expression of the heavy chain of IgG (IgGγ) and kappa light chain (Igκ) in papillary thyroid cancer cells. Using *in situ* hybridization, we detected the constant region of human IgG1 *(IGHG1)* in papillary thyroid cancer cells. With laser capture microdissection followed by RT-PCR, mRNA transcripts of *IGHG1, Igκ, recombination activating gene 1 (RAG1), RAG2,* and *activation-induced cytidine deaminase* genes were successfully amplified from isolated papillary thyroid cancer cells. We further confirmed IgG protein expression with immunohistochemistry and found that none of the IgG receptors was expressed in papillary thyroid cancer. Differences in the level of IgGγ expression between tumor size, between papillary thyroid cancer and normal thyroid tissue, as well as between papillary thyroid cancer with and without lymph node metastasis were significant. Taken together, these results indicate that IgG is produced by papillary thyroid cancer cells and that it might be positively related to the growth and metastasis of papillary thyroid cancer cells. Furthermore, it was demonstrated that IgGγ colocalized with complement proteins in the same cancer cells, which could indicate that immune complexes were formed. Such immune complexes might consist of IgG synthesized by the host against tumor surface antigens and locally produced anti-idiotypic IgG with specificity for the variable region of these 'primary' antibodies. The cancer cells might thus escape the host tumor-antigen-specific immune responses, hence promoting tumor progression (Fig 1).

▶ Belonging to humoral immunity, immunoglobulin-G (IgG) is commonly produced and secreted by plasma cells subsequent to antigen contact. Recently, however, studies have revealed that several other cell types besides plasma cells, among other different tumor entities, are capable of producing IgG. Furthermore, because of differences in in vitro studies and the correlation of tumor—IgG levels with the severity of disease in soft tissue tumors, it has been proposed that IgG has an impact on tumor growth and spread. Therefore, the authors analyzed the expression of IgG in papillary thyroid cancer in this study. They also focused on proteins that belong to the complement system, as they are supposed to be

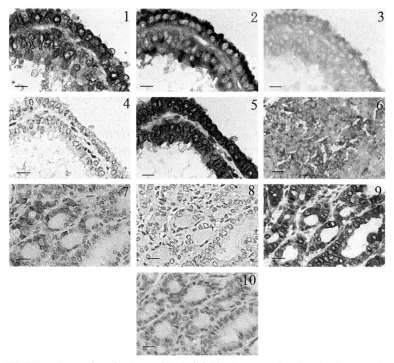

FIGURE 1.—Immunohistochemistry and *in situ* hybridization on serial sections showing expression of IgG proteins and mRNA. Figures 1—5 and 7—10 are serial sections. The signals are localized to the cytoplasm. (1) Primary antibody: polyclonal rabbit anti-human IgGγ. (2) *In situ* hybridization show *IGHG1* antisense probe. (3) Sense *IGHG1* probe, no signal with a sense probe. (4) Primary antibody: mouse anti-human CD20. (5) Primary antibody: mouse anti-human CK. (6) Human spleen as a positive control for the *IGHG1* antisense probe. (7) Primary antibody: mouse anti-human Igκ. (8) Primary antibody: mouse anti-human CD20. (9) Primary antibody: mouse anti-human CK. (10) PBS as a negative control. Scale bars, 50 μm. (Reprinted from Qiu Y, Korteweg C, Chen Z, et al. Immunoglobulin G expression and its colocalization with complement proteins in papillary thyroid cancer. *Mod Pathol.* 2012;25:36-45, Copyright 2012, with permission from Macmillan Publishers Ltd: Modern Pathology.)

involved in antitumor immune surveillance via the classical complement pathway, thus also involving IgG. Up to 80% of the papillary thyroid cancer cells were positive for IgGγ and IgGκ in contrast to normal thyroid tissue (Fig 1). This finding was also affirmed at the messenger RNA (mRNA) level. Also, complement proteins were detected, partly localizing with IgG. However, no complement mRNA was observed. The total number of positive cells besides the intensity of IgGγ staining correlated with tumor size and lymph node metastases. Moreover, IgG production was supported by detection of the *RAG1*, *RAG2*, and activation-induced cytidine deaminase genes. Since the cells were negative for IgG-specific Fc receptors, an IgG expression that resulted from uptake by receptors was unlikely. A contamination with B cells was also ruled out. On the one hand, complement factors were colocalized with IgG, indicating a possible immune reaction with cytotoxic capacity. On the other hand, the presence of IgG correlated with a worse clinical outcome. Consequently, the authors developed a very intriguing theory, proposing that IgG directed against tumor antigens is colocalized with a complement on the tumor surface, however functionally inhibited by distinct IgGs produced by the tumor that are directed against host IgG. Further studies are needed to prove this very interesting theory and also to search for similar growth factor properties of IgG. Moreover, IgG may be useful as a prognostic marker in papillary thyroid cancer.

A. Thiel, MD

M. Schott, MD, PhD

Associations between promoter polymorphism -106A/G of interleukin-11 receptor alpha and papillary thyroid cancer in Korean population

Eun YG, Shin IH, Kim M-J, et al (Sungkyunkwan Univ School of Medicine, Changwon, Republic of Korea; Kyung Hee Univ, Seoul, Republic of Korea)
Surgery 151:323-329, 2012

Background.—The interleukin11 (IL11) and IL11 receptor alpha (IL11RA) are involved in cellular growth, differentiation, invasiveness, and tumor progression in several tumors. We investigated whether coding single nucleotide polymorphisms (cSNPs) of IL11 and promoter SNP IL11RA would contribute to the development of papillary thyroid cancer (PTC). We also assessed the relationships between IL11 and IL11RA SNPs and the clinicopathologic characteristics of PTC.

Methods.—One coding SNP, designated as rs1126757, Ala82Ala, in IL11 and one promoter SNP, designated as rs1061758, −106A/G, in IL11RA were genotyped using direct sequencing in 94 patents with PTC and 213 patients without PTC (controls). Genetic data were analyzed using commercially available software. The patients with PTC were dichotomized and compared with respect to clinicopathologic characteristics of PTC.

Results.—We found an association between PTC and the coding SNP(rs1061758) in IL11RA (codominant model 1 [G/G vs A/G], odds ratio [OR] = 2.91, 95% confidence interval [CI], 1.44−5.89; $P = .003$;

codominant model 2 [G/G vs A/A], OR = 2.95, 95% CI, 1.30–6.72; P =.01; and dominant model, OR = 2.92, 95% CI, 1.47–5.80; P =.002). Moreover, SNP rs1061758 in IL11RA was associated with the multifocality of PTC (codominant model 2 [A/A vs G/G], OR = 9.56, 95% CI, 1.77–51.69; P =.009; and recessive model, OR = 7.22, 95% CI, 1.72–30.3; P =.007). Genotype and allele analyses of SNP variant rs1126757 in IL11 revealed no statistically significant differences between patients with PTC and controls.

Conclusion.—Our results suggest that an IL11RA promoter polymorphism — rs1061758 — may be associated with the risk of PTC in the Korean population. In addition, rs1061758 might be related to the multifocality of PTC.

▶ Recently, a genetic predisposition has been proposed for papillary thyroid cancer; however, possible interrelated mechanisms remain undefined. Due to a significant correlation of interleukin (IL)-11/ IL11 receptor alpha (IL-11RA) expression with tumor invasion and proliferation in different solid cancers, the authors analyzed the role of IL-11/IL-11RA in the development of papillary thyroid cancer and in the relationship to clinicopathologic features. In this study, they especially focused on single nucleotide polymorphisms, as such have been linked to cancer predisposition in other cytokines, for example, IL-6 and IL-10. The analysis revealed a significant correlation of the incidence of the IL-11RA-promotor single nucleotide polymorphism rs1061758 with the development of papillary thyroid cancer. Affected patients also exhibited augmented rs1061758 gene allele frequencies. Furthermore, the rs1061758 gene allele was associated with multifocality of papillary thyroid cancer; however, interestingly not with tumor size, location, extrathyroidal invasion, or lymph node metastasis. Actually, one would have expected different results because IL-11 being related to IL-6 has been shown to regulate cell motility, invasion, and metastasis[1,2] and because the STAT and MAPK pathways and gp130-dependent cytokines (also part of the IL11 pathway) play an important role in tumor proliferation and invasion. Nevertheless, this study represents a new and interesting approach to the subject, as to date no studies are available, proving an association of IL-11 or IL-11RA polymorphisms with the susceptibility to different cancers. Moreover, the authors emphasize the importance of the significant association to multifocality, thus, linked with indications for completion thyroidectomy and postoperative radioactive iodine ablation. Indeed, IL-11RA polymorphisms could not only be potentially involved in controlling therapeutic approaches; in fact, prevention programs are imaginable. However, further studies are obligatory to analyze the molecular in vivo effects of this single nucleotide polymorphism, especially as the allele does not seem to influence familiar elements of tumor spreading. Additionally, it would be reasonable to evaluate the incidence of single nucleotide polymorphisms in other populations besides the Korean population. Altogether, this article comprises a promising and intriguing approach to the subject.

A. Thiel, MD
M. Schott, MD, PhD

References

1. Nakayama T, Yoshizaki A, Izumida S, et al. Expression of interleukin-11 (IL-11) and IL-11 receptor alpha in human gastric carcinoma and IL- 11 upregulates the invasive activity of human gastric carcinoma cells. *Int J Oncol.* 2007;30:825-833.
2. Liu XH, Kirschenbaum A, Lu M, et al. Prostaglandin E(2) stimulates prostatic intra-epithelial neoplasia cell growth through activation of the interleukin-6/GP130/STAT-3 signaling pathway. *Biochem Biophys Res Commun.* 2002;290:249-255.

The Effects of Four Different Tyrosine Kinase Inhibitors on Medullary and Papillary Thyroid Cancer Cells

Verbeek HHG, Alves MM, de Groot J-WB, et al (Univ of Groningen, The Netherlands)
J Clin Endocrinol Metab 96:E991-E995, 2011

Context.—Medullary and papillary thyroid carcinoma (MTC and PTC) are two types of thyroid cancer that can originate from activating mutations or rearrangements in the *RET* gene. Therapeutic options are limited in recurrent disease, but because RET is a tyrosine kinase (TK) receptor involved in cellular growth and proliferation, treatment with a TK inhibitor might be promising. Several TK inhibitors have been tested in clinical trials, but it is unknown which inhibitor is most effective and whether there is any specificity for particular *RET* mutations.

Objective.—We aimed to compare the effect of four TK inhibitors (axitinib, sunitinib, vandetanib, and XL184) on cell proliferation, RET expression and autophosphorylation, and ERK activation in cell lines expressing a MEN2A (MTC-TT), a MEN2B (MZ-CRC-1) mutation, and a RET/PTC (TPC-1) rearrangement.

Design.—The three cell lines were cultured and treated with the four TK inhibitors. Effects on cell proliferation and RET and ERK expression and activation were determined.

Results.—XL184 and vandetanib most effectively inhibited cell proliferation, RET autophosphorylation in combination with a reduction of RET expression, and ERK phosphorylation in MTC-TT and MZ-CRC-1, respectively. TPC-1 cells showed a decrease in RET autophosphorylation after treatment with XL184, but no effect was observed on ERK activation.

Conclusion.—There is indeed specificity for different *RET* mutations, with XL184 being the most potent inhibitor in MEN2A and PTC and vandetanib the most effective in MEN2B *in vitro*. No TK inhibitor was superior for all the cell lines tested, indicating that mutation-specific therapies could be beneficial in treating MTC and PTC (Fig 1C).

▶ The molecular background to both the aforementioned studies is shown in this study by Verbeek and coworkers. Here, the authors investigated the role of 4 different tyrosine kinase inhibitors in medullary and dedifferentiated thyroid cancer, namely, axitinib, sunitinib, vandetanib, and XL184. The authors investigated the role of these substances on cell proliferation, RET expression and

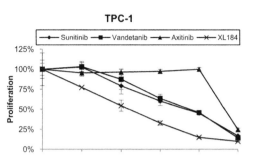

FIGURE 1.—Effect of XL184, vandetanib, sunitinib, and axitinib on cell proliferation. A–C, Dose-response curve of TPC-1. (C) cell lines incubated with different concentrations of XL184, vandetanib, sunitinib, and axitinib. (Reprinted from Verbeek HHG, Alves MM, de Groot J-WB, et al. The effects of four different tyrosine kinase inhibitors on medullary and papillary thyroid cancer cells. *J Clin Endocrinol Metab.* 2011;96:E991-E995, Copyright 2011, with permission from The Endocrine Society.)

autophosphorylation, and ERK activation in cell lines expressing an MEN2A (MTC-TT) mutation, MEN2B (MZ-CRC-1) mutation, and RET/PTC (TPC-1) rearrangement. The authors could demonstrate that all substances have a direct effect on tumor growth (Fig 1C). This is especially important for the substances vandetanib and XL184. Vandetanib has now been approved by the Food and Drug Agency as well as the European Medicines Agency for the treatment of metastatic (and growing) medullary thyroid carcinomas. Regarding XL184, an international, multicenter, placebo-controlled trial is presently ongoing. Depending on these results, endocrinologists may have in the near future 2 substances available for the treatment of patients with medullary thyroid carcinoma.

M. Schott, MD, PhD

A. Thiel, MD

Current Thyroglobulin Autoantibody (TgAb) Assays Often Fail to Detect Interfering TgAb that Can Result in the Reporting of Falsely Low/ Undetectable Serum Tg IMA Values for Patients with Differentiated Thyroid Cancer

Spencer C, Petrovic I, Fatemi S (Univ of Southern California, Los Angeles; Kaiser Permanente, Panorama City, CA)
J Clin Endocrinol Metab 96:1283-1291, 2011

Context.—Specimens have thyroglobulin antibody (TgAb) measured prior to thyroglobulin (Tg) testing because the qualitative TgAb status (positive or negative) determines risk for Tg assay interference, and the quantitative TgAb concentration serves as a surrogate tumor marker for differentiated thyroid cancer.

Objective.—This study assessed the reliability of four TgAb methods to detect interfering TgAb [as judged from abnormally low Tg immunometric assay (IMA) to TgRIA ratios] and determine whether between method conversion factors might prevent a change in method from disrupting TgAb monitoring.

Methods.—Sera from selected and unselected TgAb-negative and TgAb-positive differentiated thyroid cancer patients had serum Tg measured by both IMA and RIA and TgAb measured by a reference method and three additional methods.

Results.—The Tg IMA and Tg RIA values were concordant when TgAb was absent. Tg IMA to Tg RIA ratios below 75% were considered to indicate TgAb interference. Manufacturer-recommended cutoffs were set in the detectable range, and when used to determine the presence of TgAb misclassified many specimens displaying Tg interference as TgAb negative. False-negative misclassifications were virtually eliminated for two of four methods by using the analytical sensitivity (AS) as the detection limit for TgAb. Relationships between values for different specimens were too variable to establish between-method conversion factors.

Conclusions.—Many specimens with interfering TgAb were misclassified as TgAb negative using manufacturer-recommended cutoffs. It is recommended that assay AS limits be used to detect TgAb to minimize false-negative misclassifications. However, for two of four assays, AS limits failed to detect interfering TgAb in 20–30% of cases. TgAb methods were too qualitatively and quantitatively variable to establish conversion factors that would allow a change in method without disrupting serial TgAb monitoring.

▶ Serum thyroglobulin (Tg) is primarily measured as a postoperative tumor marker test for patients with differentiated thyroid cancer (DTC). The goals of this study were (1) to assess whether the manufacturer-recommended cutoffs (MCs) of 4 different Tg antibody (Ab) methods reliably identified TgAb-containing specimens, using a low-serum Tg immunometric assay (IMA) to Tg RIA ratio to indicate the presence of interfering TgAb, and (2) to evaluate whether fixed factors could be used to convert the TgAb values reported by different methods so that a change in TgAb method could be made without disrupting the serial monitoring pattern.

This study of 4 different TgAb methods found that the use of the MC to determine the presence of TgAb frequently led to false-negative misclassifications of specimens displaying Tg interference, as judged from the presence of discordance between Tg IMA versus Tg RIA measurements (Figs 1 and 2 in the original article). In many of these cases, the interference in this study was severe and had the potential to influence clinical management. When all values detected above the assay sensitivity (AS) limit were considered as TgAb positive, false-negative specimen misclassifications were greatly reduced, and all misclassifications of specimens displaying severe interference were eliminated for 2 of the 4 methods (assays 1 and 2). However, with methods 3 and 4, even the use of the AS limit failed to detect interfering TgAb in a high percentage of cases (21.9 and 34.3%, respectively). Although there was a general ranking of values between assays, there were wide disparities between the absolute values reported by the different methods for the same specimen and disparate relationships between the values reported for different specimens. This study suggests that TgAb assay AS limits should be used to detect TgAb to minimize false-negative misclassifications. Furthermore, it is probably not possible to harmonize the TgAb values reported by different assays or calculate between-method conversion factors that would allow changing methods without disrupting serial TgAb monitoring used as a surrogate DTC tumor marker.

M. Schott, MD, PhD

A. Thiel, MD

Mutationally Activated BRAF[V600E] Elicits Papillary Thyroid Cancer in the Adult Mouse

Charles R-P, Iezza G, Amendola E, et al (Univ of California, San Francisco; L'Istituto di Ricerche Genetiche, Italy)
Cancer Res 71:3863-3871, 2011

Mutated *BRAF* is detected in approximately 45% of papillary thyroid carcinomas (PTC). To model PTC, we bred mice with adult-onset,

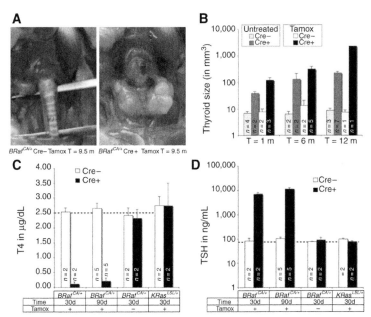

FIGURE 1.—BRAF[V600E] expression induces goiter which progresses to PTC. A, representative images of the thyroid gland from control *BRaf^{CA/+}* (left) or *Thyro::CreER^{T2}; BRaf^{CA/+}* mice (right) 9.5 months after tamoxifen administration. B, quantification of average thyroid volume of mice of the indicated genotype either untreated or treated with tamoxifen as indicated. *n*, number of mice in each group. C and D, serum concentration of T4 (C) or TSH (D) in *Thyro::CreER* mice that also carry either a Cre-activated *BRaf^{CA}* or *KRas^{LSL}* allele as indicated. Tamoxifen-treated (+Tamox) or control (−Tamox) mice were euthanized at 30 or 90 days as indicated and serum samples prepared. Serum T4 or TSH were measured by radioimmune assay as described in Materials and Methods. Dotted lines indicate the concentration of T4 (μg/dL) or TSH (ng/mL) in normal mice. *n*, number of mice in each group. (Reprinted from Charles R-P, Iezza G, Amendola E, et al. Mutationally activated BRAF[V600E] elicits papillary thyroid cancer in the adult mouse. *Cancer Res.* 2011;71:3863-3871, with permission from American Association for Cancer Research.)

thyrocyte-specific expression of BRAF^{V600E}. One month following BRAF^{V600E} expression, mice displayed increased thyroid size, widespread alterations in thyroid architecture, and dramatic hypothyroidism. Over 1 year, without any deliberate manipulation of tumor suppressor genes, all mice developed PTC displaying nuclear atypia and marker expression characteristic of the human disease. Pharmacologic inhibition of MEK1/2 led to decreased thyroid size, restoration of thyroid form and function, and inhibition of tumorigenesis. Mice with BRAF^{V600E}-induced PTC will provide an excellent system to study thyroid tumor initiation and progression and the evaluation of inhibitors of oncogenic BRAF signaling (Figs 1 and 2).

▶ The aim of this study was to establish a mouse model expression of BRAF^{V600E}. As shown in Fig 1, mice displayed increased thyroid size, widespread alterations in thyroid architecture, and dramatic hypothyroidism. Importantly, all mice also developed papillary thyroid carcinomas (PTC), as shown in Fig 2. Pharmacologic inhibition of MEK1/2 led to decreased thyroid size, restoration of thyroid form and function, and inhibition of tumorigenesis. Therefore, these data suggest that

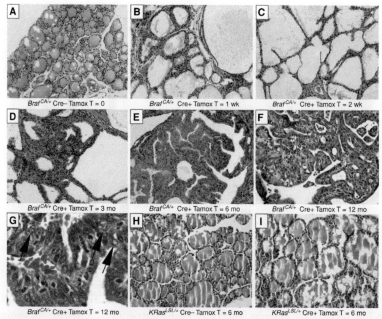

FIGURE 2.—Histologic analysis of thyroid tissue. Control (Cre-) or *Thyro::CreER* (Creþ) mice carrying either a Cre-activated *BRaf^{CA}* or *KRas^{LSL}* alleles were either untreated or treated with tamoxifen as indicated. At different times thereafter (1 week—12 months), mice were euthanized for analysis of formaldehyde-fixed, paraffin-embedded thyroid tissue by Hematoxylin and Eosin (H&E) staining. A, control *BRaf^{CA}* mice; B—G, tamoxifen-treated *Thyro::CreER; BRaf^{CA}* mice analyzed: 1 week (B); 2 weeks (C); 3 months (D); 6 months (E), or 12 months (F and G) after tamoxifen treatment. H, control *KRas^{LSL}* mice. I, *Thyro::CreER; KRas^{LSL}* mice analyzed 6 months after tamoxifen treatment. Magnification is 200× with the exception of G, which is 400×. (Reprinted from Charles R-P, Iezza G, Amendola E, et al. Mutationally activated BRAF^{V600E} elicits papillary thyroid cancer in the adult mouse. *Cancer Res.* 2011;71:3863-3871, with permission from American Association for Cancer Research.)

BRAF^{V600E}-induced PTC critically relies on MEK1/2 signaling. However, a more effective test of such agents might be in the context of BRAF^{V600E}-induced thyroid cancers with concomitant silencing of relevant tumor suppressor genes such as Trp53, Cdkn2a, or Pten. Indeed, preliminary evidence suggests that BRAF^{V600E} can cooperate with dominant-negative TP53R270H for thyroid cancer progression (as discussed by the authors). Finally, primary treatment for thyroid cancer often involves systemic radioiodide therapy. However, the effectiveness of such therapy is reportedly limited by the ability of BRAF^{V600E} to inhibit sodium-iodide symporter (NIS) expression. Hence, agents that target BRAF^{V600E} signaling might promote NIS reexpression, thereby sensitizing thyroid tumor cells to radioiodide therapy.

The authors describe a new mouse model of adult-onset thyroid cancer that displays key features of the human disease, which will complement studies on human thyrocytes and thyroid cancer lines. In addition, they show the utility of this model system to test the antitumor effects of pharmacologic inhibitors of BRAF/MEK/ERK signaling. It will be interesting to test the effects of deliberate tumor suppressor gene silencing on the propensity of BRAF^{V600E} induced PTC to progress to more aggressive disease and on the response of thyroid cancer cells to pathway-targeted therapy.

M. Schott, MD, PhD

A. Thiel, MD

Anaplastic Thyroid Cancers Harbor Novel Oncogenic Mutations of the *ALK* Gene

Murugan AK, Xing MM (Johns Hopkins Univ School of Medicine, Baltimore, MD)
Cancer Res 71:4403-4411, 2011

Thyroid cancer is the most common endocrine cancer, and targeted approaches to treat it pose considerable interest. In this study, we report the discovery of *ALK* gene mutations in thyroid cancer that may rationalize clinical evaluation of anaplastic lymphoma kinase (ALK) inhibitors in this setting. In undifferentiated anaplastic thyroid cancer (ATC), we identified two novel point mutations, C3592T and G3602A, in exon 23 of the *ALK* gene, with a prevalence of 11.11%, but found no mutations in the matched normal tissues or in well-differentiated thyroid cancers. These two mutations, resulting in L1198F and G1201E amino acid changes, respectively, both reside within the ALK tyrosine kinase domain where they dramatically increased tyrosine kinase activities. Similarly, these mutations heightened the ability of ALK to activate the phosphatidylinositol 3-kinase (PI3K)/ Akt and mitogen-activated protein (MAP) kinase pathways in established mouse cells. Further investigations showed that these two ALK mutants strongly promoted cell focus formation, anchorage-independent growth, and cell invasion. Similar oncogenic properties were observed in the neuroblastoma-associated ALK mutants K1062M and F1174L but not in wild-type ALK. Overall, our results reveal two novel gain-of-function mutations of *ALK* in certain ATCs, and they suggest efforts to clinically evaluate the use of ALK kinase inhibitors to treat patients who harbor ATCs with these mutations.

▶ Anaplastic thyroid cancer is one of the most devastating cancers. It is characterized by rapid growth and radioiodine, chemotherapy, and radiation insensitivity. Therefore, new therapy options are urgently needed.

In the present study, the authors investigated the mutation status of the anaplastic lymphoma kinase (*ALK*) gene in various thyroid cancers, including well-differentiated papillary thyroid cancer (PTC) and follicular thyroid cancer (FTC) and undifferentiated anaplastic thyroid cancer (ATC). *ALK* is a member of the insulin receptor subfamily of receptor tyrosine kinases (RTKs), with its encoding gene located on the short arm of chromosome 2. ALK was initially identified as part of an oncogenic fusion gene, *NPM1-ALK* (also known as *NPMALK*), in anaplastic large-cell non-Hodgkin lymphomas. It is also part of the fusion gene *EML4-ALK* in non—small cell lung cancer (NSCLC). There are a few other *ALK* fusion genes, such as *TMP3/4-ALK* and *RANBP2-ALK*, in inflammatory myofibroblastic tumors. The tyrosine kinase activities of these fusion ALK proteins are aberrantly activated and promote cell proliferation and survival. ALK fusion proteins have also been shown to activate various signaling pathways, among which are the phosphatidylinositol 3-kinase (PI3K)/Akt pathway and the Ras → Raf → MEK extracellular signal regulated kinase (ERK)/mitogen-activated protein (MAP) kinase pathway with multiple interaction points to mediate the ALK signaling. Mutations of the *ALK* gene have not been reported in human cancers other than neuroblastomas.

In the present study, the authors identified of novel somatic *ALK* mutations in ATC (Fig 1 in the original article). They also found increased tyrosine kinase activities of ALK mutants L1198F and G1201E and their activation of the PI3K/Akt and MAP kinase pathways (Fig 2 in the original article). These are gain-of-function mutations that cause dual activation of the PI3K/Akt and MAP kinase pathways in ATC. Development of inhibitors targeting *ALK* is an exciting current research area. Recently, it has been reported that most of the patients with NSCLC harboring *EML4-ALK* responded effectively to the treatment with an anti-*ALK* agent crizotinib,[1] which has also been recently reported to be effective in treating a patient with inflammatory myofibroblastic tumor harboring *RANBP2-ALK*. Possibly, this may be another way to establish a new therapy for ATC.

M. Schott, MD, PhD

A. Thiel, MD

Reference

1. Kwak EL, Bang YJ, Camidge DR, et al. Anaplastic lymphoma kinase inhibition in non-small-cell lung cancer. *N Engl J Med.* 2010;363:1693-1703.

Activity of XL184 (Cabozantinib), an Oral Tyrosine Kinase Inhibitor, in Patients With Medullary Thyroid Cancer

Kurzrock R, Sherman SI, Ball DW, et al (The Univ of Texas MD Anderson Cancer Ctr, Houston, TX; Univ of Chicago, IL; Sidney Kimmel Comprehensive Cancer Ctr, Baltimore, MD; et al)
J Clin Oncol 29:2660-2666, 2011

Purpose.—XL184 (cabozantinib) is a potent inhibitor of MET, vascular endothelial growth factor receptor 2 (VEGFR2), and RET, with robust antiangiogenic, antitumor, and anti-invasive effects in preclinical models. Early observations of clinical benefit in a phase I study of cabozantinib, which included patients with medullary thyroid cancer (MTC), led to expansion of an MTC-enriched cohort, which is the focus of this article.

Patients and Methods.—A phase I dose-escalation study of oral cabozantinib was conducted in patients with advanced solid tumors. Primary end points included evaluation of safety, pharmacokinetics, and maximum-tolerated dose (MTD) determination. Additional end points included RECIST (Response Evaluation Criteria in Solid Tumors) response, pharmacodynamics, *RET* mutational status, and biomarker analyses.

Results.—Eighty-five patients were enrolled, including 37 with MTC. The MTD was 175 mg daily. Dose-limiting toxicities were grade 3 palmar plantar erythrodysesthesia (PPE), mucositis, and AST, ALT, and lipase elevations and grade 2 mucositis that resulted in dose interruption and reduction. Ten (29%) of 35 patients with MTC with measurable disease had a confirmed partial response. Overall, 18 patients experienced tumor shrinkage of 30% or more, including 17 (49%) of 35 patients with MTC with measurable disease. Additionally, 15 (41%) of 37 patients with MTC had stable disease (SD) for at least 6 months, resulting in SD for 6 months or longer or confirmed partial response in 68% of patients with MTC.

Conclusion.—Cabozantinib has an acceptable safety profile and is active in MTC. Cabozantinib may provide clinical benefit by simultaneously targeting multiple pathways of importance in MTC, including MET, VEGFR2, and RET. A global phase III pivotal study in MTC is ongoing (ClinicalTrials.gov number NCT00215605) (Fig 1).

▶ The development of antiangiogenic agents targeting the vascular endothelial growth factor (VEGF)/VEGF receptor (VEGFR) signaling pathway has led to key advances in the treatment of cancer. For example, the monoclonal antibody bevacizumab and small-molecule multitargeted VEGFR tyrosine kinase inhibitors sorafenib and sunitinib have produced statistically significant survival improvements in some cancers. Cabozantinib is a potent inhibitor of proinvasive receptor tyrosine kinases, including MET, VEGFR2, and RET. In preclinical studies, cabozantinib exhibited significant antiangiogenic and antitumor activity in a broad range of tumor models, including a model of medullary thyroid cancer (MTC) with an activating RET mutation. Importantly, it has also been shown in preclinical studies that treatment with cabozantinib results in decreased tumor invasiveness and decreased metastasis compared with either vehicle control or agents targeting

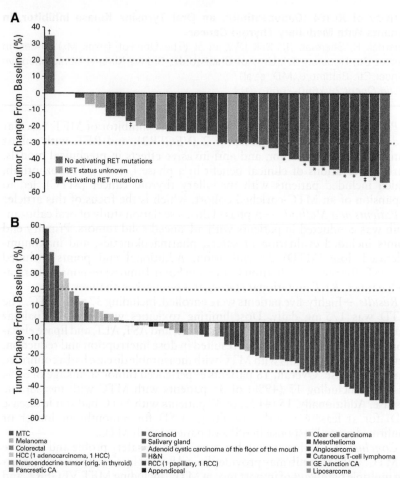

FIGURE 1.—(A) Best radiologic response in patients with medullary thyroid cancer (MTC) with one or more postbaseline scans (n = 34). Scan data available for 34 patients with MTC with measurable disease and at least one postbaseline scan. Two patients had nonmeasurable disease, and one patient had no postbaseline scan. (*) Confirmed partial response per Response Evaluation Criteria in Solid Tumors (RECIST). (†) Patient with MTC and G469A BRAF mutation. (‡) Germline RET mutation. (B) Best radiologic response in all patients with one or more postbaseline scan (n = 70). Scan data available for all patients with measurable disease and with at least one postbaseline scan. Eight patients had nonmeasurable disease and are not represented in this graph. An additional seven patients had no postbaseline scan and are also not represented in this graph. HCC, hepatocellular; CA, carcinoma; H&N, head and neck; RCC, renal cell carcinoma; GE, gastroesophageal. (Reprinted from Kurzrock R, Sherman SI, Ball DW, et al. Activity of XL184 (Cabozantinib), an oral tyrosine kinase inhibitor, in patients with medullary thyroid cancer. *J Clin Oncol.* 2011;29:2660-2666, Copyright 2011, with permission from American Society of Clinical Oncology. All rights reserved.)

VEGF signaling without MET inhibition. This report focuses on results from a phase I open-label dose-escalation study of cabozantinib in patients with a wide range of advanced malignancies, including an expanded cohort of patients with advanced MTC. Activating mutations in RET play a central role in tumorigenesis in both inherited and sporadic forms of MTC.

The present phase I dose-escalation study of oral cabozantinib was conducted in patients with advanced solid tumors. Primary end points included evaluation of safety, pharmacokinetics, and maximum tolerated dose (MTD) determination. Additional end points included Response Evaluation Criteria in Solid Tumors response and so forth. Of 35 patients with MTC with measurable disease, 29% had a confirmed partial response. Overall, 18 patients experienced tumor shrinkage of 30% or more, including 17 (49%) of 35 patients with MTC with measurable disease (Fig 1). Additionally, 15 (41%) of 37 patients with MTC had stable disease (SD) for at least 6 months, resulting in SD for 6 months or longer or confirmed partial response in 68% of patients with MTC. In summary, these phase I results indicate that cabozantinib is active in patients with MTC, including those who harbor somatic RET mutations and are potentially at high risk for progression and death. Cabozantinib has an acceptable safety profile and dose-dependent exposure and half-life supporting once-daily dosing, with only moderate interindividual variability. Future studies will evaluate the need for administration of the drug in a fasting state. Furthermore, cabozantinib is active in patients who have progressed while receiving prior therapies, including other inhibitors of RET and VEGFR2. In parallel to the present study, an international phase III study of cabozantinib is ongoing in patients with progressive MTC, which will hopefully show equal encouraging results.

M. Schott, MD, PhD

Sunitinib-Induced Hypothyroidism Is due to Induction of Type 3 Deiodinase Activity and Thyroidal Capillary Regression

Kappers MHW, van Esch JHM, Smedts FMM, et al (Erasmus Med Ctr, Rotterdam, The Netherlands)
J Clin Endocrinol Metab 96:3087-3094, 2011

Context.—Anticancer treatment with the tyrosine kinase inhibitor sunitinib causes thyroid dysfunction.

Objective.—Our objective was to investigate the time course and underlying mechanisms of sunitinib-induced thyroid dysfunction.

Design.—Thyroid function tests of 83 patients on sunitinib were collected retrospectively for their total treatment duration between January 2006 and November 2009 and prospectively in 15 patients on sunitinib for 10 wk. Additionally, thyroid function and histology were assessed in rats on sunitinib (8 d; n = 10) and after sunitinib withdrawal (11 d; n = 7) and compared with controls (n = 7).

Setting.—Patients were seen at a university outpatient oncology clinic.

Patients and Animals.—Patients with metastatic renal cell carcinoma or gastrointestinal stromal tumors participated in the clinical study and Wistar Kyoto rats were used in the rat study.

Intervention.—Sunitinib was taken according to a 4 wk "on," 2 wk "off" treatment regimen. Blood samples for measurement of thyroid function were collected at baseline and at wk 4 and 10. In rats, blood, liver, and thyroid were collected to assess thyroid hormones, deiodinase activity, and thyroid histology.

Main Outcome Measures.—TSH and free T_4 levels, deiodinase activity, and thyroid histology were assessed.

Results.—Forty-two percent of patients in the retrospective study developed elevated TSH levels. Prospective analysis showed increased TSH levels within 10 wk of treatment, accompanied by a decreased T_3/rT_3 ratio. In rats, serum T_4 and T_3 decreased, hepatic type 3 deiodinase activity increased, and thyroid histology showed marked capillary regression, which all but thyroid hormones reversed after sunitinib withdrawal.

Conclusion.—Sunitinib induces hypothyroidism due to alterations in T_4/T_3 metabolism as well as thyroid capillary regression.

▶ The multikinase inhibitor, sunitinib, is broadly used in anticancer therapy, including in renal cell cancer but also in endocrine malignancies such as dedifferentiated thyroid cancer and neuroendocrine cancer. The aim of this study was to obtain more insight into the time course, incidence, and mechanisms involved in sunitinib-associated thyroid dysfunction. In agreement with previous reports, the authors found that sunitinib-induced hypothyroidism, as reflected by increased serum thyroid-stimulating hormone (TSH) values, develops in a substantial proportion of patients. Prospective evaluation of the time course of ensuing thyroid dysfunction showed an increase in TSH levels already within 10 weeks of treatment, although values at this time were still within the normal reference range. In the past, it has been proposed that hypothyroidism in patients receiving sunitinib might be due to the induction of an autoimmune process. Here the increase in TSH was, however, not accompanied by increased circulating antithyroid peroxidase antibodies. Second, the incidence of autoimmune-mediated thyroiditis is much higher in women than in men. The observation that the incidence of transiently elevated TSH levels was similar in women and men in this study makes an autoimmune-mediated mechanism less likely. Third, histologic examination of the thyroid of rats exposed to sunitinib did not show an inflammatory reaction that would have been suggestive for immune-mediated damage. Based on a rat model, the authors found das serum T_4 and T_3 decreased and hepatic type 3 deiodinase activity increased, and thyroid histology showed marked capillary regression (Figs 3 and 4 in the original article), which all but thyroid hormones reversed after sunitinib withdrawal. This article describes for the first time the mechanistic background of sunitinib-induced hypothyroidism.

A. Thiel, MD

M. Schott, MD, PhD

Neuropilin-2 Expression in Papillary Thyroid Carcinoma: Correlation with VEGF-D Expression, Lymph Node Metastasis, and VEGF-D-Induced Aggressive Cancer Cell Phenotype

Yasuoka H, Kodama R, Hirokawa M, et al (Wakayama Med Univ, Japan; Kuma Hosp, Kobe, Japan)

J Clin Endocrinol Metab 96:E1857-E1861, 2011

Context.—Neuropilin-2 (Nrp2) is a coreceptor for vascular endothelial growth factor-D (VEGF-D) that is expressed on the surface of endothelial cells. Recently, Nrp2 was shown to play a role in lymph node metastasis and promotion of cancer cell migration. VEGF-D also promotes lymphangiogenesis, which in turn promotes tumor metastasis.

Objective.—The aim was to study the role of neuropilin-2 in lymph node metastasis in human papillary thyroid carcinoma (PTC).

Design.—Expression of Nrp2 was studied by immunohistochemistry and the relationship between Nrp2 expression and lymph node metastasis, VEGF-D expression and other established clinicopathological variables were analyzed in PTC. The effects of neutralizing anti-Nrp2 antibody on VEGF-D-induced invasion and migration were assessed in PTC cell lines.

Results.—Nrp2 expression was observed in 64.3% (36 of 56) of the PTC patients. Nrp2 expression was significantly correlated with lymph node metastasis $(P = 0.0216)$ and VEGF-D expression $(P = 0.0034)$. VEGF-D was shown to promote filopodia formation and cancer cell migration and invasion by K1 and B-CPAP cells. These responses were significantly blocked by neutralizing anti-Nrp2 antibody.

Conclusion.—Nrp2 expression was correlated with lymph node metastasis and VEGF-D expression in PTC. Our data also showed a role for Nrp2 in regulating VEGF-D-induced invasion and migration in vitro (Table 1).

▶ Neuropilin-2 (Nrp2) is a nontyrosine kinase transmembrane glycoprotein and was first identified on neurons. Recently, Nrp2 was additionally detected on endothelial and tumor cells acting as a coreceptor for vascular endothelial growth factor-D (VEGF-D). Furthermore, it appeared to be involved in tumor migration in breast cancer and promoted growth and angiogenesis in pancreatic adenocarcinoma. Moreover, in breast cancer Nrp2 significantly correlated with lymph node metastasis and a poor prognosis.[1] VEGF-D has previously been shown to support lymph node metastasis in papillary thyroid carcinoma, among other human cancers. In this study, the authors reveal a correlation between Nrp2 expression, lymph node metastasis, and VEGF-D expression in papillary thyroid carcinoma (Table 1). Furthermore, they demonstrate that VEGF-D promotes filopodia formation in cell lines in vitro, and that VEGF-D action is dependent on Nrp2. As the papillary thyroid carcinoma route of spreading mainly occurs via the lymphatic channels, it seems reasonable to unravel the nebulous pathomechanisms involved in disease progress. Recently, it has been proposed that VEGF-D expression and increased lymph vessel density play a key role.[2] However, the role of Nrp2 expression in papillary thyroid carcinoma has not yet been investigated. Therefore, this work may contribute to the revelation of pathways leading to metastasis and

TABLE 1.—Clinicopathological Data for 56 PTC Cases and Relationship Between Nrp2 Expression and Covariates

Factors	Nrp2 Expression		P Value
	Negative	Positive	
Age			
<45 yr	8 (38%)	13 (62%)	0.7815
≥45 yr	12 (34%)	23 (66%)	
Sex			
Male	2 (29%)	5 (71%)	0.6733
Female	18 (37%)	31 (63%)	
Histology			
Common	16 (33%)	33 (67%)	0.2350
Follicular variant	3 (75%)	1 (25%)	
Tall cell variant	1 (33%)	2 (67%)	
Tumor size			
pT1	3 (43%)	4 (57%)	0.4042
pT2	12 (32%)	25 (68%)	
pT3	3 (75%)	1 (25%)	
pT4	2 (25%	6 (75%)	
Lymph node metastasis			
pN0	9 (64%)	5 (36%)	0.0216
pN1	11 (26%)	31 (74%)	
VEGF-D expression			
Negative	18 (50%)	18 (50%)	0.0034
Positive	2 (10%)	18 (90%)	

Tumor size (T), lymph node metastasis (N), and distant metastasis (M) were classified according to the TNM classification of the Union for International Cancer Control, 2002. Fisher's exact test or χ^2 test was used to examine the association between Nrp2 expression and covariates.

tumor invasion. Filopodia formation, which is clearly linked to VEGF-D and thus Nrp2, has especially been shown to have an important impact on tumor metastasis.[3] Further studies of interest would be to investigate whether Nrp2 also has an impact on migration controlled by CXCR4, as previously demonstrated in breast cancer. Additionally, in vivo studies are needed to analyze the effect of anti-Nrp2-antibodies on tumor metastasis, as already successfully demonstrated in a model for lung metastasis. Altogether, this work hopefully will present potential alternative therapeutic approaches for papillary thyroid cancer. Larger studies and preclinical trials will have to prove the possible clinical benefit of these findings.

M. Schott, MD, PhD

References

1. Yasuoka H, Kodama R, Tsujimoto M, et al. Neuropilin-2 expression in breast cancer: correlation with lymph node metastasis, poor prognosis, and regulation of CXCR4 expression. *BMC Cancer.* 2009;9:220.
2. Yasuoka H, Nakamura Y, Zuo H, et al. VEGF-D expression and lymph vessels play an important role for lymph node metastasis in papillary thyroid carcinoma. *Mod Pathol.* 2005;18:1127-1133.
3. Machesky LM. Lamellipodia and filopodia in metastasis and invasion. *FEBS Lett.* 2008;582:2102-2111.

Glucagon Like Peptide-1 Receptor Expression in the Human Thyroid Gland

Gier B, Butler PC, Lai CK, et al (David Geffen School of Medicine at the Univ of California, Los Angeles)
J Clin Endocrinol Metab 97:121-131, 2012

Background.—Glucagon like peptide-1 (GLP-1) mimetic therapy induces medullary thyroid neoplasia in rodents. We sought to establish whether C cells in human medullary thyroid carcinoma, C cell hyperplasia, and normal human thyroid express the GLP-1 receptor.

Methods.—Thyroid tissue samples with medullary thyroid carcinoma (n = 12), C cell hyperplasia (n = 9), papillary thyroid carcinoma (n = 17), and normal human thyroid (n = 15) were evaluated by immunofluorescence for expression of calcitonin and GLP-1 receptors.

Results.—Coincident immunoreactivity for calcitonin and GLP-1 receptor was consistently observed in both medullary thyroid carcinoma and C cell hyperplasia. GLP-1 receptor immunoreactivity was also detected in 18% of papillary thyroid carcinoma (three of 17 cases). Within normal human thyroid tissue, GLP-1 receptor immunoreactivity was found in five of 15 of the examined cases in about 35% of the total C cells assessed.

Conclusions.—In humans, neoplastic and hyperplastic lesions of thyroid C cells express the GLP-1 receptor. GLP-1 receptor expression is detected in 18% papillary thyroid carcinomas and in C cells in 33% of control thyroid lobes. The consequence of long-term pharmacologically increased GLP-1 signaling on these GLP-1 receptor-expressing cells in the thyroid gland in humans remains unknown, but appropriately powered prospective studies to exclude an increase in medullary or papillary carcinomas of the thyroid are warranted.

▶ The aim of this study was to investigate the glucagon like peptide-1 (GLP-1) receptor expression on thyroid tissue, especially on thyroid tumors. The GLP-1 receptor expression was consistently observed in both medullary thyroid cancer and C cell hyperplasia. One example of a patient with medullary thyroid cancer is given in Fig 2 in the original article. Importantly, GLP-1 receptor expression was also detected in 18% of papillary thyroid carcinomas. These results are, therefore, in broad agreement with the work of Korner et al,[1] who found GLP-1 receptor expression in approximately 30% of medullary thyroid carcinomas by use of GLP-1 receptor scintigraphy, and Bjerre Knudsen et al,[2] who reported that GLP-1 receptors are rarely present in normal human thyroid C cells. The data lend mechanistic plausibility to the apparent signal of increased reported thyroid tumors in patients treated with exenatide in the US Food and Drug Administration Adverse Event Reporting database.[3] Such a signal would seem unlikely to arise exclusively from medullary thyroid cancer, given the rarity of this tumor, but it would be less surprising if long-term pharmacologic exposure to GLP-1—based therapy was to promote the growth of the relatively common small papillary thyroid carcinomas present in the general population.

M. Schott, MD, PhD

A. Thiel, MD

References

1. Körner M, Stöckli M, Waser B, Reubi JC. GLP-1 receptor expression in human tumors and human normal tissues: potential for in vivo targeting. *J Nucl Med.* 2007;48:736-743.
2. Bjerre Knudsen L, Madsen LW, Andersen S, et al. Glucagon-like Peptide-1 receptor agonists activate rodent thyroid C-cells causing calcitonin release and C-cell proliferation. *Endocrinology.* 2010;151:1473-1486.
3. Elashoff M, Matveyenko AV, Gier B, Elashoff R, Butler PC. Pancreatitis, pancreatic, and thyroid cancer with glucagon-like peptide-1-based therapies. *Gastroenterology.* 2011;141:150-156.

Thyroid Disease in Pregnancy

Antenatal Thyroid Screening and Childhood Cognitive Function

Lazarus JH, Bestwick JP, Channon S, et al (Cardiff Univ School of Medicine, Wales, UK; Queen Mary Univ of London, UK; St David's Hosp, Cardiff, UK; et al)

N Engl J Med 366:493-501, 2012

Background.—Children born to women with low thyroid hormone levels have been reported to have decreased cognitive function.

Methods.—We conducted a randomized trial in which pregnant women at a gestation of 15 weeks 6 days or less provided blood samples for measurement of thyrotropin and free thyroxine (T_4). Women were assigned to a screening group (in which measurements were obtained immediately) or a control group (in which serum was stored and measurements were obtained shortly after delivery). Thyrotropin levels above the 97.5th percentile, free T_4 levels below the 2.5th percentile, or both were considered a positive screening result. Women with positive findings in the screening group were assigned to 150 μg of levothyroxine per day. The primary outcome was IQ at 3 years of age in children of women with positive results, as measured by psychologists who were unaware of the group assignments.

Results.—Of 21,846 women who provided blood samples (at a median gestational age of 12 weeks 3 days), 390 women in the screening group and 404 in the control group tested positive. The median gestational age at the start of levothyroxine treatment was 13 weeks 3 days; treatment was adjusted as needed to achieve a target thyrotropin level of 0.1 to 1.0 mIU per liter. Among the children of women with positive results, the mean IQ scores were 99.2 and 100.0 in the screening and control groups, respectively (difference, 0.8; 95% confidence interval [CI], −1.1 to 2.6; $P = 0.40$ by intention-to-treat analysis); the proportions of children with an IQ of less than 85 were 12.1% in the screening group and 14.1% in the control group (difference, 2.1 percentage points; 95% CI, −2.6 to 6.7; $P = 0.39$). An on-treatment analysis showed similar results.

Conclusions.—Antenatal screening (at a median gestational age of 12 weeks 3 days) and maternal treatment for hypothyroidism did not result in improved cognitive function in children at 3 years of age. (Funded

TABLE 2.—Standardized Full-Scale Child IQ and Scores on the Child Behavior Checklist (CBCL) and the Behavior Rating Inventory of Executive Function, Preschool Version (Brief-P), According to Study Group*

Test	Screening Group (N = 390)	Control Group (N = 404)	Difference (95% CI) (Control Group − Screening Group)[†]	P Value
IQ				
Mean	99.2±13.3	100.0±13.3	0.8 (−1.1 to 2.6)	0.40
<85 (% of children)	12.1	14.1	2.1 (−2.6 to 6.7)	0.39
CBCL T score[‡]				
Mean	44.4±12.4	45.1±13.6	0.7 (−1.2 to 2.5)	0.49
Brief-P T score[§]				
Median	40	40	0	0.59
Interquartile range	47–55	47–55		

*Plus—minus values are means ± SD. The full-scale child IQ test was standardized so that for each psychologist, the mean score among the children in the control group whom they tested was 100. In the screening group, the women were assigned to treatment with levothyroxine.
[†]For percentages of children with an IQ below 85, the absolute (percentage-point) differences are shown.
[‡]For the CBCL, a T score above the 98th percentile is indicative of a clinically significant problem.
[§]For the Brief-P, a T score above 65 is indicative of a clinically significant problem.

by the Wellcome Trust UK and Compagnia di San Paulo, Turin; Current Controlled Trials number, ISRCTN46178175.) (Table 2).

▶ In 1999, Haddow et al[1] reported on a lower IQ score in children (at age 7 to 9) of untreated pregnant women with hypothyroidism compared with children from euthyroid mothers.[2] The mean (±SD) serum thyroid-stimulating hormone (TSH) level in the women with hypothyroidism was 13.2 ± 0.3 mU/L compared with 1.4 ± 0.2 mU/L in control euthyroid mothers (P < .001), with 9 of 62 women having TSH values greater than 30 mU/L. Serum free thyroxine (T_4) and free T_4 were also significantly different between hypothyroid and euthyroid women. In the current study by Lazarus et al, the median serum TSH in women with hypothyroidism was 3.8 mIU/L in the screening group and 3.2 mIU/L in the women in the control group (not treated) (interquartile ranges, 1.5 to 4.7 and 1.2 to 4.2, respectively). Here, the authors did not find any significant differences in IQ (Table 2). Figs 2 and 3 in the original article show the relative risk of an IQ score according to the intention-to-treat analysis and the on-treatment analysis. This is an excellent study showing that slightly elevated maternal TSH levels may not influence outcome of children in terms of IQ (at least in the younger age). Nonetheless, there are still open questions. Additional randomized studies are needed to answer 3 important clinical questions. (1) Does starting L-T_4 therapy early in pregnancy in women with subclinical hypothyroidism—and also in euthyroid women with chronic thyroiditis—prevent obstetric or long-term complications in offspring? (2) If so, is universal or case finding early in pregnancy cost effective in preventing such complications? (3) What initial screening tests should be performed: TSH, free T_4 or equivalent, or anti-thyroid peroxidase antibodies? In the meantime, physicians treating women of reproductive age should be aware that a significant number of them have symptoms that could indicate thyroid disease that prompt assessment of thyroid status, and, if there is evidence of hypothyroidism, L-T$_4$ therapy is of potential benefit not only to the patient during the current pregnancy but also if there is a subsequent pregnancy. At this point, once a woman is pregnant, whether to perform universal screening or case finding is a decision based on personal experience.[2]

A. Thiel, MD

M. Schott, MD, PhD

References

1. Haddow JE, Palomaki GE, Allan WC, et al. Maternal thyroid deficiency during pregnancy and subsequent neuropsychological development of the child. *N Engl J Med*. 1999;341:549-555.
2. Mestman JH. The evidence of performing universal screening for detection of thyroid disease in pregnancy continues to be "soft" [commentary]. *Clin Thyroid*. 2012;24:5-7.

Thyroid Nodules

On the prevalence of the *PAX8-PPARG* fusion resulting from the chromosomal translocation t(2;3)(q13;p25) in adenomas of the thyroid
Klemke M, Drieschner N, Laabs A, et al (Univ of Bremen, Germany; et al)
Cancer Genet 204:334-339, 2011

The chromosomal translocation t(2;3)(q13;p25) characterizes a subgroup of tumors originating from the thyroid follicular epithelium and was initially discovered in a few cases of adenomas. Later, a fusion of the genes *PAX8* and *PPARG* resulting from this translocation was frequently observed in follicular carcinomas and considered as a marker of follicular thyroid cancer. According to subsequent studies, however, this rearrangement is not confined to carcinomas but also occurs in adenomas, with considerably varying frequencies. Only five cases of thyroid adenomas with this translocation detected by conventional cytogenetics have been documented. In contrast, studies using reverse-transcription polymerase chain reaction (RT-PCR) detected fusion transcripts resulting from that translocation in an average of 8.2% of adenomas. The aim of this study was to determine the frequency of the *PAX8-PPARG* fusion in follicular adenomas and to use the *HMGA2* mRNA level of such tumors as an indicator of malignancy. In cytogenetic studies of 192 follicular adenomas, the t(2;3)(q13;p25) has been identified in only two cases described herein. Histopathology revealed no evidence of malignancy in either case, and, concordantly, *HMGA2* mRNA levels were not elevated. In summary, the fusion is a rare event in follicular adenomas and its prevalence may be overestimated in many RT-PCR—based studies.

▶ Distinguishing follicular thyroid carcinomas (FTC) from adenomas cytologically represents a major diagnostic challenge because of their similar appearance, so there is a need for specific markers. The chromosomal t(2;3)(q13;p25) is a recurrent cytogenetic aberration in follicular neoplasias of the thyroid leading to a fusion of the genes encoding the thyroid-specific transcription factor PAX8 and the peroxisome proliferator-activated receptor gamma (PPARG). Although the translocation had been reported before in adenomas as well, the PAX8-PPARG rearrangement was considered a marker of FTC in a study by Kroll et al[1] who detected PAX8-PPARG fusion transcripts in 5/8 FTCs but in none of 20 follicular adenomas, 10 papillary carcinomas, and 10 multinodular hyperplasias. In recent studies of fine-needle aspiration biopsy material, the PAX8-PPARG rearrangement has also been studied. It was found in 1 of 84 biopsies in 1 study with the pathology showing a follicular carcinoma,[2] but it was not was found in any of 235 samples in another biopsy study.[3] These 2 studies were done by reverse-transcription polymerase chain reaction (RT-PCR), the method that could lead to false-positive results according to the current report. However, because of the rarity of the PAX8-PPARG rearrangement, only 8.2% when detected by RT-PCR, it is probably appropriate to send patients who have this molecular marker to surgery, although the data from this study suggest that false-positive results are lower than previously reported, even by RT-PCR. Some believe that large follicular adenomas are precursors to follicular carcinoma. The presence of the PAX8-PPARG rearrangement provides some evidence for this concept. Nevertheless, the RT-PCR may result in a 4-fold increase of false-positive diagnosis of follicular carcinoma when the pathologic diagnosis is follicular adenoma.[4]

M. Schott, MD, PhD

References

1. Kroll TG, Sarraf P, Pecciarini L, et al. PAX8-PPARgamma1 fusion oncogene in human thyroid carcinoma [corrected]. *Science.* 2000;289:1357-1360.
2. Nikiforov YE, Steward DL, Robinson-Smith TM, et al. Molecular testing for mutations in improving the fine-needle aspiration diagnosis of thyroid nodules. *J Clin Endocrinol Metab.* 2009;94:2092-2098.
3. Cantara S, Capezzone M, Marchisotta S, et al. Impact of proto-oncogene mutation detection in cytological specimens from thyroid nodules improves the diagnostic accuracy of cytology. *J Clin Endocrinol Metab.* 2010;95:1365-1369.
4. Hershman JM. On the prevalence of the PAX8-PPARG fusion resulting from the chromosomal translocation t(2;3)(q13;p25) in adenomas of the thyroid. *Clin Thyroidology.* 2011;23:11-12.

Delta-Like 4/Notch Pathway Is Differentially Regulated in Benign and Malignant Thyroid Tissues
Geers C, Colin IM, Gérard A-C (Vrij Univ of Brussels (VUB), Belgium; Catholic Univ of Louvain (UCL), Brussels, Belgium)
Thyroid 21:1323-1330, 2011

Background.—Angiogenesis plays an essential role in embryonic and tumoral developments. Vascular endothelial growth factor (VEGF), one of the best known proangiogenic factors, is increased in thyroid cancers, especially in papillary carcinomas (PC). However, other regulating mechanisms refine VEGF-induced cellular changes, such as the Notch family of ligands and receptors. Their role has not yet been investigated in the thyroid. The purpose of our study was to analyze the expression of Notch1, Notch4, and Delta-like 4 (DLL4) in benign and malignant thyroid lesions.

Methods.—The expression of Notch1, Notch4, and DLL4 was analyzed by immunohistochemistry, quantitative reverse transcriptase—polymerase chain reaction (qRT-PCR), and Western-blot in normal thyroids (NTs), hyperplasic thyroids from patients with Graves' disease (GD), microcarcinomas, PC, and follicular carcinomas.

Results.—The immunohistochemical expression of Notch1, Notch4, and DLL4 was highly variable in thyrocytes from NTs and GD. In contrast, the staining in tumors was homogeneous and often intense. The increased expression of Notch1, Notch4, and DLL4 in carcinomas compared with the neighboring normal tissue was confirmed by qRT-PCR and Western-blot. However, only capillary endothelial cells from GD samples were positive for DLL4, the expression being restricted to large vessels in carcinomas and NTs.

Conclusions.—The detection of Notch1, Notch4, and DLL4 in thyrocytes and their regulation in various pathologies suggest that this pathway may play a role in thyroid carcinogenesis and angiogenesis.

▶ Proangiogenic factors significantly contribute to the development of different tumor entities.[1] Vascular endothelial growth factor (VEGF) is one of the best known proangiogenic factors and has been well established in thyroid cancer. However, factors modulating proangiogenic molecules, including the Notch family and its ligands, have not been well defined in the thyroid.[1,2] As several tumors show a resistance toward therapies targeting VEGF, the identification of additional regulators of angiogenesis is required to develop alternative therapeutic strategies. The Notch family has been proposed to be one of the main regulators of VEGF signaling. In this study, the authors provide evidence for the expression of Notch1, Notch4, and Delta-like 4 (DLL4) in the thyroid besides their regulation in different thyroid diseases. The Notch receptor is a transmembrane protein, which partly translocates into the nucleus and triggers the transcription of different genes subsequent to stimulation. The DLL4 ligand is the specific ligand for Notch1 and Notch4 and is thought to play a central role in the regulation of angiogenesis. DLL4 is induced by VEGF and decreases VEGF-R expression by activating Notch1. Furthermore, DLL4 also prevents excessive vessel proliferation and has been shown to block the growth of anti-VEGF—resistant tumors. In this study it was demonstrated that DLL4 mRNA and DLL4 protein expression in thyroid papillary carcinoma (PC) was significantly higher than in normal tissues (NT) and colloid nodules. The number of DLL4-positive cells was also higher in follicular carcinomas and in microcarcinomas than in normal, although less than in PC. Immunohistologic staining found that in addition to thyrocytes, DLL-4 was also detected in vessels. Endothelial staining for DLL4 was restricted to large vessels in NTs and in cancers, whereas small vessels were only positive in Graves disease (GD). Thyroid PC also revealed a significantly higher Notch1 and Notch4 expression compared with NT tissues and colloid nodules. In GD thyroids, the number of highly positive cells for Notch1 was significantly decreased compared with NTs. Altogether, the authors demonstrate an overexpression of DLL4, Notch1, and Notch4 in thyroid cancer. Interestingly, the 3 proteins are expressed in both thyrocytes and endothelial cells. The observation that DLL4 is absent in small vessels of neoplastic thyroids along with a high VEGF expression may be interpreted as a loss of finely tuned angiogenesis in malignant lesions. Conversely, in hyperplastic benign thyroids, although the vasculature is hypertrophic, DLL4 expression is present in the microvessels, thus suggesting that the growing vasculature is controlled to a certain extent. These findings may blaze a trail for new therapeutic approaches in thyroid cancer and autoimmune diseases.

M. Schott, MD, PhD

A. Thiel, MD

References

1. Sakurai T, Kudo M. Signaling pathways governing tumor angiogenesis. *Oncology.* 2011;81:24-29.
2. Kacer D, McIntire C, Kirov A, et al. Regulation of non-classical FGF1 release and FGF-dependent cell transformation by CBF1-mediated notch signaling. *J Cell Physiol.* 2011;226:3064-3075.

Thyrotoxicosis

A Hidden Solution

Pramyothin P, Leung AM, Pearce EN, et al (Boston Med Ctr and Boston Univ School of Medicine, MA; et al)

N Engl J Med 365:2123-2127, 2011

Background.—The thyroid gland maintains normal thyroid function in the presence of excess iodine through a transient decline in thyroid hormone synthesis. If the effect persists, however, excess iodine can produce hypothyroidism or hyperthyroidism.

Case Report.—Woman, 51, reported a 6-month history of intermittent palpitations, fast but regular heart rate, and recent worsening fatigue, heat intolerance, and weight loss despite a good appetite. She had suffered a spinal cord injury at T12 at age 21 years, leaving her paraplegic with associated fecal and urinary incontinence. She underwent a colostomy and urinary diversion with a Koch pouch that required self-catheterization several times a day. She developed urinary tract infections intermittently and was receiving recombinant human parathyroid hormone, calcium, and vitamin D for osteoporosis. She was independent in a wheelchair, was able to drive, and maintained a full-time job. Physical examination revealed a pulse of 99 beats per minute, normal blood pressure, and a slightly enlarged, nontender thyroid gland that was firm on palpation and exhibited a pebbly surface with no discrete nodules. She had no exophthalmos, extraocular muscle weakness, or lid lag, and the results of her cardiovascular and abdominal examinations were normal. Her serum thyrotropin level was undetectable. Her serum thyroxine (T_4) level was 14.2 $\mu g/dl$, triiodothyronine (T_3) level was 97 ng/dl, T_4 resin uptake was 37%, and free T_4 index was 4.9. Tests of thyroid peroxidase antibodies, thyroglobulin antibodies, and thyroid-stimulating immunoglobulin were negative. Her thyroid ultrasound study revealed a slightly enlarged but diffusely hypoechoic thyroid gland with no marked increase in intraglandular vascular flow. The iodine-123 uptake at 24 hours was 1.8%, with poor images because of this low level.

The patient denied the use of exogenous thyroid hormone, thyroid extract, or other iodine-rich dietary supplements. She had not had any recent radiographic studies using iodine-containing contrast agents. However, she had used povidone-iodine swabs for many years before urinary self-catheterization four to five times daily. Her serum thyroglobulin level was 69.9 ng/mL. Serum inorganic iodide concentration was markedly elevated (57 $\mu g/L$) shortly after she performed a povidone-iodine swabbing and self-catheterization. She was diagnosed with thyrotoxicosis related to excess iodine exposure.

The patient was asked to stop using povidone-iodine swabs and substituted chlorhexidine swabs. She was given a beta-adrenergic blocker to manage her tachycardia. After 8 weeks, she had normal thyroid hormone levels and a detectable thyrotropin level. At 12 weeks, her 24-hour thyroid uptake of iodine-123 was normal. All symptoms of thyrotoxicosis had abated.

Conclusions.—The widely used antiseptic povidone-iodine 10% topically can be absorbed systemically through mucosal surfaces and at areas of skin breakage. The excess iodine in this patient probably resulted from absorption at the mucosal opening of her ileal pouch during self-catheterization. The low thyroid uptake of iodine-123 was extremely useful in this diagnosis, since few disorders cause low uptake (Table 1).

▶ Multiple etiological factors can potentially be involved in the development of thyrotoxicosis, and often diagnosis is challenging in daily routine. In this article, the authors approach the subject in the form of a dialogue, presenting clinical facts in stages to an expert clinician, who responds to the information, integrating the reader into his approach and conclusions. The patient introduced in the dialogue presents with thyrotoxicosis combined with a complicated medical history and eventually, during evaluation, a contamination with iodine emerges as the cause of thyrotoxicosis.

Chronologically, anamnesis presents the reader with an oligosymptomatic hyperthyroidism and a spinal cord injury in the past, necessitating daily self-catheterizations. The examination was inconspicuous and an electrocardiogram

TABLE 1.—Differential Diagnosis of Thyrotoxicosis and Tests That May Help Distinguish among the Various Causes

Cause	Thyroid Iodine-123 Uptake	Thyroid Peroxidase Antibodies	Thyroid-Stimulating Immunoglobulin	Thyroglobulin
Graves' disease	Elevated	Usually positive	Usually positive	Increased
Toxic nodular goiter	Elevated	Negative	Negative	Increased
Thyrotropin-secreting pituitary adenoma	Elevated	Negative	Negative	Increased
Trophoblastic tumor	Elevated	Negative	Negative	Increased
Hyperemesis gravidarum	Elevated	Negative	Negative	Increased
Painful thyroiditis	Low	Negative	Negative	Increased
Silent lymphocytic thyroiditis	Low	Usually positive	Negative	Increased
Drugs (amiodarone, interferon alfa, and lithium)	Low	Usually negative	Negative	Increased
Iodine-induced hyperthyroidism	Low	Usually negative	Negative	Increased
Struma ovarii	Low	Negative	Negative	Increased
Thyrotoxicosis factitia	Low	Negative	Negative	Decreased

revealed sinus tachycardia without other abnormalities. After ruling out an infection besides metabolic disorders, thyrotoxicosis is suspected at this point in the text and underlined by presentation of laboratory parameters. The most common cause of this condition in a woman of this age (Graves disease) is discussed in the dialogue and also ruled out by laboratory parameters and ultrasonography. There was no evidence for toxic nodular goiter, and the uptake of radioactive iodine was low. The authors discuss this part of the dialogue as an important crossroad in diagnosing, as medications associated with low-uptake thyrotoxicosis could be ruled out and the negative tests for thyroid peroxidase and thyroglobulin antibodies provided further evidence against silent lymphocytic thyroiditis. Furthermore, slightly elevated thyroglobulin levels in the absence of thyroglobulin antibodies essentially ruled out thyrotoxicosis factitia, so contamination with iodine remained the most likely cause. Subsequent to further systematic evaluation, use of povidone iodine for self- catheterizations was presented as the cause of thyrotoxicosis.

Later in the article, the authors also provide background information and discuss the Wolff-Chaikoff effect in different pathophysiological settings. The authors emphasize the necessity of an accurate medical history, the importance of a logical approach to the subject, and the special status of iodine-123 uptake in the differential diagnosis of thyrotoxicosis (Table 1). This article is a valuable contribution to the clinical management of thyrotoxicosis.

A. Thiel, MD

M. Schott, MD, PhD

5 Calcium and Bone Metabolism

Introduction

A variety of interesting clinical studies were published in the area of calcium and bone disorders during the last year. Several of the studies presented in this section describe results of major clinical trials or pathophysiology studies published this past year in the clinically important area of osteoporosis. The rest of the papers evaluate various aspects of mineral and vitamin D metabolism and metabolic bone disease. These studies focus attention on many of the major advances in our understanding of calcium and bone disorders. These studies are collectively impacting clinical endocrine practice significantly already. As with any review of selected papers from the literature, there were many other significant papers published this past year that could not be included in this short chapter.

The first section focuses on current issues in osteoporosis therapy. One of the major unresolved questions regarding bisphosphonate therapies is the optimum duration of therapy for each agent. The first report (5-1) evaluated the effects of zoledronic acid given once yearly over 6 years to postmenopausal osteoporotic women compared to effects seen when zoledronic acid was given once yearly over 3 years, followed by placebo for 3 years. This study is similar to the FLEX trial with alendronate, except that zoledronic acid was given for 3 years rather than 5 years. The findings suggested that many osteoporotic women may be able to complete 3 years of yearly zoledronic acid infusions, and then stop therapy for at least 3 years without adversely affecting their fracture risk. However, the findings also suggested that patients at high risk of fracture, especially vertebral fracture, should probably continue to receive therapy, rather than taking a drug holiday, because of the increased risk of vertebral fracture in those who stopped therapy at 3 years.

The next article (5-2) reported that discontinuation of risedronate treatment for 1 year in patients who had received 2 to 7 years of continuous risedronate therapy led to increases in the bone resorption marker NTx-telopeptide, corrected for creatinine, toward the baseline pretreatment level, and was associated with decreases in femoral trochanter and total hip bone mineral density (BMD). These findings suggested that discontinuation of risedronate leads to onset of bone loss more rapidly than discontinuation of alendronate or zoledronic acid. The implication is that duration of antiresorptive effect varies between bisphosphonates, and that not all bisphosphonates may be stopped for 3 years or 5 years without increased fracture risk.

The next 5 papers (5-3 through 5-7) summarize findings of major clinical trials with the new antiresorptive osteoporosis agent denosumab. Denosumab is a fully human monoclonal antibody that is a first-in-class inhibitor of receptor activator of nuclear factor κB (RANK) ligand (RANKL). Denosumab acts as an antiresorptive agent by potently suppressing osteoclast activity by blocking the interaction of RANKL with RANK on the surface of osteoclasts and osteoclast precursors. This agent was approved for treatment of postmenopausal osteoporosis in the United States on June 1, 2010. The first paper (5-3) reported the effects of treatment of postmenopausal women with osteoporosis with 5 years of continuous therapy with denosumab, as part of a 2-year extension study to the original 3-year pivotal fracture trial. The women in this study continued to have reduced markers of bone turnover and increased BMD over 5 years, as well as low fracture rates and a favorable risk/benefit profile. No new or worsened risks were seen over 5 years of continuous therapy, including risks of serious infections or malignancies. The next paper (5-4) reported that, unlike other antiresorptive therapies, a major part of the fracture risk reduction due to denosumab resulted from improvement in BMD. The study concluded that previous patient-level studies may have underestimated the strength of the relationship between BMD change and treatment effect on fracture risk, or that this relationship may be unique to denosumab. The following study (5-5) reported that denosumab 60 mg administered subcutaneously every 6 months for 3 years to postmenopausal women with osteoporosis caused reduced risk of new vertebral fractures to a similar degree in all subgroups in the study population. However, the effect of denosumab on nonvertebral fracture risk differed by femoral neck BMD, body mass index (BMI), and prevalent vertebral fracture at baseline. These findings indicated that denosumab is different from other antiresorptive drugs, where efficacy of vertebral fracture reduction differs by patient characteristics, such as age, BMD, and fracture history. The next paper (5-6) demonstrated that denosumab reduced the incidence of new vertebral and hip fractures in postmenopausal women with osteoporosis who were at higher risk for fracture, highlighting the consistent antifracture efficacy of denosumab in patients with varying degrees of fracture risk. Denosumab effectively prevented fractures in women with baseline multiple and/or moderate or severe prevalent vertebral fractures, those aged 75 years or older, and those with femoral neck BMD T-scores of -2.5 or less. The final study (5-7) evaluated the benefits and risks of denosumab in subjects with chronic kidney disease (CKD) that participated in the Fracture Reduction Evaluation of Denosumab in Osteoporosis Every 6 Months (FREEDOM) Study. The study contained 73 women with an estimated glomerular filtration rate (eGFR) of 15 to 29 mL/min (stage IV CKD), 2817 between 30 to 59 mL/min (stage III CKD), 4069 between 60 to 89 mL/min (stage II CKD), and 842 above 90 mL/min (stage I CKD). None of the subjects had stage 5 CKD. The study concluded that denosumab was effective at reducing fracture risk in subjects regardless of the stage of CKD and was not associated with an increase in adverse events at any stage of renal dysfunction.

The following study (5-8) reported that ronacaleret, a new small molecule calcium-sensing receptor antagonist that stimulates endogenous parathyroid hormone (PTH) release from the parathyroid glands, did not function as an oral osteoanabolic agent for the treatment of osteoporosis. Despite the fact that this was a negative study, ronacaleret was able to cause temporary increases in PTH secretion, similar to those previously demonstrated with teriparatide. However, the prolonged stimulation of PTH secretion in the context of the BMD findings and increased bone turnover suggested that ronacaleret induced mild hyperparathyroidism. Ronacaleret only modestly increased lumbar spine BMD and was unable to prevent decreased BMD at the hip sites. Other agents with shorter-acting effects on PTH stimulation may eventually be found that will be able to serve as effective bone anabolic agents.

The next article (5-9) demonstrated that alendronate and concurrent PPI use was associated with a dose-dependent loss of alendronate protection against hip fracture in elderly patients. This observational study did not provide formal proof of causality, but the dose-response relationship and the lack of impact of prior PPI use provided reasonable grounds for concluding that routine use of PPIs for control of upper gastrointestinal tract complaints should be discouraged in patients treated with oral bisphosphonates for osteoporosis.

The final study of this section is a meta-analysis (5-10) that evaluated whether use of calcium supplements with or without vitamin D increased the risk of cardiovascular events, especially myocardial infarction, in the Women's Health Initiated (WHI) calcium + vitamin D study and 7 other studies. This study analyzed the risk of cardiovascular events only in women in the WHI who did not take personal calcium supplements. Fifty-four percent of the women in the WHI took personal calcium supplements during the course of the 7-year study. The meta-analysis found that calcium and vitamin D supplements increased the risk of myocardial infarction in postmenopausal women. The study claims that this finding was obscured in the original WHI Ca + D Study by the widespread use of personal calcium supplements. The investigators recommended that a reassessment of the role of calcium supplements in osteoporosis management is warranted.

The next section of this chapter discusses a variety of studies offering insight into the epidemiology and pathophysiology of osteoporosis. The first study (5-11) showed that survival of postmenopausal women with hip fractures was similar 1 year after fracture to survival of age-matched controls without hip fracture, except in those aged 65 to 69 years, who continued to have increased mortality. Short-term mortality over 1 year was increased after hip fracture in women aged 65 to 79 years, and in exceptionally healthy women 80 years or older. Women 70 years or older returned to previous risk levels by 1 year after fracture. The study concluded that interventions are needed to decrease mortality in the first year after hip fracture, when mortality risk is highest.

The next article (5-12) reported that antiresorptive treatments reduced all types of nonvertebral fractures regardless of degree of trauma or special groupings. Study-level data were combined from 5 randomized fracture prevention trials of antiresorptive agents that reduced the risk of nonvertebral fracture in postmenopausal women, including 30 118 women, with 2997 having had at least 1 nonvertebral fracture. These studies evaluated the effects of alendronate, clodronate, denosumab, lasofoxifene, or zoledronic acid. The study concluded that all nonvertebral fractures should be used as a standard endpoint of osteoporosis trials, and that these fractures should be used as the basis for estimating the benefits and cost-effectiveness of future treatments for osteoporosis.

The following paper (5-13) demonstrated that femoral neck BMD T-score and FRAX® score were associated with hip and nonspine fracture risk among older adults with type 2 diabetes mellitus. Type 2 diabetes mellitus is associated with higher BMD and paradoxically with increased fracture risk, but it was not previously known if low BMD, central to fracture prediction in older adults, identified fracture risk in patients with type 2 diabetes mellitus. In subjects with type 2 diabetes mellitus, compared with participants without diabetes, the fracture risk was higher for a given T-score and age or for a given FRAX® score. These findings provide further evidence that patients with type 2 diabetes mellitus have higher fracture risk for a given age, BMD, or FRAX® score.

The subsequent study (5-14) provided evidence that effectiveness of fracture prevention among men with prostate cancer may be limited because advanced-stage disease and pathologic fractures accounted for most of the excess fracture risk. This population-based study showed that overall fracture risk in men with early stage prostate cancer was elevated 1.9-fold, with an absolute increase in risk of 9.0%. Relative to rates among community-dwelling men, fracture risk was increased even among men not on androgen deprivation therapy (ADT), but was elevated a further 1.7-fold among ADT-treated compared with untreated men with prostate cancer. The increased risk of fracture following various forms of ADT was accounted for mainly by pathologic fractures (14% of all fractures). Among the 62% of men not on ADT in the study cohort, more traditional osteoporosis risk factors were implicated in causation of fractures.

It has been known for many years that high BMD protects against fractures in general. However, high BMD may also increase the risk of other adverse outcomes, such as prostate cancer as described above. For example, women with higher BMD have been reported to have a higher risk of breast cancer. The next article (5-15) showed that women with invasive breast cancer did not have a higher risk of overall fractures or osteoporotic fractures, despite therapies that might be expected to increase the risk of fracture. Nevertheless, these women had the expected rate of fracture for age- and sex-matched controls, indicating that higher BMD did not protect them from fracture. This finding suggests that increased

BMD may not always protect against fractures as it is assumed to, similar to the findings in type 2 diabetes mellitus described above.

Previous studies using dual-energy x-ray absorptiometry (DXA) have shown that age is a major predictor of bone fragility and fracture risk, independent of areal bone mineral density (aBMD). While the aBMD-independent effect of age has been attributed to poor bone "quality," the structural basis for poor bone quality remains unclear. The following paper (5-16) reported that younger and older women and men matched for DXA aBMD have similar radial trabecular microarchitecture, but clearly different cortical microstructure. The study concluded that future studies will be necessary to define the extent to which this deterioration in cortical microstructure contributes to the aBMD-independent effect of age on bone fragility and fracture risk at the distal radius and other sites of osteoporotic fractures.

The next study (5-17) reported that a cohort of young and old men and women matched by femoral neck aBMD had relatively similar femoral strength and load-to-strength ratio because of the offsetting effects of bone size and volumetric BMD (vBMD). Using combined DXA and quantitative computed tomography (QCT), the study demonstrated that men matched with women for femoral neck aBMD had lower vBMD, higher bone cross-sectional area, and relatively similar values for finite element analysis-derived bone strength. Given that aBMD by DXA is widely used to identify patients at risk for osteoporotic fractures, and that this measurement is influenced by bone size (ie, matched for vBMD, larger bones have higher aBMD), increasing evidence indicates that absolute aBMD predicts a similar risk of fracture in men and women.

The next article (5-18) identified key determinants of ultradistal radius strength and evaluated their relationships with age, sex steroid levels, and measures of habitual skeletal loading. The findings demonstrated that ultradistal radius bone strength, as quantified by microfinite element analysis (μFE), can be predicted from variables obtained by high-resolution peripheral quantitative computed tomography (HRpQCT), and that predicted bone strength declines with age and with changes in ultradistal radius trabecular vBMD and cortical area, which is related in turn to reduced skeletal loading and sex steroid levels.

The undercarboxylated form of the osteoblast-secreted protein osteocalcin (ucOC) has favorable effects on fat and glucose metabolism in mice. In human subjects, cross-sectional studies have also suggested a relevant association. The following paper (5-19) showed that changes in ucOC induced by PTH(1-84) and alendronate were associated with beneficial changes in a variety of metabolic indices. These associations are consistent with observations from animal models and support a role for ucOC in the skeletal regulation of energy metabolism in humans.

Patients with an activating mutation of the low-density lipoprotein receptor-related protein 5 (Lrp5) gene exhibit high bone mass (HBM). Limited information is available regarding compartment-specific changes in bone in this genetic disorder, and the relationship between the high bone mass phenotype and serum serotonin is not well documented. The final study of this section (5-20) evaluated bone, serum serotonin, and bone turnover markers in 19 Lrp5-HBM patients with the T253I mutation, and compared them to findings in 19 age- and sex-matched controls. The study showed that increased bone mass in Lrp5-HBM patients seemed to be caused primarily by changes in trabecular and cortical bone mass and structure. In addition, the phenotype appeared to progress with age, but bone turnover markers did not suggest increased bone formation. These findings give further insight into the mechanisms behind the high bone mass skeletal phenotype.

The next section of this chapter reviews 2 studies that shed light on issues in mineral and vitamin D metabolism. Little consensus exists on the link between vitamin D levels and muscle mass or strength. The first paper in this section (5-21) reported that the association between low serum 25-hydroxyvitamin D and increased fall risk may be due to factors that affect neuromuscular function, rather than factors affecting muscle strength. This study investigated the association of serum 25-hydroxyvitamin D, 1,25-dihydroxyvitamin D, and PTH levels with skeletal muscle mass and strength in 311 men (mean age, 56 years) and 356 women (mean age, 57 years) in an age-stratified, random sample of community-dwelling adults. The findings indicated an association between low serum 1,25-dihydroxyvitamin D and low skeletal mass and low knee extension strength, particularly in younger people, but did not find an association between these characteristics and low serum 25-hydroxyvitamin D levels. These findings call into question whether serum 25-hydroxyvitamin D directly influences muscle mass or strength.

Previous studies have shown that low serum 25-hydroxyvitamin D levels are associated with many different diseases and conditions. In patients with lung diseases, low serum 25-hydroxyvitmain D levels have been associated with lower FEV(1), impaired immunologic control, and increased airway inflammation. Because many patients with chronic obstructive pulmonary disease (COPD) have vitamin D deficiency, effects of vitamin D supplementation may extend beyond prevention of osteoporosis. The final study in this section (5-22) showed that high-dose vitamin D supplementation in a group of patients with COPD did not reduce the incidence of COPD exacerbations, but that in participants with severe vitamin D deficiency at baseline, supplementation may reduce exacerbations. The study was unable to identify reasons for lack of benefit in this study population.

The final section in this chapter reviews several studies clarifying current issues in metabolic bone disease. The first article (5-23) described results showing that PTH is a regulator of sclerostin in human disorders of parathyroid function. Sclerostin, a protein encoded by the *SOST* gene in osteocytes and an antagonist of the Wnt signaling pathway in osteoblasts and osteoblast precursors, is down-regulated by PTH administration. The premise of this study was that disorders of parathyroid function might be useful clinical settings in which to study this relationship. The study showed that increased PTH levels in primary hyperparathyroidism decreased sclerostin production, and that decreased PTH levels in hypoparathyroidism increased sclerostin levels. This study also showed that bone mineral content may be a factor that influences sclerostin production by osteocytes.

Hypoparathyroidism is associated with abnormal structural and dynamic skeletal properties. The next study (5-24) hypothesized that PTH(1-84) treatment would restore skeletal properties toward normal in patients with hypoparathyroidism. Sixty-four subjects with hypoparathyroidism were treated with PTH(1-84) for 2 years. The study showed that these patients developed increases in histomorphometric and biochemical indices of skeletal dynamics. Structural changes were consistent with an increased remodeling rate in both trabecular and cortical compartments, with tunneling resorption in the trabecular compartment. The study concluded that PTH(1-84) improves abnormal skeletal properties in hypoparathyroidism and restores bone metabolism toward normal euparathyroid levels.

Two trials have shown that a single 5-mg infusion of zoledronic acid achieves much higher response rates in patients with Paget's disease of bone than risedronate. The duration of this effect of zoledronic acid is unknown. The final paper presented in this section (5-25) was an open follow-up study of responders from the 2 trials, in which 152 subjects were originally treated with zoledronic acid, and 115 with risedronate. Subjects were followed for up to 6.5 years without further intervention. The study showed that a single infusion of zoledronic acid causes an unprecedented duration of remission of Paget's disease of bone, as well as an improved quality of life in affected patients.

In summary, these selected papers give a sampling of the variety of excellent clinical studies published in calcium and bone disorders during the last year. It is readily acknowledged that many other significant papers are not included in this review due to space constraints. Some of the studies included verify long-held views regarding calcium and bone disorders based on previous observations, whereas others demonstrate previously unsuspected physiological functions of the skeleton. Future clinical studies will continue to clarify recent findings that do not fit within the classical paradigms of skeletal function in health and disease.

Bart L. Clarke, MD

Current Issues in Osteoporosis Therapy

Calcium supplements with or without vitamin D and risk of cardiovascular events: reanalysis of the Women's Health Initiative limited access dataset and meta-analysis

Bolland MJ, Grey A, Avenell A, et al (Univ of Auckland, New Zealand; Univ of Aberdeen, Scotland)

BMJ 342:d2040, 2011

Objectives.—To investigate the effects of personal calcium supplement use on cardiovascular risk in the Women's Health Initiative Calcium/ Vitamin D Supplementation Study (WHI CaD Study), using the WHI dataset, and to update the recent meta-analysis of calcium supplements and cardiovascular risk.

Design.—Reanalysis of WHI CaD Study limited access dataset and incorporation in meta-analysis with eight other studies.

Data source.—WHI CaD Study, a seven year, randomised, placebo controlled trial of calcium and vitamin D (1g calcium and 400 IU vitamin D daily) in 36 282 community dwelling postmenopausal women.

Main Outcome Measures.—Incidence of four cardiovascular events and their combinations (myocardial infarction, coronary revascularisation, death from coronary heart disease, and stroke) assessed with patient-level data and trial-level data.

Results.—In the WHI CaD Study there was an interaction between personal use of calcium supplements and allocated calcium and vitamin D for cardiovascular events. In the 16 718 women (46%) who were not taking personal calcium supplements at randomisation the hazard ratios for cardiovascular events with calcium and vitamin D ranged from 1.13 to 1.22 ($P=0.05$ for clinical myocardial infarction or stroke, $P=0.04$ for clinical myocardial infarction or revascularisation), whereas in the women taking personal calcium supplements cardiovascular risk did not alter with allocation to calcium and vitamin D. In meta-analyses of three placebo controlled trials, calcium and vitamin D increased the risk of myocardial infarction (relative risk 1.21 (95% confidence interval 1.01 to 1.44), $P=0.04$), stroke (1.20 (1.00 to 1.43), $P=0.05$), and the composite of myocardial infarction or stroke (1.16 (1.02 to 1.32), $P=0.02$). In metaanalyses of placebo controlled trials of calcium or calcium and vitamin D, complete trial-level data were available for 28 072 participants from eight trials of calcium supplements and the WHI CaD participants not taking personal calcium supplements. In total 1384 individuals had an incident myocardial infarction or stroke. Calcium or calcium and vitamin D increased the risk of myocardial infarction (relative risk 1.24 (1.07 to 1.45), $P=0.004$) and the composite of myocardial infarction or stroke (1.15 (1.03 to 1.27), $P=0.009$).

Conclusions.—Calcium supplements with or without vitamin D modestly increase the risk of cardiovascular events, especially myocardial infarction, a finding obscured in the WHI CaD Study by the widespread use of personal calcium supplements. A reassessment of the role of calcium supplements in osteoporosis management is warranted.

▶ Recent studies have raised concern that calcium supplementation used to treat or prevent osteoporosis may increase cardiovascular risk, including the risk of myocardial infarction, in at least some patients.[1-3] Three recent studies by the same group have found increased cardiovascular risk associated with calcium supplementation, whereas previous studies by different groups have not shown evidence of increased risk.[4-6] This study re-analyzed a limited access dataset from the Women's Health Initiative (WHI) Calcium + D (CaD) study, and incorporated these data into a meta-analysis with 8 other studies. Data from the WHI CaD study was obtained from 36 282 community-dwelling postmenopausal women taking either 1000 mg elemental calcium and 400 IU vitamin D, or placebo, each day for 7 years. The analysis of the limited access dataset from the WHI CaD study showed an interaction between personal use of calcium supplements and calcium and vitamin D supplementation assigned for the trial. In fact, 54% of women enrolled in the WHI CaD study took personal calcium supplements in addition to the study calcium supplement. In the 16 718 women not taking personal calcium supplements at the start of the WHI CaD trial, risk of cardiovascular events, including clinical myocardial infarction and stroke or clinical myocardial infarction and revascularization, increased significantly by 13% to 22% in the women assigned to receive calcium and vitamin D. This increased risk was not seen in the women assigned to receive calcium and vitamin D who were taking personal calcium supplements.

The meta-analysis incorporated the limited access WHI CaD study data from the women not taking personal calcium supplements at baseline with data from 8 other placebo-controlled studies and found a 24% increased risk of myocardial infarction and 15% increased composite risk of myocardial infarction or stroke. The study concluded that calcium supplements with or without vitamin D modestly increased the risk of cardiovascular events, especially myocardial infarction. The authors noted that they believed that the previously published negative WHI CaD study findings were obscured by use of personal calcium supplements in 54% of the women enrolled in this study.

These findings suggest that calcium supplementation with or without vitamin D may increase the risk of cardiovascular events in postmenopausal women taking calcium and vitamin D supplementation to prevent osteoporosis. The initial analysis of the complete WHI CaD trial dataset by the WHI investigators reported no improvement or worsening of cardiovascular endpoints. If it is true that calcium supplementation increases the risk of cardiovascular events, especially myocardial infarction, it is not evident why women in the WHI CaD study who were taking personal calcium supplements beyond their assigned calcium and vitamin D supplementation did not have an even higher risk of cardiovascular events. Perhaps subjects with higher risk of cardiovascular events, such as those with chronic kidney disease or diabetes, may explain the increased risk of cardiovascular events seen in this study. This debate will likely continue for some time and may never be completely resolved due to ethical restrictions limiting conduct of a definitive trial to settle the question.

B. L. Clarke, MD

References

1. Bolland MJ, Grey A, Gamble GD, Reid IR. Calcium and vitamin D supplements and health outcomes: a reanalysis of the Women's Health Initiative (WHI) limited-access data set. *Am J Clin Nutr.* 2011;94:1144-1149.
2. Bolland MJ, Avenell A, Baron JA, et al. Effect of calcium supplements on risk of myocardial infarction and cardiovascular events: meta-analysis. *BMJ.* 2010;341: c3691.
3. Bolland MJ, Barber PA, Doughty RN, et al. Vascular events in healthy older women receiving calcium supplementation: randomised controlled trial. *BMJ.* 2008;336:262-266.
4. LaCroix AZ, Kotchen J, Anderson G, et al. Calcium plus vitamin D supplementation and mortality in postmenopausal women: the Women's Health Initiative calcium-vitamin D randomized controlled trial. *J Gerontol A Biol Sci Med Sci.* 2009;64:559-567.
5. Hsia J, Heiss G, Ren H, et al; Women's Health Initiative Investigators. Calcium/ vitamin D supplementation and cardiovascular events. *Circulation.* 2007;115: 846-854.
6. Wang L, Manson JE, Song Y, Sesso HD. Systematic review: vitamin D and calcium supplementation in prevention of cardiovascular events. *Ann Intern Med.* 2010; 152:315-323.

Proton Pump Inhibitor Use and the Antifracture Efficacy of Alendronate

Abrahamsen B, Eiken P, Eastell R (Univ of Southern Denmark, Odense, Denmark; Hillerød Hosp, Denmark; Univ of Sheffield, England)
Arch Intern Med 171:998-1004, 2011

Background.—Proton pump inhibitors (PPIs) are widely used in elderly patients and are frequently coadministered in users of oral bisphosphonates. Biologically, PPIs could affect the absorption of calcium, vitamin B_{12}, and bisphosphonates and could affect the osteoclast proton pump, thus interacting with bisphosphonate antifracture efficacy. Moreover, PPIs themselves have been linked to osteoporotic fractures.

Methods.—Population-based, national register—based, open cohort study of 38 088 new alendronate sodium users with a mean duration of follow-up of 3.5 years. We related risk of hip fracture to recent pharmacy records of refill of prescriptions for alendronate.

Results.—For hip fractures, there was statistically significant interaction with alendronate for PPI use ($P< .05$). The treatment response associated with complete refill compliance to alendronate was a 39% risk reduction (hazard ratio [HR], 0.61; 95% confidence interval [CI], 0.52-0.71; $P< .001$) in patients who were not PPI users, while the risk reduction in concurrent PPI users was not significant (19%; HR, 0.81; 95% CI, 0.64-1.01; $P = .06$). The attenuation of the risk reduction was dose and age dependent. In contrast, there was no significant impact of concurrent use of histamine H_2 receptor blockers.

Conclusions.—Concurrent PPI use was associated with a dose-dependent loss of protection against hip fracture with alendronate in elderly patients. This is an observational study, so a formal proof of causality cannot be made, but the dose-response relationship and the lack of impact of prior PPI use provides reasonable grounds for discouraging the use of PPIs to control upper gastrointestinal tract complaints in patients treated with oral bisphosphonates.

▶ Previous studies have found increased hip fracture risk in patients taking proton pump inhibitors (PPIs).[1-5] Some of these studies have found dose-response relationships between PPI use and fracture risk. It has been presumed that PPIs decrease stomach acid secretion sufficiently to reduce intestinal absorption of calcium carbonate due to lack of solubilization of calcium carbonate tablets in reduced or minimal stomach acid.[1] PPIs may also possibly affect absorption of oral bisphosphonates by reducing conversion of bisphosphonate salts to bisphosphonate acids in stomach acid, as normally occurs. Finally, PPIs theoretically could have direct effects on osteoclast proton pumps, leading to decreased acidification of bone resorption lacunae.

This population-based national register open cohort study evaluated fracture risk in a large number of new alendronate sodium users over a mean follow-up of 3.5 years. National pharmacy records were used to verify alendronate prescription refills, and hip fractures were assessed based on national hospital discharge records. For subjects not taking PPIs who refilled all their alendronate prescriptions over the study interval, hip fracture risk was reduced by 39%, similar to previously published studies. For subjects who took PPIs concurrently and refilled all alendronate prescriptions, hip fracture risk reduction was only 19%, but this change was nonsignificant. The increase in hip fracture risk seen with PPI use was both dose dependent and age dependent, with elderly patients having the greatest loss of hip fracture protection from alendronate. This study also showed no effect on hip fracture reduction with histamine 2 receptor (H_2)-blockers. The study concluded that PPI use concurrent with oral bisphosphonate use may reduce hip fracture protection in the elderly.

These findings raise concern that hip fracture risk reduction associated with oral bisphosphonate therapy may be minimized by simultaneous PPI therapy. Because many patients taking oral bisphosphonates also take PPIs for gastroesophageal reflux symptoms, it is possible that the bisphosphonate therapy is not benefiting these patients as much as previously thought. In some patients, PPI therapy has been prescribed to minimize gastroesophageal irritation resulting from bisphosphonate use. These findings suggest that patients requiring PPI therapy for treatment of gastroesophageal irritation may be better served by taking their bisphosphonate therapy by an intravenous route or by taking a nonbisphosphonate type of medication to treat their osteoporosis. Alternatively, H_2-blocker therapy might be considered in place of PPI therapy to reduce reflux symptoms in patients taking oral bisphosphonate therapy.

B. L. Clarke, MD

References

1. Yang YX, Lewis JD, Epstein S, Metz DC. Long-term proton pump inhibitor therapy and risk of hip fracture. *JAMA.* 2006;296:2947-2953.
2. Gray SL, LaCroix AZ, Larson J, et al. Proton pump inhibitor use, hip fracture, and change in bone mineral density in postmenopausal women: results from the Women's Health Initiative. *Arch Intern Med.* 2010;170:765-771.
3. Corley DA, Kubo A, Zhao W, Quesenberry C. Proton pump inhibitors and histamine-2 receptor antagonists are associated with hip fractures among at-risk patients. *Gastroenterology.* 2010;139:93-101.
4. Pouwels S, Lalmohamed A, Souverein P, et al. Use of proton pump inhibitors and risk of hip/femur fracture: a population-based case-control study. *Osteoporos Int.* 2011;22:903-910.
5. Ngamruengphong S, Leontiadis GI, Radhi S, Dentino A, Nugent K. Proton pump inhibitors and risk of fracture: a systematic review and meta-analysis of observational studies. *Am J Gastroenterol.* 2011;106:1209-1218.

Effect of Stopping Risedronate after Long-Term Treatment on Bone Turnover

Eastell R, Hannon RA, Wenderoth D, et al (Univ of Sheffield, UK; Warner Chilcott Deutschland GmbH, Weiterstadt, Germany; et al)
J Clin Endocrinol Metab 96:3367-3373, 2011

Context.—Determining how quickly bisphosphonate treatment effects begin to regress is crucial when considering termination of treatment.

Objective.—Our objective was to assess the effects of 1 yr discontinuation of risedronate use in postmenopausal women with osteoporosis who had previously received risedronate for 2 or 7 yr.

Design and Setting.—Before initiation of the current study, placebo/5-mg-risedronate patients had received placebo for 5 yr and risedronate for 2 yr, whereas 5-mg-risedronate patients had received risedronate for a total of 7 yr. Risedronate was then discontinued for 1 yr (yr 8).

Patients.—Postmenopausal women with osteoporosis who had previously completed the 3-yr Vertebral Efficacy with Risedronate Therapy Multi National (VERT-MN) pivotal trial, plus a 2-yr extension comparing risedronate or placebo for a total of 5 yr, followed by 2 yr of open-label risedronate treatment were enrolled in these trial extensions.

Main Outcome Measures.—Evaluations included changes in type I collagen cross-linked N-telopeptide (NTX)/creatinine (Cr) and bone mineral density (BMD) values, fracture incidence, and adverse events.

Results.—After 1 yr of risedronate discontinuation, NTX/Cr levels increased toward baseline in both patient groups vs. the values at the end of yr 7. In both treatment groups, off-treatment total hip and femoral trochanter BMD values decreased, whereas lumbar spine and femoral neck BMD were maintained or slightly increased. The adverse event profiles were similar between the two treatment groups during yr 8.

Conclusions.—One year of discontinuation of risedronate treatment in patients who had received 2 or 7 yr of risedronate therapy led to increases in NTX/Cr levels toward baseline and decreases in femoral trochanter and total hip BMD.

▶ Because of concerns regarding long-term safety and efficacy of bisphosphonate therapy, including risks related to jaw osteonecrosis and atypical subtrochanteric femoral fractures, the US Food and Drug Administration (FDA) has recommended that patients not be treated with continuous therapy with bisphosphonates for more than 5 years.[1] It has been assumed that all bisphosphonates share the same degree of long-term risk. Based on FLEX trial data with alendronate,[2,3] new HORIZON trial data with zoledronic acid,[4] and older data with risedronate,[5] it is assumed that most patients given a drug holiday after long-term treatment with bisphosphonate therapy should remain off treatment for at least 1, and perhaps as long as 5 years. No studies have addressed fracture risk after risedronate or ibandronate have been stopped.

This extension study gives insight into fracture risk in the first year after stopping risedronate after long-term therapy. Postmenopausal women with osteoporosis in the original VERT-MN pivotal fracture trial received treatment with risedronate for 3 years followed by a 2-year extension of risedronate treatment, and then 2 more years of open-label risedronate for a maximum cumulative exposure of 7 years, before they stopped treatment for 1 year.[6,7] The study showed that 24-hour urinary NTx-telopeptide recovered toward baseline over the year off treatment, suggesting wearing off of the antiresorptive effect of the previous long-term risedronate therapy. In addition, total hip and greater trochanteric bone mineral density (BMD) decreased, whereas lumbar spine and femoral neck BMD remained stable or slightly increased. Fractures did not increase during the year off treatment. The study concluded that stopping risedronate for 1 year after 2 to 7 years of continuous therapy led to urinary NTx-telopeptide increasing toward baseline after 1 year off therapy, with loss of total hip and greater trochanteric BMD, but without increased risk of fracture.

These findings suggest differences between the duration of antiresorptive effect of risedronate and longer-acting alendronate and zoledronic acid. The antiresorptive effect of longer-acting alendronate may take up to 5 years to wear off, whereas zoledronic acid takes at least 3 years to wear off. Why risedronate treatment effect appears to wear off so much more quickly is not clear, but it may have to do with avidity of binding of the drug to hydroxyapatite or other properties unique to risedronate. These findings reinforce the fact that not all bisphosphonates are the same, and that bone density protective effects of some bisphosphonates last longer than for other bisphosphonates.

B. L. Clarke, MD

References

1. Traynor K. FDA advisers uneasy about long-term bisphosphonate use. *Am J Health Syst Pharm.* 2011;68:2006-2008.
2. Black DM, Schwartz AV, Ensrud KE, et al; FLEX Research Group. Effects of continuing or stopping alendronate after 5 years of treatment: the Fracture Intervention Trial Long-term Extension (FLEX): a randomized trial. *JAMA.* 2006;296:2927-2938.

3. Schwartz AV, Bauer DC, Cummings SR, et al; FLEX Research Group. Efficacy of continued alendronate for fractures in women with and without prevalent vertebral fracture: the FLEX trial. *J Bone Miner Res.* 2010;25:976-982.
4. Black DM, Reid IR, Boonen S, et al. The effect of 3 versus 6 years of zoledronic acid treatment of osteoporosis: a randomized extension to the HORIZON-Pivotal Fracture Trial (PFT). *J Bone Miner Res.* 2012;27:243-254.
5. Watts NB, Chines A, Olszynski WP, et al. Fracture risk remains reduced one year after discontinuation of risedronate. *Osteoporos Int.* 2008;19:365-372.
6. Harris ST, Watts NB, Genant HK, et al; Effects of risedronate treatment on vertebral and nonvertebral fractures in women with postmenopausal osteoporosis: a randomized controlled trial. Vertebral Efficacy With Risedronate Therapy (VERT) Study Group. *JAMA.* 1999;282:1344-1352.
7. Reginster J, Minne HW, Sorensen OH, et al; Randomized trial of the effects of risedronate on vertebral fractures in women with established postmenopausal osteoporosis. Vertebral Efficacy with Risedronate Therapy (VERT) Study Group. *Osteoporos Int.* 2000;11:83-91.

The Effect of 3 Versus 6 Years of Zoledronic Acid Treatment of Osteoporosis: A Randomized Extension to the HORIZON-Pivotal Fracture Trial (PFT)

Black DM, Reid IR, Boonen S, et al (Univ of California, San Francisco; Univ of Auckland, New Zealand; Katholieke Universiteit Leuven, Belgium; et al)
J Bone Miner Res 27:243-254, 2012

Zoledronic acid 5 mg (ZOL) annually for 3 years reduces fracture risk in postmenopausal women with osteoporosis. To investigate long-term effects of ZOL on bone mineral density (BMD) and fracture risk, the Health Outcomes and Reduced Incidence with Zoledronic acid Once Yearly–Pivotal Fracture Trial (HORIZON-PFT) was extended to 6 years. In this international, multicenter, double-blind, placebo-controlled extension trial, 1233 postmenopausal women who received ZOL for 3 years in the core study were randomized to 3 additional years of ZOL (Z6, $n = 616$) or placebo (Z3P3, $n = 617$). The primary endpoint was femoral neck (FN) BMD percentage change from year 3 to 6 in the intent-to-treat (ITT) population. Secondary endpoints included other BMD sites, fractures, biochemical bone turnover markers, and safety. In years 3 to 6, FN-BMD remained constant in Z6 and dropped slightly in Z3P3 (between-treatment difference = 1.04%; 95% confidence interval 0.4 to 1.7; $p = 0.0009$) but remained above pretreatment levels. Other BMD sites showed similar differences. Biochemical markers remained constant in Z6 but rose slightly in Z3P3, remaining well below pretreatment levels in both. New morphometric vertebral fractures were lower in the Z6 ($n = 14$) versus Z3P3 ($n = 30$) group (odds ratio = 0.51; $p = 0.035$), whereas other fractures were not different. Significantly more Z6 patients had a transient increase in serum creatinine >0.5 mg/dL (0.65% versus 2.94% in Z3P3). Nonsignificant increases in Z6 of atrial fibrillation serious adverse events (2.0% versus 1.1% in Z3P3; $p = 0.26$) and stroke (3.1% versus 1.5% in Z3P3; $p = 0.06$) were seen. Post-dose symptoms were similar in both groups. Reports of hypertension were significantly lower in Z6 versus Z3P3 (7.8% versus 15.1%, $p < 0.001$). Small differences in bone density and markers in those who continued versus those who stopped treatment suggest residual effects, and therefore, after 3 years of annual ZOL, many patients may discontinue therapy up to 3 years. However, vertebral fracture reductions suggest that those at high fracture risk, particularly vertebral fracture, may benefit by continued treatment. (ClinicalTrials.gov identifier: NCT00145327) (Fig 4).

▶ The optimal duration of treatment of osteoporosis with oral or intravenous bisphosphonate therapies remains a major concern. Most clinical trials with bisphosphonates evaluated the safety and efficacy of these drugs over only 3 to 5 years. It is not yet clear that these drugs are safe or efficacious when used for longer than 5 years. Because of concerns regarding rare risks of serious adverse effects, such as atypical subtrochanteric femur fractures and osteonecrosis of the jaw, many physicians are treating patients with osteoporosis with alendronate for no longer than 5 years and then recommending a drug holiday of up to five years, based on the results of the FLEX trial.[1] This multicenter extension study of the original Health Outcomes and Reduced Incidence with Zoledronic acid Once yearly—Pivotal Fracture Trial (HORIZON-PFT)[2] extended the original 3-year study to 6 years. Of the 1233 women who had received zoledronic acid 5 mg intravenously once a year for 3 years, half were randomly assigned to receive the same dose of zoledronic acid for another 3 years (n = 616) and the other half placebo (n = 617). Femoral neck bone mineral density (BMD) remained stable in those who received another 3 years of zoledronic acid, whereas it decreased slightly in those receiving placebo. BMD at other skeletal sites showed similar changes. Markers of bone turnover remained stable in those receiving zoledronic acid but increased slightly in those receiving placebo. The zoledronic acid—treated group experienced 14 vertebral morphometric fractures, whereas the placebo group developed 30 fractures (Fig 4). Significantly more zoledronic acid—treated subjects had an increase in serum creatinine compared with the placebo group (2.94% vs 0.6%). Nonsignificant increases in atrial fibrillation and stroke were also seen in the zoledronic acid group. The study concluded that some subjects may be treated with zoledronic acid for 3 years before safely stopping therapy for 3 years, whereas subjects at high fracture risk, particularly of vertebral fracture, may benefit from continued treatment.

This study provides clarification of the optimal duration of therapy for osteoporosis with zoledronic acid, the most potent bisphosphonate therapy available today. As with alendronate, some patients continue to benefit sufficiently from previous therapy that zoledronic acid can be safely discontinued for 3 years after receiving zoledronic acid once a year continuously for 3 years, whereas other patients require therapy indefinitely for continued fracture reduction benefit. Long-acting bisphosphonate therapies are different in this respect than short-acting biological therapies such as teriparatide[3,4] or denosumab,[5] which must be continued indefinitely for continued fracture reduction benefit.

B. L. Clarke, MD

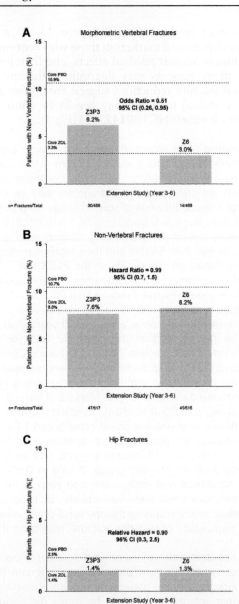

FIGURE 4.—Incidence of fractures by treatment in the extension for morphometric vertebral fractures (*A*), nonvertebral fractures (*B*), and hip fractures (*C*). The dashed lines indicate the incidence in the core trial by core treatment for the corresponding fracture types. For *B* and *C*, the percentages given are the event rate from the Kaplan–Meier estimate at month 36 in the extension (bars) or core study (dashed lines). (Reprinted from Black DM, Reid IR, Boonen S, et al. The effect of 3 versus 6 years of Zoledronic acid treatment of osteoporosis: a randomized extension to the HORIZON-Pivotal Fracture Trial (PFT). *J Bone Miner Res.* 2012;27:243-254, with permission from American Society for Bone and Mineral Research.)

References

1. Schwartz AV, Bauer DC, Cummings SR, et al. Efficacy of continued alendronate for fractures in women with and without prevalent vertebral fracture: the FLEX trial. *J Bone Miner Res.* 2010;25:976-982.
2. Lyles KW, Colón-Emeric CS, Magaziner JS, et al; HORIZON Recurrent Fracture Trial. Zoledronic Acid and clinical fractures and mortality after hip fracture. *New Engl J Med.* 2007;357:1799-1809.
3. Leder BZ, Neer RM, Wyland JJ, et al. Effects of teriparatide treatment and discontinuation in postmenopausal women and eugonadal men with osteoporosis. *J Clin Endocrinol Metab.* 2009;94:2915-2921.
4. Eastell R, Christiansen C, Grauer A, et al. Effects of denosumab on bone turnover markers in postmenopausal osteoporosis. *J Bone Miner Res.* 2011;26:530-537.
5. Cummings SR, San Martin J, McClung MR, et al; FREEDOM Trial. Denosumab for prevention of fractures in postmenopausal women with osteoporosis. *N Engl J Med.* 2009;361:756-765.

Effect of Denosumab Treatment on the Risk of Fractures in Subgroups of Women With Postmenopausal Osteoporosis

McClung M, Boonen S, Törring O, et al (Oregon Osteoporosis Ctr, Portland; Leuven Univ, Belgium; Karolinska Institutet Sodersjukhuset, Stockholm, Sweden; et al)

J Bone Miner Res 27:211-218, 2012

Denosumab reduces the risk of new vertebral and nonvertebral fractures. Previous trials suggest that the efficacy of antiresorptives on fractures might differ by patients' characteristics, such as age, bone mineral density (BMD), and fracture history. In the FREEDOM study, 7808 women aged 60 to 90 years with osteoporosis were randomly assigned to receive subcutaneous injections of denosumab (60 mg) or placebo every 6 months for 3 years. New vertebral and nonvertebral fractures were radiologically confirmed. Subgroup analyses described in this article were prospectively planned before study unblinding to evaluate the effect of denosumab on new vertebral and nonvertebral fractures across various subgroups. Compared with placebo, denosumab decreased the risk of new vertebral fractures in the overall study population over 3 years. This effect did not significantly differ for any of the nine subgroups analyzed ($p > 0.09$ for all potential interactions). Denosumab also reduced all nonvertebral fractures by 20% in the full study cohort over 3 years. This risk reduction was statistically significant in women with a baseline femoral neck BMD *T*-score ≤ -2.5 but not in those with a *T*-score > -2.5; in those with a body mass index (BMI) <25 kg/m^2 but not ≥ 25 kg/m^2; and in those without but not with a prevalent vertebral fracture. These differential treatment effects were not explained by differences in BMD responses to denosumab. Denosumab 60 mg administered every 6 months for 3 years in women with osteoporosis reduced the risk of new vertebral fractures to a similar degree in all subgroups. The effect of denosumab on nonvertebral fracture risk differed by femoral neck BMD, BMI, and prevalent vertebral fracture at baseline.

▶ Previous studies have found that antiresorptive and anabolic agents have different fracture reduction effects in postmenopausal osteoporotic women with different baseline characteristics. For example, these drugs may have a greater effect in women of different ages, baseline bone mineral density (BMD), or history of fractures.[1-6] These observations are biologically plausible in that certain patients are at higher risk of fracture, and antiresorptive agents such as denosumab likely have greater effect in those at highest risk of fracture.[7] This study found that denosumab decreased the risk of new vertebral fractures by 70% compared with placebo in 9 predetermined study subgroups in the 3-year phase III, randomized, placebo-controlled FREEDOM Trial.[8] Denosumab also reduced the risk of non-vertebral fractures by 20% in the whole study population over 3 years, but in this case, risk reduction varied by baseline characteristics. Nonvertebral risk reduction was significant in those women with baseline femoral neck T-score less than -2.5 but not above, women with body mass index less than 25.0 kg/m^2 but not above, and women without prevalent vertebral fracture but not those with prevalent vertebral fracture. It is not evident why fracture risk reduction was different in these different groups, because fracture risk reduction did not correlate with differences in BMD response to denosumab.

These findings illustrate some of the challenges in translating results from the large osteoporosis clinical trials into clinical practice. Subgroups within the study cohorts may have different responses to therapy based on their baseline characteristics, and these differences must be kept in mind when selecting patients for treatment with different agents. Baseline characteristics of patients must be kept in mind when selecting antiresorptive therapies for postmenopausal women with osteoporosis.

B. L. Clarke, MD

References

1. Delmas PD, Genant HK, Crans GG, et al. Severity of prevalent vertebral fractures and the risk of subsequent vertebral and nonvertebral fractures: results from the MORE trial. *Bone.* 2003;33:522-532.
2. Marcus R, Wang O, Satterwhite J, Mitlak B. The skeletal response to teriparatide is largely independent of age, initial bone mineral density, and prevalent vertebral fractures in postmenopausal women with osteoporosis. *J Bone Miner Res.* 2003; 18:18-23.
3. Ensrud KE, Black DM, Palermo L, et al. Treatment with alendronate prevents fractures in women at highest risk: results from the Fracture Intervention Trial. *Arch Intern Med.* 1997;157:2617-2624.
4. Kanis JA, Barton IP, Johnell O. Risedronate decreases fracture risk in patients selected solely on the basis of prior vertebral fracture. *Osteoporos Int.* 2005;16: 475-482.
5. Seibel MJ, Naganathan V, Barton I, Grauer A. Relationship between pretreatment bone resorption and vertebral fracture incidence in postmenopausal osteoporotic women treated with risedronate. *J Bone Miner Res.* 2004;19:323-329.
6. Roux C, Reginster JY, Fechtenbaum J, et al. Vertebral fracture risk reduction with strontium ranelate in women with postmenopausal osteoporosis is independent of baseline risk factors. *J Bone Miner Res.* 2006;21:536-542.

7. Boonen S, Adachi JD, Man Z, et al. Treatment with denosumab reduces the incidence of new vertebral and hip fractures in postmenopausal women at high risk. *J Clin Endocrinol Metab.* 2011;96:1727-1736.
8. Cummings SR, San Martin J, McClung MR, et al. Denosumab for prevention of fractures in postmenopausal women with osteoporosis. *N Engl J Med.* 2009; 361:756-765.

Treatment with Denosumab Reduces the Incidence of New Vertebral and Hip Fractures in Postmenopausal Women at High Risk

Boonen S, Adachi JD, Man Z, et al (Leuven Univ Division of Geriatric Medicine, Belgium; Charlton Med Centre, Hamilton, Ontario, Canada; Centro T.I.E.M.P.O., Buenos Aires, Argentina; et al)
J Clin Endocrinol Metab 96:1727-1736, 2011

Context.—The FREEDOM (Fracture REduction Evaluation of Denosumab in Osteoporosis every 6 Months) trial showed denosumab significantly reduced the risk of fractures in postmenopausal women with osteoporosis.

Objective.—We evaluated the effect of denosumab on the incidence of new vertebral and hip fractures in subgroups of women at higher risk for these fractures.

Design.—FREEDOM was a 3-yr, randomized, double-blind, placebo-controlled, phase 3 trial.

Participants and Setting.—Postmenopausal women (N = 7808) with osteoporosis were enrolled at 213 study sites worldwide.

Interventions.—Subjects received sc denosumab (60 mg) or placebo every 6 months and daily supplements of calcium ($\geq$1000 mg) and vitamin D ($\geq$400 IU).

Main Outcome Measures.—This *post hoc* analysis evaluated fracture incidence in women with known risk factors for fractures including multiple and/or moderate or severe prevalent vertebral fractures, aged 75 yr or older, and/or femoral neck bone mineral density T-score of −2.5 or less.

Results.—Compared with placebo, denosumab significantly reduced the risk of new vertebral fractures in women with multiple and/or severe prevalent vertebral fractures (16.6% placebo *vs.* 7.5% denosumab; $P < 0.001$). Similarly, denosumab significantly reduced the risk of hip fractures in subjects aged 75 yr or older (2.3% placebo vs. 0.9% denosumab; $P < 0.01$) or with a baseline femoral neck bone mineral density T-score of −2.5 or less (2.8% placebo *vs.* 1.4% denosumab; $P = 0.02$). These risk reductions in higher-risk individuals were consistent with those seen in patients at lower risk of fracture.

Conclusions.—Denosumab reduced the incidence of new vertebral and hip fractures in postmenopausal women with osteoporosis at higher risk for fracture. These results highlight the consistent antifracture efficacy of denosumab in patients with varying degrees of fracture risk.

▶ Antiresorptive and anabolic agents effectively reduce fractures in postmenopausal osteoporotic women who are at increased risk of fractures. However, not all agents reduce fractures with equal efficacy in this population. All approved antiresorptive and anabolic agents reduce the risk of vertebral fractures but not all reduce the risk of hip or nonvertebral fractures. The efficacy of some antiresorptive and anabolic agents in postmenopausal women depends on their baseline risk factors for osteoporotic fracture.[1-6]

This post-hoc analysis evaluated the effect of denosumab on the incidence of new vertebral and hip fractures in subpopulations in the overall study cohort in the large phase III, randomized, double-blind, placebo-controlled FREEDOM Trial.[7] Women at high risk of fracture, including women with multiple or moderate or severe prevalent vertebral fractures, age over 75 years, or femoral neck bone mineral density T-scores less than -2.5 were assessed for their treatment response to denosumab. Compared with placebo, denosumab decreased new vertebral and hip fracture risk in women with these high-risk characteristics similarly to women at lower risk of fracture. The study concluded that denosumab has consistent antifracture efficacy in postmenopausal women with varying degrees of fracture risk.

This study confirms the consistent antifracture efficacy of denosumab in different types of patients with different degrees of fracture risk. Even though other antiresorptive and anabolic agents show variance in their fracture reduction efficacy depending on baseline risk factors, this new biological agent does not. This may make denosumab more broadly applicable in the treatment of patients with postmenopausal osteoporosis.

B. L. Clarke, MD

References

1. Harris ST, Watts NB, Genant HK, et al. Effects of risedronate treatment on vertebral and nonvertebral fractures in women with postmenopausal osteoporosis: a randomized controlled trial. Vertebral Efficacy With Risedronate Therapy (VERT) Study Group. *JAMA.* 1999;282:1344-1352.
2. Ettinger B, Black DM, Mitlak BH, et al. Reduction of vertebral fracture risk in postmenopausal women with osteoporosis treated with raloxifene: results from a 3-year randomized clinical trial. Multiple Outcomes of Raloxifene Evaluation (MORE) Investigators. *JAMA.* 1999;282:637-645.
3. Chesnut CH 3rd, Silverman S, Andriano K, et al. A randomized trial of nasal spray salmon calcitonin in postmenopausal women with established osteoporosis: the prevent recurrence of osteoporotic fractures study. PROOF Study Group. *Am J Med.* 2000;109:267-276.
4. Chesnut CH III, Skag A, Christiansen C, et al; Oral Ibandronate Osteoporosis Vertebral Fracture Trial in North America and Europe (BONE). Effects of oral ibandronate administered daily or intermittently on fracture risk in postmenopausal osteoporosis. *J Bone Miner Res.* 2004;19:1241-1249.
5. Greenspan SL, Bone HG, Ettinger MP, et al; Treatment of Osteoporosis with Parathyroid Hormone Study Group. Effect of recombinant human parathyroid hormone (1-84) on vertebral fracture and bone mineral density in postmenopausal women with osteoporosis: a randomized trial. *Ann Intern Med.* 2007;146:326-339.
6. Silverman SL, Christiansen C, Genant HK, et al. Efficacy of bazedoxifene in reducing new vertebral fracture risk in postmenopausal women with osteoporosis: results from a 3-year, randomized, placebo-, and active-controlled clinical trial. *J Bone Miner Res.* 2008;23:1923-1934.
7. Cummings SR, San Martin J, McClung MR, et al. Denosumab for prevention of fractures in postmenopausal women with osteoporosis. *N Engl J Med.* 2009; 361:756-765.

Effects of Denosumab on Fracture and Bone Mineral Density by Level of Kidney Function

Jamal SA, Ljunggren Ö, Stehman-Breen C, et al (Univ of Toronto, Ontario, Canada; Uppsala Univ Hosp, Sweden; Amgen, Inc, Thousand Oaks, CA; et al)
J Bone Miner Res 26:1829-1835, 2011

The incidences of osteoporosis and chronic kidney disease (CKD) both increase with increasing age, yet there is a paucity of data on treatments for osteoporosis in the setting of impaired kidney function. We examined the efficacy and safety of denosumab (DMAb) among subjects participating in the Fracture Reduction Evaluation of Denosumab in Osteoporosis Every 6 Months (FREEDOM) Study. We estimated creatinine clearance (eGFR) using Cockcroft-Gault and classified levels of kidney function using the modified National Kidney Foundation classification of CKD. We examined incident fracture rates; changes in bone mineral density (BMD), serum calcium, and creatinine; and the incidence of adverse events after 36 months of follow-up in subjects receiving DMAb or placebo, stratified by level of kidney function. We used a subgroup interaction term to determine if there were differences in treatment effect by eGFR. Most (93%) women were white, and the mean age was 72.3 ± 5.2 years; 73 women had an eGFR of 15 to 29 mL/min; 2817, between 30 to 59 mL/min; 4069, between 60 to 89 mL/min, and 842 had an eGFR of 90 mL/min or greater. None had stage 5 CKD. Fracture risk reduction and changes in BMD at all sites were in favor of DMAb. The test for treatment by subgroup interaction was not statistically significant, indicating that treatment efficacy did not differ by kidney function. Changes in creatinine and calcium and the incidence of adverse events were similar between groups and did not differ by level of kidney function. It is concluded that DMAb is effective at reducing fracture risk and is not associated with an increase in adverse events among patients with impaired kidney function.

▶ One of the most frequent reasons that limit the use of antiresorptive or anabolic therapies in patients with osteoporosis is chronic kidney disease (CKD).[1] This is particularly true for oral or intravenous bisphosphonates but also true for teriparatide due to the secondary or tertiary hyperparathyroidism that accompanies late-stage chronic kidney disease. Most of the clinical trials for approved osteoporosis drugs contained relatively small numbers of subjects with estimated glomerular filtration rate (GFR) less than 60 mL/min, in the range of stage 3 or 4 CKD, but post-hoc analysis showed no evidence of worsening renal function or other adverse events, equal fracture reduction, and equal improvement in bone mineral density (BMD) compared with subjects with normal renal function.[2-5] Newer nonbisphosphonate therapies may potentially have this same limitation.[6]

This study evaluated the effects of denosumab on subjects with CKD in the FREEDOM Trial by using the Cockcroft-Gault equation to estimate creatinine clearance as a surrogate for measured GFR. Study subjects were then classified using the National Kidney Foundation definition of CKD based on estimated GFR. Twenty-nine subjects were identified with estimated GFR between 15 and 29 mL/min (stage 4 CKD) and 2817 subjects with estimated GFR between 30 and 59 mL/min (stage 3 CKD). No subjects were included in the trial with stage 5 CKD, with estimated GFR of less than 15 mL/min. Denosumab treatment effect did not differ by level of renal function, either by fracture risk reduction or improvement in BMD at all skeletal sites. Changes in serum calcium and creatinine level and incidence of adverse events did not differ by level of renal function. The study concluded that denosumab reduced fracture risk regardless of the level of renal function and that denosumab did not cause increased adverse events in subjects with CKD.

This study shows that denosumab is likely to be safe when used in subjects with stage 3 or 4 CKD. There is no evidence that denosumab causes more adverse events or is less effective therapeutically when used in subjects with late-stage renal disease. However, this study does not show that denosumab is less likely to convert high-turnover hyperparathyroid bone disease to low-turnover or adynamic disease than other potent antiresorptive drugs such as bisphosphonates, because bone histomorphometry was not done in subjects with late-stage CKD. All antiresorptive and anabolic agents must be used with caution in patients with stage 3–5 CKD.

B. L. Clarke, MD

References

1. McCarthy JT, Rule AD, Achenbach SJ, Bergstralh EJ, Khosla S, Melton LJ 3rd. Use of renal function measurements for assessing fracture risk in postmenopausal women. *Mayo Clin Proc.* 2008;83:1231-1239.
2. Ishani A, Blackwell T, Jamal SA, Cummings SR; MORE Investigators. The effect of raloxifene treatment in postmenopausal women with CKD. *J Am Soc Nephrol.* 2008;19:1430-1438.
3. Miller PD, Schwartz EN, Chen P, Misurski DA, Krege JH. Teriparatide in postmenopausal women with osteoporosis and mild or moderate renal impairment. *Osteoporos Int.* 2007;18:59-68.
4. Jamal SA, Bauer DC, Ensrud KE, et al. Alendronate treatment in women with normal to severely impaired renal function: an analysis of the fracture intervention trial. *J Bone Miner Res.* 2007;22:503-508.
5. Miller PD, Roux C, Boonen S, Barton IP, Dunlap LE, Burgio DE. Safety and efficacy of risedronate in patients with age-related reduced renal function as estimated by the Cockcroft and Gault method: a pooled analysis of nine clinical trials. *J Bone Miner Res.* 2005;20:2105-2115.
6. Cummings SR, San Martin J, McClung MR, et al. Denosumab for prevention of fractures in postmenopausal women with osteoporosis. *N Engl J Med.* 2009; 361:756-765.

Relationship Between Bone Mineral Density Changes With Denosumab Treatment and Risk Reduction for Vertebral and Nonvertebral Fractures
Austin M, for the FREEDOM Trial (Amgen Inc, Thousand Oaks, CA; et al)
J Bone Miner Res 27:687-693, 2012

Dual-energy X-ray absorptiometric bone mineral density (DXA BMD) is a strong predictor of fracture risk in untreated patients. However, previous patient-level studies suggest that BMD changes explain little of the fracture risk reduction observed with osteoporosis treatment. We investigated the relevance of DXA BMD changes as a predictor for fracture risk reduction using data from the FREEDOM trial, which randomly assigned placebo or denosumab 60 mg every 6 months to 7808 women aged 60 to 90 years with a spine or total hip BMD *T*-score < −2.5 and not < −4.0. We took a standard approach to estimate the percent of treatment effect explained using percent changes in BMD at a single visit (months 12, 24, or 36). We also applied a novel approach using estimated percent changes in BMD from baseline at the time of fracture occurrence (time-dependent models). Denosumab significantly increased total hip BMD by 3.2%, 4.4%, and 5.0% at 12, 24, and 36 months, respectively. Denosumab decreased the risk of new vertebral fractures by 68% ($p < 0.0001$) and nonvertebral fracture by 20% ($p = 0.01$) over 36 months. Regardless of the method used, the change in total hip BMD explained a considerable proportion of the effect of denosumab in reducing new or worsening vertebral fracture risk (35% [95% confidence interval (CI): 20%−61%] and 51% [95% CI: 39%−66%] accounted for by percent change at month 36 and change in time-dependent BMD, respectively) and explained a considerable amount of the reduction in nonvertebral fracture risk (87% [95% CI: 35%−>100%] and 72% [95% CI: 24%−>100%], respectively). Previous patient-level studies may have underestimated the strength of the relationship between BMD change and the effect of treatment on fracture risk or this relationship may be unique to denosumab.

▶ Bone mineral density (BMD) is the best clinical predictor of fracture risk in individual patients. Most antiresorptive and anabolic agents increase BMD moderately, yet previous analyses have shown that these agents do not reduce fracture risk primarily by increasing BMD.[1-5] Instead, fracture reduction with these agents largely results from preservation of bone microarchitecture.[6]

This study evaluated the effects of denosumab on hip fracture risk reduction in the large phase III, randomized, placebo-controlled FREEDOM Trial.[7] Fracture risk reduction was evaluated by the standard approach, using percentage of change in BMD from baseline at the 12-, 24-, and 36-month visits but also by a new approach using estimated percentage of change in BMD from baseline at the time of fracture occurrence in a time-dependent model. Unlike previous analyses of other antiresorptive agents, both methods unexpectedly showed that the change in total hip BMD explained a significant portion of the denosumab treatment effect in reducing new or worsening vertebral and nonvertebral fracture risk. This study concluded that previous studies of antiresorptive and anabolic drugs may have underestimated the strength of the relationship between BMD change and effect of treatment on fracture risk but acknowledged that denosumab may be different from other antiresorptive drugs in this respect.

Re-analysis of previous studies using time-dependent models will be required to clarify this issue, but it is clear that denosumab may function differently from other antiresorptive agents such as bisphosphonates or raloxifene, or anabolic agents such as teriparatide. If so, this may be due to the unique biological effects of denosumab as a monoclonal antibody specific for RANKL. It is not immediately evident why denosumab should be different from other agents, but further studies should clarify whether the apparent difference in the mechanism by which denosumab reduces fracture risk is verified.

B. L. Clarke, MD

References

1. Sarkar S, Mitlak BH, Wong M, Stock JL, Black DM, Harper KD. Relationships between bone mineral density and incident vertebral fracture risk with raloxifene therapy. *J Bone Miner Res.* 2002;17:1-10.
2. Chapurlat RD, Palermo L, Ramsay P, Cummings SR. Risk of fracture among women who lose bone density during treatment with alendronate. The Fracture Intervention Trial. *Osteoporos Int.* 2005;16:842-848.
3. Watts NB, Geusens P, Barton IP, Felsenberg D. Relationship between changes in BMD and nonvertebral fracture incidence associated with risedronate: reduction in risk of nonvertebral fracture is not related to change in BMD. *J Bone Miner Res.* 2005;20:2097-2104.
4. Chen P, Miller PD, Delmas PD, Misurski DA, Krege JH. Change in lumbar spine BMD and vertebral fracture risk reduction in teriparatide-treated postmenopausal women with osteoporosis. *J Bone Miner Res.* 2006;21:1785-1790.
5. Bruyere O, Roux C, Detilleux J, et al. Relationship between bone mineral density changes and fracture risk reduction in patients treated with strontium ranelate. *J Clin Endocrinol Metab.* 2007;92:3076-3081.
6. Hochberg MC, Greenspan S, Wasnich RD, Miller P, Thompson DE, Ross PD. Changes in bone density and turnover explain the reductions in incidence of nonvertebral fractures that occur during treatment with antiresorptive agents. *J Clin Endocrinol Metab.* 2002;87:1586-1592.
7. Cummings SR, San Martin J, McClung MR, et al. Denosumab for prevention of fractures in postmenopausal women with osteoporosis. *N Engl J Med.* 2009; 361:756-765.

Five Years of Denosumab Exposure in Women With Postmenopausal Osteoporosis: Results From the First Two Years of the FREEDOM Extension

Papapoulos S, Chapurlat R, Libanati C, et al (Leiden Univ Med Ctr, The Netherlands; Université de Lyon, France; Amgen Inc, Thousand Oaks, CA; et al)

J Bone Miner Res 27:694-701, 2012

The 3-year FREEDOM trial assessed the efficacy and safety of 60 mg denosumab every 6 months for the treatment of postmenopausal women with osteoporosis. Participants who completed the FREEDOM trial were eligible to enter an extension to continue the evaluation of denosumab efficacy and safety for up to 10 years. For the extension results presented here, women from the FREEDOM denosumab group had 2 more years of denosumab treatment (long-term group) and those from the FREEDOM placebo group had 2 years of denosumab exposure (cross-over group). We report results for bone turnover markers (BTMs), bone mineral density (BMD), fracture rates, and safety. A total of 4550 women enrolled in the extension (2343 long-term; 2207 cross-over). Reductions in BTMs were maintained (long-term group) or occurred rapidly (cross-over group) following denosumab administration. In the long-term group, lumbar spine and total hip BMD increased further, resulting in 5-year gains of 13.7% and 7.0%, respectively. In the cross-over group, BMD increased at the lumbar spine (7.7%) and total hip (4.0%) during the 2-year denosumab treatment. Yearly fracture incidences for both groups were below rates observed in the FREEDOM placebo group and below rates projected for a "virtual untreated twin" cohort. Adverse events did not increase with long-term denosumab administration. Two adverse events in the cross-over group were adjudicated as consistent with osteonecrosis of the jaw. Five-year denosumab treatment of women with postmenopausal osteoporosis maintained BTM reduction and increased BMD, and was associated with low fracture rates and a favorable risk/benefit profile.

▶ Denosumab is a fully human monoclonal antibody against receptor activator of nuclear factor kappa B (RANK) ligand (RANKL) that was approved for treatment of postmenopausal osteoporosis in June 2010.[1] RANKL is critical for the formation, function, and survival of osteoclasts and is synthesized and expressed extracellularly by osteoblasts and osteoblast precursors.[2,3] Denosumab binds RANKL secreted by osteoblasts and osteoblast precursors and prevents its interaction with the receptor RANK on osteoclasts and osteoclast precursors.[4] The antibody reversibly inhibits osteoclast-mediated bone resorption and has been shown to prevent bone loss and fractures.[1,5] This 2-year extension of the initial 3-year FREEDOM treatment trial of postmenopausal osteoporotic women with denosumab[1] was performed to obtain long-term safety and efficacy data in subjects for up to 5 years and will be continued to obtain 10-year data. All 4550 subjects in this study received denosumab. Women who had received denosumab in the initial 3-year trial continued denosumab for another 2 years (n = 2343), whereas women who had received placebo in the 3-year trial were crossed over to denosumab for 2 years (n = 2207). Markers of bone turnover remained decreased in the continued treatment group and decreased rapidly in the crossover group. Bone mineral density (BMD) continued to increase further in the continued treatment group, and increased significantly in the crossover group. Fractures were reduced in both groups below the placebo rate in the FREEDOM trial. Adverse events did not increase further in the continued treatment group, and 2 subjects in the crossover group had findings consistent with jaw osteonecrosis. The investigators concluded that treatment of postmenopausal osteoporotic women with denosumab for 5 years maintains reduction in markers of bone turnover, increases BMD, and reduces fractures, with a low risk of side effects.

These findings suggest that the monoclonal antibody denosumab continues to potently suppress bone turnover, improve BMD, and prevent fractures in postmenopausal women with osteoporosis for up to 5 years. This study also shows that 5 years of continuous treatment with denosumab does not increase the risk of serious adverse events in those who continue therapy. The optimal duration of therapy with denosumab is not yet known, but because of its rapid off-set of action, it is likely that long-term treatment will be necessary to maximize its bone protection effects.[6]

B. L. Clarke, MD

References

1. Cummings SR, San Martin J, McClung MR, et al. Denosumab for prevention of fractures in postmenopausal women with osteoporosis. *N Engl J Med.* 2009; 361:756-765.
2. Lacey DL, Timms E, Tan HL, et al. Osteoprotegerin ligand is a cytokine that regulates osteoclast differentiation and activation. *Cell.* 1998;93:165-176.
3. Lacey DL, Tan HL, Lu J, et al. Osteoprotegerin ligand modulates murine osteoclast survival in vitro and in vivo. *Am J Pathol.* 2000;157:435-448.
4. Hsu H, Lacey DL, Dunstan CR, et al. Tumor necrosis factor receptor family member RANK mediates osteoclast differentiation and activation induced by osteoprotegerin ligand. *Proc Natl Acad Sci U S A.* 1999;96:3540-3545.
5. McClung MR, Lewiecki EM, Cohen SB, et al. Denosumab in postmenopausal women with low bone mineral density. *N Engl J Med.* 2006;354:821-831.
6. Bone HG, Bolognese MA, Yuen CK, et al. Effects of denosumab treatment and discontinuation on bone mineral density and bone turnover markers in postmenopausal women with low bone mass. *J Clin Endocrinol Metab.* 2011;96:972-980.

The Effects of Ronacaleret, a Calcium-Sensing Receptor Antagonist, on Bone Mineral Density and Biochemical Markers of Bone Turnover in Postmenopausal Women with Low Bone Mineral Density

Fitzpatrick LA, Dabrowski CE, Cicconetti G, et al (King of Prussia, PA; et al)
J Clin Endocrinol Metab 96:2441-2449, 2011

Context.—Ronacaleret, a calcium-sensing receptor antagonist that stimulates PTH release from the parathyroid glands, was evaluated as an oral osteoanabolic agent for the treatment of osteoporosis.

Objective.—Our objective was to compare the effects of ronacaleret, teriparatide, and alendronate on bone mineral density (BMD) and markers of bone turnover.

Design and Setting.—In this randomized, placebo-controlled, dose-ranging trial, spine and hip BMD were assessed by dual-energy x-ray absorptiometry and bone turnover markers were measured.

Patients.—Patients included 569 postmenopausal women with low BMD.

Interventions.—Subjects were offered open-label 20 μg teriparatide sc once daily or were randomized to 100, 200, 300, or 400 mg oral ronacaleret once daily, 70 mg alendronate once weekly, or placebo and were followed for up to 12 months.

Main Outcome Measure.—Percentage change from baseline in lumbar spine BMD was assessed at month 12.

Results.—With ronacaleret, the increases in lumbar spine BMD at 12 months (0.3–1.6%) were significantly lower than those attained with teriparatide (9.1%) or alendronate (4.5%). There were small decreases in total hip, femoral neck, and trochanter BMD at month 12 with ronacaleret compared with increases in the teriparatide and alendronate arms. Bone turnover markers increased in the ronacaleret and teriparatide arms and decreased in the alendronate arm. PTH elevations with ronacaleret were prolonged relative to those previously reported with teriparatide.

Conclusion.—The densitometric findings in the context of prolonged PTH elevation and increased bone turnover suggest ronacaleret induces mild hyperparathyroidism. Ronacaleret only modestly increased lumbar spine BMD and decreased BMD at hip sites.

▶ The search for new anabolic agents to treat osteoporosis has made continued progress in recent years. The only currently approved anabolic agent, teriparatide (human recombinant parathyroid hormone [PTH] 1−34) is given as a once-daily bolus subcutaneous injection.[1] The recognition that intermittent PTH bolus injections cause increased bone density, whereas continuous PTH oversecretion causes bone loss, has led to efforts to stimulate endogenous PTH secretion intermittently by indirect means. Certain new agents, such as antisclerostin monoclonal antibody, cathepsin K inhibitors, and Dkk inhibitors appear to have anabolic properties in addition to their antiresorptive effects. Some of these agents may act in part by stimulating endogenous PTH secretion. Ronacaleret is a member of a new class of calcium-sensing receptor (CaSR) antagonists with short half-lives that stimulate intermittent PTH secretion due to transient blockade of the CaSR.[2,3] Transient inhibition of the CaSR causes parathyroid cells to sense lower ambient ionized calcium than present in interstitial fluid, which causes them to transiently increase PTH secretion.

This study evaluated the effects of ronacaleret, teriparatide, alendronate, and placebo on bone mineral density (BMD) and bone turnover markers in postmenopausal osteoporotic women. Subjects were randomly assigned to receive standard doses of daily teriparatide and weekly alendronate, varying doses of ronacaleret, or placebo for up to 1 year. Ronacaleret caused mild increases in lumbar spine BMD but was associated with mild decreases in total hip, femoral neck, and greater trochanter BMD over 12 months of therapy. The other 2 agents caused significant increases in BMD at these same skeletal sites, as expected. Bone turnover markers increased in the ronacaleret and teriparatide groups and decreased in subjects treated with alendronate. Serum PTH increased in the ronacaleret group longer than teriparatide levels increased in the teriparatide group (Fig 4 in the original article). These findings are interpreted to indicate that ronacaleret caused mild hyperparathyroidism, while mildly improving lumbar spine BMD but not protecting against hip bone loss.

This study demonstrates that therapeutic agents that stimulate PTH secretion will require pharmacokinetics similar to teriparatide to stimulate increased BMD. Agents that stimulate PTH secretion in a more prolonged fashion that more closely approximates chronic hyperparathyroidism will likely cause increased bone turnover leading to bone loss. Previous clinical trials with PTH 1−84 caused more hypercalcemia than with teriparatide (recombinant human PTH 1−34), resulting in disapproval of PTH 1−84 for treatment of postmenopausal osteoporosis in the United States.[4,5] Newer drugs are being sought that will stimulate PTH secretion with a more favorable kinetic profile, leading to increased BMD and reduced fracture risk.

B. L. Clarke, MD

References

1. Neer RM, Arnaud CD, Zanchetta JR, et al. Effect of parathyroid hormone (1-34) on fractures and bone mineral density in postmenopausal women with osteoporosis. *N Engl J Med.* 2001;344:1434-1441.
2. Fitzpatrick LA, Dabrowski CE, Cicconetti G, et al. Ronacaleret, a calcium-sensing receptor antagonist, increases trabecular but not cortical bone in postmenopausal women. *J Bone Miner Res.* 2011;96:2441-2449.
3. Fitzpatrick LA, Smith PL, McBride TA, et al. Ronacaleret, a calcium-sensing receptor antagonist, has no significant effect on radial fracture healing time: results of a randomized, double-blinded, placebo-controlled Phase II clinical trial. *Bone.* 2011;49:845-852.
4. Black DM, Bouxsein ML, Palermo L, et al; PTH Once-Weekly Research (POWR) Group. Randomized trial of once-weekly parathyroid hormone (1-84) on bone mineral density and remodeling. *J Clin Endocrinol Metab.* 2008;93:2166-2172.
5. Bauer DC, Garnero P, Bilezikian JP, et al. Short-term changes in bone turnover markers and bone mineral density response to parathyroid hormone in postmenopausal women with osteoporosis. *J Clin Endocrinol Metab.* 2006;91:1370-1375.

Epidemiology and Pathophysiology of Osteoporosis

Hip Fracture and Increased Short-term but Not Long-term Mortality in Healthy Older Women

LeBlanc ES, Hillier TA, Pedula KL, et al (Kaiser Permanente Northwest, Portland, OR; et al)
Arch Intern Med 171:1831-1837, 2011

Background.—Fractures have been associated with subsequent increases in mortality, but it is unknown how long that increase persists.

Methods.—A total of 5580 women from a large community-based, multicenter US prospective cohort of 9704 (Study of Osteoporotic Fractures) were observed prospectively for almost 20 years. We age-matched 1116 hip fracture cases with 4 control participants (n = 4464). To examine the effect of health status, we examined a healthy older subset (n = 960) 80 years or older who attended the 10-year follow-up examination and reported good or excellent health. Incident hip fractures were adjudicated from radiology reports by study physicians. Death was confirmed by death certificates.

Results.—Hip fracture cases had 2-fold increased mortality in the year after fracture compared with controls (16.9% vs 8.4%; multivariable adjusted odds ratio [OR], 2.4; 95% CI, 1.9-3.1]. When examined by age and health status, short-term mortality was increased in those aged 65 to 69 years (16.3% vs 3.7%; OR, 5.0; 95% CI, 2.6-9.5), 70 to 79 years (16.5% vs 8.9%; OR, 2.4; 95% CI, 1.8-3.3), and only in those 80 years or older with good or excellent health (15.1% vs 7.2%; multivariable adjusted OR, 2.8; 95% CI, 1.5-5.2). After the first year, survival of hip fracture cases and controls was similar except in those aged 65 to 69 years, who continued to have increased mortality.

Conclusions.—Short-term mortality is increased after hip fracture in women aged 65 to 79 years and in exceptionally healthy women 80 years or older. Women 70 years or older return to previous risk levels after a year. Interventions are needed to decrease mortality in the year after hip fracture, when mortality risk is highest.

▶ Low- to moderate-trauma osteoporotic fractures, particularly hip and vertebral fractures, have been associated with increased mortality, especially for the first 3 to 6 months after fracture, with some studies showing prolonged increased mortality for several years.[1-6] Wrist and other nonvertebral fractures have not been reported to be associated with increased mortality in most studies. Men appear to have increased mortality after hip fracture longer than women.[2] Hip fractures may be a sign of increased age and morbidity that might be expected to lead to increased morality, but this is less so for vertebral fractures. How long the increased risk of mortality persists after hip fracture depends on age and sex of the patient as well as other factors.[3,5,6]

This study evaluated 5580 women from the Study of Osteoporotic Fractures, who were followed up for over almost 20 years, obtained from the larger cohort of 9704 women enrolled in this large prospective, community-based, multicenter US study. Of the 5580 women evaluated, 1116 hip fracture cases were matched for age to 4464 control subjects without hip fracture. The health status of fracture subjects and case controls was compared with 960 women age 80 or older who attended the 10-year follow-up study examination and reported good or excellent health. Incident hip fractures in the cohort were confirmed by review of radiology reports by study physicians, and deaths were confirmed by review of death certificates. Mortality rate increased 2.4-fold in the year after hip fracture compared with that in control subjects, and short-term mortality increased in all subjects aged 65–79 years but only in subjects 80 years or older who were in good or excellent health. One year after hip fracture, however, mortality remained increased only in subjects 65–69 years old. The study concluded that mortality after hip fracture in older women is increased for 1 year in those aged 70–79 years old and for exceptionally healthy women 80 years or older, but that mortality remains increased for longer than 1 year in those aged 65–69 years.

These findings indicate that mortality risk after hip fracture in older women occurs mainly during the first year after fracture, except for those in their later 60s, where increased mortality risk continues for longer. The implications of this study are that efforts to decrease mortality after hip fracture should be focused primarily during the first year after hip fracture for most postmenopausal women, except for those 65–69 years old, where longer-term interventions may be required. This study did not evaluate mortality risk after vertebral, nonvertebral, or other fractures, so it is not clear that mortality risk after other types of common osteoporotic fracture follows the same trend over time.

B. L. Clarke, MD

References

1. Empana JP, Dargent-Molina P, Bréart G; EPIDOS Group. Effect of hip fracture on mortality in elderly women: the EPIDOS prospective study. *J Am Geriatr Soc.* 2004;52:685-690.
2. Haentjens P, Magaziner J, Colón-Emeric CS, et al. Meta-analysis: excess mortality after hip fracture among older women and men. *Ann Intern Med.* 2010;152: 380-390.

3. Forsén L, Sogaard AJ, Meyer HE, Edna T, Kopjar B. Survival after hip fracture: short- and long-term excess mortality according to age and gender. *Osteoporos Int.* 1999;10:73-78.
4. Ensrud KE, Ewing SK, Taylor BC, et al; Study of Osteoporotic Fractures Research Group. Frailty and risk of falls, fracture, and mortality in older women: the study of osteoporotic fractures. *J Gerontol A Biol Sci Med Sci.* 2007;62:744-751.
5. Bliuc D, Nguyen ND, Milch VE, Nguyen TV, Eisman JA, Center JR. Mortality risk associated with low-trauma osteoporotic fracture and subsequent fracture in men and women. *JAMA.* 2009;301:513-521.
6. Ioannidis G, Papaioannou A, Hopman WM, et al. Relation between fractures and mortality: results from the Canadian Multicentre Osteoporosis study. *CMAJ.* 2009;181:265-271.

Association of Hip Strength Estimates by Finite-Element Analysis With Fractures in Women and Men

Amin S, Kopperdhal DL, Melton LJ III, et al (Mayo Clinic, Rochester, MN; ON Diagnostics, Berkeley, CA)
J Bone Miner Res 26:1593-1600, 2011

Finite-element analysis (FEA) of quantitative computed tomography (QCT) scans can estimate site-specific whole-bone strength. However, it is uncertain whether the site-specific detail included in FEA-estimated proximal femur (hip) strength can determine fracture risk at sites with different biomechanical characteristics. To address this question, we used FEA of proximal femur QCT scans to estimate hip strength and load-to-strength ratio during a simulated sideways fall and measured total hip areal and volumetric bone mineral density (aBMD and vBMD) from QCT images in an age-stratified random sample of community-dwelling adults age 35 years or older. Among 314 women (mean age ± SD: 61 ± 15 years; 235 postmenopausal) and 266 men (62 ± 16 years), 139 women and 104 men had any prevalent fracture, whereas 55 Women and 28 men had a prevalent osteoporotic fracture that had occurred at age 35 years or older. Odds ratios by age-adjusted logistic regression analysis for prevalent overall and osteoporotic fractures each were similar for FEA hip strength and load-to-strength ratio, as well as for total hip aBMD and vBMD. C-statistics (estimated areas under *ROC* curves) also were similar [eg, 0.84 to 0.85 (women) and 0.75 to 0.78 (men) for osteoporotic fractures]. In women and men, the association with prevalent osteoporotic fractures increased below an estimated hip strength of approximately 3000 N. Despite its site-specific nature, FEA-estimated hip strength worked equally well at predicting prevalent overall and osteoporotic fractures. Furthermore, an estimated hip strength below 3000 N may represent a critical level of systemic skeletal fragility in both sexes that warrants further investigation.

▶ Estimation of bone strength by finite element analysis has been used to predict forearm strength.[1] Finite element analysis may be applied to findings from quantitative computed tomography (CT) scans to derive estimates of whole-bone strength by incorporating the relevant bone mineral density (BMD) and geometry information from the scans. This type of analysis has also been applied to the proximal femur to evaluate fracture risk.[2,3]

This study evaluated whether finite element analysis-estimated proximal femur strength and load-to-strength ratio during a sideways-simulated fall could determine fracture risk at sites with different biomechanical characteristics. Proximal femur quantitative CT scan data from 314 women and 266 men from an age-stratified random sample of community-dwelling adults age 35 years or older were analyzed. Of these subjects, 139 women and 104 men had prevalent fractures of any type at the time of study, whereas 55 women and 28 men had prevalent osteoporotic fractures that had occurred at age 35 years or older. The odds ratios by age-adjusted logistic regression analysis for prevalent overall and osteoporotic fractures were similar for finite element analysis hip strength and load-to-strength ratio as well as for total hip areal BMD and volumetric BMD. The estimated areas under the receiver-operator curves were also similar. The association with prevalent osteoporotic fractures increased below an estimated hip strength of 3000 Newtons. Even though this analysis was specific to the proximal femur, finite element analysis-estimated hip strength predicted prevalent overall and osteoporotic fractures equally well. The study concluded that estimated proximal femur strength predicted fracture risk at other sites in the skeleton with different biomechanical characteristics and that an estimated hip strength below 3000 Newtons may predict a significant level of systemic skeletal fragility.

These findings show that estimates of proximal femur strength using finite element analysis of quantitative CT scan images can predict fracture risk at the hip, as well as other sites in the skeleton, in both women and men. This result is analogous to previous studies showing that total hip dual-energy X-ray absorptiometry areal BMD and volumetric BMD predict fracture risk at the hip and other skeletal sites in both sexes.[4,5] It is not intrinsically obvious that this should be the case for proximal femur strength estimates, as 3-dimensional proximal femur shape, femoral neck BMD, and spatial distribution of BMD within the femur may be biomechanically meaningful primarily at the hip. Typical traumatic loading conditions, most often a sideways fall on the hip, are specific for hip fracture and may not predict other factures. Nevertheless, the study reports an estimated hip strength of 3000 Newtons below which fracture risk is increased in both women and men,[6] analogous to previous studies that showed an absolute BMD threshold below which fracture risk was increased.

B. L. Clarke, MD

References

1. Melton LJ 3rd, Riggs BL, Müller R, et al. Determinants of forearm strength in postmenopausal women. *Osteoporos Int.* 2011;22:3047-3054.
2. Melton LJ 3rd, Riggs BL, Keaveny TM, et al. Structural determinants of vertebral fracture risk. *J Bone Miner Res.* 2007;22:1885-1892.
3. Melton LJ 3rd, Riggs BL, van Lenthe GH, et al. Contribution of in vivo structural measurements and load/strength ratios to the determination of forearm fracture risk in postmenopausal women. *J Bone Miner Res.* 2007;22:1442-1448.
4. Riggs BL, Melton LJ 3rd, Robb RA, et al. Population-based analysis of the relationship of whole bone strength indices and fall-related loads to age- and sex-specific patterns of hip and wrist fractures. *J Bone Miner Res.* 2006;21:315-323.

5. Keyak JH, Sigurdsson S, Karlsdottir G, et al. Male-female differences in the association between incident hip fracture and proximal femoral strength: a finite element analysis study. *Bone.* 2011;48:1239-1245.
6. Keaveny TM, Bouxsein ML. Theoretical implications of the biomechanical fracture threshold. *J Bone Miner Res.* 2008;23:1541-1547.

Relationship of femoral neck areal bone mineral density to volumetric bone mineral density, bone size, and femoral strength in men and women

Srinivasan B, Kopperdahl DL, Amin S, et al (Mayo Clinic, Rochester, MN; O. N. Diagnostics, Berkeley, CA; et al)

Osteoporos Int 23:155-162, 2012

Summary.—Using combined dual-energy X-ray absorptiometry (DXA) and quantitative computed tomography, we demonstrate that men matched with women for femoral neck (FN) areal bone mineral density (aBMD) have lower volumetric BMD (vBMD), higher bone cross-sectional area, and relatively similar values for finite element (FE)-derived bone strength.

Introduction.—aBMD by DXA is widely used to identify patients at risk for osteoporotic fractures. aBMD is influenced by bone size (i.e., matched for vBMD, larger bones have higher aBMD), and increasing evidence indicates that absolute aBMD predicts a similar risk of fracture in men and women. Thus, we sought to define the relationships between FN aBMD (assessed by DXA) and vBMD, bone size, and FE-derived femoral strength obtained from quantitative computed tomography scans in men versus women.

Methods.—We studied men and women aged 40 to 90 years and not on osteoporosis medications.

Results.—In 114 men and 114 women matched for FN aBMD, FN total cross-sectional area was 38% higher ($P<0.0001$) and vBMD was 16% lower ($P<0.0001$) in the men. FE models constructed in a subset of 28 women and 28 men matched for FN aBMD showed relatively similar values for bone strength and the load-to-strength ratio in the two groups.

Conclusions.—In this cohort of young and old men and women from Rochester, MN, USA who are matched by FN aBMD, because of the offsetting effects of bone size and vBMD, femoral strength and the load-to-strength ratio tended to be relatively similar across the sexes.

▶ Age-related bone loss results in increased fracture risk in both women and men, but the mechanisms for bone loss appear to be different between women and men.[1-5] Trabecular bone loss begins in both women and men in the third decade, whereas cortical bone loss begins in both in the sixth decade.[6] Aging women predominantly have a decrease in trabecular number, whereas men lose trabecular thickness while maintaining trabecular number.[7] The net effect of these changes leads to decreased bone mineral density (BMD) with age, with greater loss of bone strength in women compared with men, and corresponding increased fracture risk in women compared with men.

This study evaluated women and men matched for femoral neck areal BMD by dual-energy x-ray absorptiometry (DXA) and assessed volumetric BMD, bone cross-sectional area, and finite element analysis—derived bone strength. Areal BMD by DXA is currently used clinically to predict fracture risk in patients. This parameter is influenced heavily by bone cross-sectional area, with larger bones having higher BMD when matched for volumetric BMD. The study attempted to define relationships between femoral neck BMD by DXA and volumetric BMD, bone size, and finite element—derived femoral strength from quantitative computed tomography (CT) scans in women and men. None of the subjects in this cohort of 114 women and 114 men from age 40 to 90 years was taking osteoporosis medications. When matched for femoral neck areal BMD, femoral neck cross-sectional area was almost 40% higher, and volumetric BMD 16% lower in men. Finite element analysis of CT scan results from a subset of 28 women and 28 men matched for femoral neck areal BMD showed relatively similar values for bone strength and load-to-strength ratio in the 2 groups, implying that bone size and volumetric BMD have offsetting effects on femoral neck strength and the load-to-strength ratio.

These findings imply that the skeleton is able to model to compensate for sex-specific differences in skeletal size to ensure that bone strength is adequate to prevent fractures throughout life. Sexual dimorphism in the skeleton is largely determined by gonadal sex steroid secretion beginning at puberty and continuing throughout life, until menopause in women.[8] Men acquire larger bone size due primarily to the effect of testosterone on periosteal apposition. These findings suggest that the male skeleton adapts to larger bone size by developing lower volumetric BMD and that the female skeleton compensates for smaller bone size by developing higher volumetric BMD. In both cases, the skeleton is able to maintain bone strength to prevent fracture. These findings support the assumption in the World Health Organization fracture risk assessment tool (FRAX®) that fracture risk is similar in men and women with the same femoral neck areal BMD.

B. L. Clarke, MD

References

1. Szulc P, Munoz F, Duboeuf F, Marchand F, Delmas PD. Low width of tubular bones is associated with increased risk of fragility fracture in elderly men—the MINOS study. *Bone*. 2006;38:595-602.
2. Peacock M, Buckwalter KA, Persohn S, Hangartner TN, Econs MJ, Hui S. Race and sex differences in bone mineral density and geometry at the femur. *Bone*. 2009;45:218-225.
3. Sheu Y, Zmuda JM, Boudreau RM, et al; Osteoporotic Fractures in Men MrOS Research Group. Bone strength measured by peripheral quantitative computed tomography and the risk of nonvertebral fractures: the osteoporotic fractures in men (MrOS) study. *J Bone Miner Res*. 2011;26:63-71.
4. Khoo BC, Brown K, Cann C, et al. Comparison of QCT-derived and DXA-derived areal bone mineral density and T scores. *Osteoporos Int*. 2009;20:1539-1545.
5. Riggs BL, Melton LJ 3rd, Robb RA, et al. Population-based analysis of the relationship of whole bone strength indices and fall-related loads to age- and sex-specific patterns of hip and wrist fractures. *J Bone Miner Res*. 2006;21:315-323.
6. Riggs BL, Melton LJ, Robb RA, et al. A population-based assessment of rates of bone loss at multiple skeletal sites: evidence for substantial trabecular bone loss in young adult women and men. *J Bone Miner Res*. 2008;23:205-214.

7. Riggs BL, Melton LJ 3rd, Robb RA, et al. Population-based study of age and sex differences in bone volumetric density, size, geometry, and structure at different skeletal sites. *J Bone Miner Res.* 2004;19:1945-1954.
8. Duan Y, Beck TJ, Wang XF, Seeman E. Structural and biomechanical basis of sexual dimorphism in femoral neck fragility has its origins in growth and aging. *J Bone Miner Res.* 2003;18:1766-1774.

Relationship of Age to Bone Microstructure Independent of Areal Bone Mineral Density

Nicks KM, Amin S, Atkinson EJ, et al (Mayo Clinic, Rochester, MN)
J Bone Miner Res 27:637-644, 2011

Previous studies using dual-energy X-ray absorptiometry (DXA) have demonstrated that age is a major predictor of bone fragility and fracture risk independent of areal bone mineral density (aBMD). Although this aBMD-independent effect of age has been attributed to poor bone "quality," the structural basis for this remains unclear. Because high-resolution peripheral quantitative computed tomography (HRpQCT) can assess bone microarchitecture, we matched younger and older subjects for aBMD at the ultradistal radius and assessed for possible differences in trabecular or cortical microstructure by HRpQCT. From an age-stratified, random sample of community adults, 44 women aged <50 years (mean age 41.0 years) were matched to 44 women aged ≥50 years (mean age 62.7 years) by ultradistal radius aBMD (mean ± SEM, younger and older aBMD 0.475 ± 0.011 and 0.472 ± 0.011 g/cm^2, respectively), and 57 men aged <50 years (mean age 41.3 years) were matched to 57 men aged ≥50 years (mean age 68.1 years; younger and older aBMD both 0.571 ± 0.008 g/cm^2). In these matched subjects, there were no sex-specific differences in trabecular microstructural parameters. However, significant differences were noted in cortical microstructure (all $p < 0.05$): Older women and men had increased cortical porosity (by 91% and 56%, respectively), total cortical pore volume (by 77% and 61%, respectively), and mean cortical pore diameter (by 9% and 8%, respectively) compared with younger subjects. These findings indicate that younger and older women and men matched for DXA aBMD have similar trabecular microarchitecture but clearly different cortical microstructure, at least at an appendicular site represented by the radius. Further studies are needed to define the extent to which this deterioration in cortical microstructure contributes to the aBMD-independent effect of age on bone fragility and fracture risk at the distal radius and other sites of osteoporotic fractures.

▶ Previous studies have shown that DXA bone mineral density (BMD) and age are independent predictors of fracture risk.[1-6] The independent effect of age is likely because of decreases in bone "quality" that lead to increased fractures, but previous studies have not clearly defined the changes that affect bone quality adversely.

This study evaluated bone microarchitecture at the ultradistal radius using high-resolution peripheral quantitative CT scans in young and old subjects matched for areal BMD in an attempt to elicit factors explaining the decrease in bone quality with age. In an age-stratified random sample of community-dwelling adults, 44 women with a mean age of 41.0 years were matched with 44 women with a mean age of 62.7 years for ultradistal radius BMD. From the same sample, 57 men with a mean age of 41.3 years and 57 men with a mean age of 68.1 years were matched for ultradistal radius BMD. The matched subjects showed no differences in trabecular microstructural parameters between women and men, but significant changes were seen in cortical microstructure. Older subjects had increased cortical porosity, total cortical pore volume, and mean cortical pore diameter compared with younger subjects. The study concluded that younger and older women and men matched for DXA areal BMD at the ultra-distal radius have similar trabecular microarchitecture but very different cortical microstructure. Whether this is representative of other skeletal sites is not yet clear.

These findings demonstrate that deterioration in cortical microarchitecture contributes to the areal BMD-independent effect of age on fracture risk at an appendicular site. Further studies will be necessary to determine if this occurs at other appendicular or central skeletal sites. Changes in cortical porosity may explain age-related changes in skeletal strength in at least some skeletal sites.

B. L. Clarke, MD

References

1. Szulc P, Boutroy S, Vilayphiou N, et al. Cross-sectional analysis of the association between fragility fractures and bone microarchitecture in older men: the STRAMBO study. *J Bone Miner Res.* 2011;26:1358-1367.
2. Sornay-Rendu E, Boutroy S, Munoz F, Delmas PD. Alterations of cortical and trabecular architecture are associated with fractures in postmenopausal women, partially independent of decreased BMD measured by DXA: the OFELY study. *J Bone Miner Res.* 2007;22:425-433.
3. Stein EM, Liu XS, Nickolas TL, et al. Abnormal microarchitecture and reduced stiffness at the radius and tibia in postmenopausal women with fractures. *J Bone Miner Res.* 2010;25:2572-2581.
4. Liu XS, Stein EM, Zhou B, et al. Individual trabecula segmentation (ITS)-based morphological analyses and micro finite element analysis of HR-pQCT images discriminate postmenopausal fragility fractures independent of DXA measurements. *J Bone Miner Res.* 2011;26:2184-2193.
5. Hansen S, Jensen JE, Ahrberg F, Hauge EM, Brixen K. The combination of structural parameters and areal bone mineral density improves relation to proximal femur strength: an in vitro study with high-resolution peripheral quantitative computed tomography. *Calcif Tissue Int.* 2011;89:335-346.
6. Srinivasan B, Kopperdahl DL, Amin S, et al. Relationship of femoral neck areal bone mineral density to volumetric bone mineral density, bone size, and femoral strength in men and women. *Osteoporos Int.* 2012;23:155-162.

Determinants of forearm strength in postmenopausal women

Melton LJ III, Riggs BL, Müller R, et al (Mayo Clinic, Rochester, MN; ETH Zurich, Switzerland; et al)

Osteoporos Int 22:3047-3054, 2011

Summary.—Bone strength at the ultradistal radius, quantified by micro-finite element modeling, can be predicted by variables obtained from high-resolution peripheral quantitative computed tomography scans. The specific formula for this bone strength surrogate ($-555.2+8.1\times$[trabecular vBMD]$+19.6\times$[cortical area]$+4.2\times$[total cross-sectional area]) should be validated and tested in fracture risk assessment.

Introduction.—The purpose of this study was to identify key determinants of ultradistal radius (UDR) strength and evaluate their relationships with age, sex steroid levels, and measures of habitual skeletal loading.

Methods.—UDR failure load ($\sim$strength) was assessed by micro-finite element (μFE) modeling in 105 postmenopausal controls from an earlier forearm fracture case-control study. Predictors of bone strength obtained by high-resolution peripheral quantitative computed tomography (HRpQCT) in this group were then evaluated in a population-based cohort of 214 postmenopausal women. Sex steroids were measured by mass spectrometry.

Results.—A surrogate variable ($-555.2+8.1\times$[trabecular vBMD]$+19.6\times$[cortical area]$+4.2\times$[total cross-sectional area]) predicted UDR strength modeled by μFE ($R^2 = 0.81$), and all parameters except total cross-sectional area declined with age. Evaluated cross-sectionally, the 21% fall in predicted bone strength between ages 40–49 years and 80+years more resembled the change in trabecular volumetric bone mineral density (vBMD) (-15%) than that in cortical area (-41%). In multivariable analyses, measures of body composition and physical activity were stronger predictors of UDR trabecular vBMD, cortical area, total cross-sectional area, and predicted bone strength than were sex steroid levels, but bio-available estradiol and testosterone were correlated with body mass.

Conclusions.—Bone strength at the UDR, as quantified by μFE, can be predicted from variables obtained by HRpQCT. Predicted bone strength declines with age with changes in UDR trabecular vBMD and cortical area, related in turn to reduced skeletal loading and sex steroid levels. The predicted bone strength formula should be validated and tested in fracture risk assessment.

▶ Bone strength at the wrist, as at other skeletal sites, can be predicted from variables obtained from high-resolution quantitative computed tomography (CT) scans using micro-finite element modeling. A previous study evaluating postmenopausal women with a distal forearm (Colles') fractures compared with postmenopausal women without previous osteoporotic fracture showed that the ratio of applied bone load to bone failure load was 24% higher in fracture cases.[1] Each standard deviation increase in this ratio led to a 3-fold increase in risk of fracture, but the applied bone load, defined as the estimated impact force on the upper extremity during a fall forward on the outstretched arm, was the same in the 2 groups, and falls were not more common among cases compared with controls. The difference in the ratio was due to a 20% reduction in failure load of the ultradistal radius as assessed by micro-finite element modeling of data from high-resolution peripheral quantitative CT scans. Other investigators previously showed that more than half of forearm fracture risk was determined by microfinite element-estimated failure load, bone density, and bone geometry.[2]

This study attempted to determine the key components of ultradistal radius strength and to evaluate their correlations with age, gonadal sex steroid levels, and measures of habitual skeletal loading. Ultradistal radius strength was assessed by micro-finite element modeling in 105 postmenopausal women, and predictors of bone strength obtained by high-resolution peripheral quantitative CT scans in these women were then evaluated in a population-based cohort of 214 postmenopausal women. A surrogate variable predicted ultradistal radius strength modeled by micro-finite element analysis, and trabecular volumetric bone mineral density (BMD) and cortical area decreased with age, but total cross-sectional area did not. Cross-sectional study showed that predicted bone strength decreased by 21% between ages 40 and greater than 80 years, resembling the decrease in trabecular volumetric BMD more than the decrease in cortical area. Multivariate analysis showed that measures of body composition and physical activity were stronger predictors of ultradistal radius trabecular volumetric BMD, cortical area, total cross-sectional area, and predicted bone strength than sex steroid levels, but that bioavailable estradiol and testosterone correlated with body mass. The study concluded that predicted bone strength decreases with age with changes in ultradistal radius trabecular volumetric BMD and cortical area, which are related to reduced skeletal loading and sex steroid levels.

These findings suggest that predicted bone strength by micro-finite element analysis assesses bone strength at the ultradistal radius better than areal BMD by dual-energy X-ray absorptiometry, and that skeletal loading variables have a greater influence on predicted bone strength and its key determinants than gonadal sex steroid levels. The study found that the age-related decrease in predicted bone strength was not nearly as rapid as the decrease in ultradistal radius or total wrist areal BMD in postmenopausal women,[3] raising the possibility that the decrease in wrist areal BMD may overestimate the loss in ultradistal radius strength with aging.[4,5] This is quite different from the proximal femur, in which the age-related decrease in femoral strength assessed by micro-finite element analysis is much greater than the decrease in areal BMD among women age 35 to 80 years.[6] The results of this study imply that different risk factors for bone loss within specific compartments of bone may reflect different osteoporosis phenotypes.

B. L. Clarke, MD

References

1. Melton LJ 3rd, Riggs BL, van Lenthe GH, et al. Contribution of in vivo structural measurements and load/strength ratios to the determination of forearm fracture risk in postmenopausal women. *J Bone Miner Res.* 2007;22:1442-1448.
2. Boutroy S, Van Rietbergen B, Sornay-Rendu E, Munoz F, Bouxsein ML, Delmas PD. Finite element analysis based on in vivo HR-pQCT images of the distal radius is

associated with wrist fracture in postmenopausal women. *J Bone Miner Res.* 2008; 23:392-399.

3. Melton LJ 3rd, Khosla S, Atkinson EJ, Oconnor MK, Ofallon WM, Riggs BL. Cross-sectional versus longitudinal evaluation of bone loss in men and women. *Osteoporos Int.* 2000;11:592-599.

4. Riggs BL, Melton LJ 3rd, Robb RA, et al. Population-based analysis of the relationship of whole bone strength indices and fall-related loads to age- and sex-specific patterns of hip and wrist fractures. *J Bone Miner Res.* 2006;21:315-323.

5. Ahlborg HG, Johnell O, Turner CH, Rannevik G, Karlsson MK. Bone loss and bone size after menopause. *N Engl J Med.* 2003;349:327-334.

6. Keaveny TM, Kopperdahl DL, Melton LJ 3rd, et al. Age-dependence of femoral strength in white women and men. *J Bone Miner Res.* 2010;25:994-1001.

Effects of Antiresorptive Treatment on Nonvertebral Fracture Outcomes

Mackey DC, Black DM, Bauer DC, et al (California Pacific Med Ctr, San Francisco; Univ of California San Francisco; et al)
J Bone Miner Res 26:2411-2418, 2011

Various definitions of nonvertebral fracture have been used in osteoporosis trials, precluding comparisons of efficacy. Using only subgroups of nonvertebral fractures for trial outcomes may underestimate the benefits and cost-effectiveness of treatments. The objectives of this study were to determine (1) the effect of antiresorptive treatment on various nonvertebral fracture outcomes, (2) whether risk reduction from antiresorptive treatment is greater for nonvertebral fractures that have stronger associations with low BMD, and (3) sample size estimates for clinical trials of osteoporosis treatments. Study-level data were combined from five randomized fracture-prevention trials of antiresorptive agents that reduce the risk of nonvertebral fracture in postmenopausal women: alendronate, clodronate, denosumab, lasofoxifene, and zoledronic acid. Pooled effect estimates were calculated with random-effects models. The five trials included 30,118 women; 2997 women had at least one nonvertebral fracture. There was no significant heterogeneity between treatments for any outcome (all $p > 0.10$). Antiresorptive treatment had similar effects on all fractures (summary hazard ratio [HR] = 0.76, 95% CI 0.70—0.81), high-trauma fractures (HR = 0.74, 95% CI 0.57—0.96), low-trauma fractures (HR = 0.77, 95% CI 0.71—0.83), nonvertebral six (ie, hip, pelvis, leg, wrist, humerus, and clavicle) fractures (HR = 0.73, 95% CI 0.66—0.80), other than nonvertebral six fractures (HR = 0.78, 95% CI 0.70—0.87), and all fractures other than finger, face, and toe (HR = 0.75, 95% CI 0.70—0.81). Risk reduction was not greater for fractures with stronger associations with low BMD ($p = 0.77$). A trial of all nonvertebral fractures would require fewer participants ($n = 2641$ per arm) than one of a subgroup of six fractures ($n = 3289$), for example. In summary, antiresorptive treatments reduced all nonvertebral fractures regardless of degree of trauma or special groupings, supporting the use of all nonvertebral fractures as a standard endpoint of osteoporosis trials and the basis for estimating the benefits and cost-effectiveness of treatments.

▶ The large majority of low- to moderate-trauma osteoporotic fractures are nonvertebral fractures, yet clinical trials have focused on prevention of hip and vertebral fractures.[1-6] This has been necessary for a variety of reasons, including the fact that, in most cases, vertebral and hip fractures are easily verifiable clinically or by x-ray. Furthermore, different clinical trials have used different definitions for nonvertebral fractures, making direct comparisons of efficacy between the available therapeutic agents very difficult.

This study attempted to estimate the effect of antiresorptive treatment on nonvertebral fracture outcomes, determine whether fracture risk reduction is greater for nonvertebral fractures associated with low bone mineral density (BMD), and estimate sample sizes required to show treatment efficacy for nonvertebral fractures in osteoporosis clinical trials. Data from 5 randomized fracture prevention trials with alendronate, clodronate, zoledronic acid, denosumab, and lasofoxifene that showed efficacy for nonvertebral fractures were pooled to derive efficacy estimates using random effects models. These 5 trials included 30 118 postmenopausal women, of whom, 2997 had at least 2 nonvertebral fractures. The analysis showed that each agent reduced all nonvertebral fractures by 24% on average, and reduced high- or low-trauma fractures, 6 common types of nonvertebral fractures (hip, pelvis, leg, wrist, humerus, and clavicle), nonvertebral fractures other than the 6 most common types, and all fractures other than finger, toe, or face fractures. These agents did not cause greater risk reduction of nonvertebral fractures associated with lower BMD. Clinical trials of drug efficacy for all nonvertebral fractures would require 2641 subjects per arm, whereas proving efficacy in a subgroup of nonvertebral fractures would require more subjects. The study concluded that these 5 antiresorptive agents reduced all nonvertebral fractures regardless of severity of trauma or subcategorization of fractures.

These important findings show that several currently available antiresorptive agents effectively reduce nonvertebral fractures of all types, albeit with reduced efficacy compared with vertebral or hip fractures. In addition, future clinical trials should assess efficacy of new agents for reduction of all nonvertebral fractures rather than subsets of nonvertebral fractures unique to each clinical trial to allow direct comparison of efficacy between agents.

B. L. Clarke, MD

References

1. Watts NB, Geusens P, Barton IP, Felsenberg D. Relationship between changes in BMD and nonvertebral fracture incidence associated with risedronate: reduction in risk of nonvertebral fracture is not related to change in BMD. *J Bone Miner Res.* 2005;20:2097-2104.
2. Hochberg MC, Greenspan S, Wasnich RD, Miller P, Thompson DE, Ross PD. Changes in bone density and turnover explain the reductions in incidence of nonvertebral fractures that occur during treatment with antiresorptive agents. *J Clin Endocrinol Metab.* 2002;87:1586-1592.
3. Siris ES, Harris ST, Eastell R, et al; Continuing Outcomes Relevant to Evista (CORE) Investigators. Skeletal effects of raloxifene after 8 years: results from

the continuing outcomes relevant to Evista (CORE) study. *J Bone Miner Res.* 2005;20:1514-1524.

4. Langsetmo LA, Morin S, Richards JB, et al; CaMos Research Group. Effectiveness of antiresorptives for the prevention of nonvertebral low-trauma fractures in a population-based cohort of women. *Osteoporos Int.* 2009;20:283-290.

5. Cadarette SM, Katz JN, Brookhart MA, Stürmer T, Stedman MR, Solomon DH. Relative effectiveness of osteoporosis drugs for preventing nonvertebral fracture. *Ann Intern Med.* 2008;148:637-646.

6. McCloskey EV, Beneton M, Charlesworth D, et al. Clodronate reduces the incidence of fractures in community-dwelling elderly women unselected for osteoporosis: results of a double-blind, placebo-controlled randomized study. *J Bone Miner Res.* 2007;22:135-141.

Association of BMD and FRAX Score With Risk of Fracture in Older Adults With Type 2 Diabetes

Schwartz AV, for the Study of Osteoporotic Fractures (SOF), the Osteoporotic Fractures in Men (MrOS), and the Health, Aging, and Body Composition (Health ABC) Research Groups (Univ of California, San Francisco; et al)
JAMA 305:2184-2192, 2011

Context.—Type 2 diabetes mellitus (DM) is associated with higher bone mineral density (BMD) and paradoxically with increased fracture risk. It is not known if low BMD, central to fracture prediction in older adults, identifies fracture risk in patients with DM.

Objective.—To determine if femoral neck BMD T score and the World Health Organization Fracture Risk Algorithm (FRAX) score are associated with hip and nonspine fracture risk in older adults with type 2 DM.

Design, Setting, and Participants.—Data from 3 prospective observational studies with adjudicated fracture outcomes (Study of Osteoporotic Fractures [December 1998-July 2008]; Osteoporotic Fractures in Men Study [March 2000-March 2009]; and Health, Aging, and Body Composition study [April 1997-June 2007]) were analyzed in older community-dwelling adults (9449 women and 7436 men) in the United States.

Main Outcome Measure.—Self-reported incident fractures, which were verified by radiology reports.

Results.—Of 770 women with DM, 84 experienced a hip fracture and 262 a nonspine fracture during a mean (SD) follow-up of 12.6 (5.3) years. Of 1199 men with DM, 32 experienced a hip fracture and 133 a nonspine fracture during a mean (SD) follow-up of 7.5 (2.0) years. Age-adjusted hazard ratios (HRs) for 1-unit decrease in femoral neck BMD T score in women with DM were 1.88 (95% confidence interval [CI], 1.43-2.48) for hip fracture and 1.52 (95% CI, 1.31-1.75) for nonspine fracture, and in men with DM were 5.71 (95% CI, 3.42-9.53) for hip fracture and 2.17 (95% CI, 1.75-2.69) for nonspine fracture. The FRAX score was also associated with fracture risk in participants with DM (HRs for 1-unit increase in FRAX hip fracture score, 1.05; 95% CI, 1.03-1.07, for women with DM and 1.16; 95% CI, 1.07-1.27, for men with DM; HRs for 1-unit increase in FRAX osteoporotic fracture score, 1.04; 95% CI, 1.02-1.05, for women with DM and 1.09; 95% CI, 1.04-1.14, for men with DM). However, for a given T score and age or for a given FRAX score, participants with DM had a higher fracture risk than those without DM. For a similar fracture risk, participants with DM had a higher T score than participants without DM. For hip fracture, the estimated mean difference in T score for women was 0.59 (95% CI, 0.31-0.87) and for men was 0.38 (95% CI, 0.09-0.66).

Conclusions.—Among older adults with type 2 DM, femoral neck BMD T score and FRAX score were associated with hip and nonspine fracture risk; however, in these patients compared with participants without DM, the fracture risk was higher for a given T score and age or for a given FRAX score.

▶ Previous studies have found increased fracture risk in adults with type 2 diabetes mellitus despite having higher bone mineral density (BMD) than age-matched controls.[1-3] These studies did not determine whether low BMD in adults with type 2 diabetes mellitus predicts fracture risk as it does in postmenopausal women or older men.[4-6]

This study evaluated whether femoral neck BMD T-score and the World Health Organization FRAX 10-year absolute fracture risk algorithm predict hip and nonvertebral fractures in older adults with type 2 diabetes mellitus. To do this, data from 3 prospective observational studies with adjudicated fracture outcomes were combined to obtain sufficient numbers of type 2 diabetic subjects. Data from the Study of Osteoporotic Fractures in postmenopausal women were obtained from December 1998 through July 2008; the Osteoporotic Fractures in Men Study from March 2000 through March 2009; and the Health, Aging, and Body Composition Study in women and men from April 1997 through June 2007. The analysis was done on 9449 community-dwelling women and 7436 community-dwelling men in the United States. Fractures identified by self-report were verified by radiology reports. In 770 women with type 2 diabetes mellitus, 84 hip fractures and 262 nonvertebral fractures were identified over 12.6 ± 5.6 years of follow-up. In 1199 men with type 2 diabetes mellitus, 32 hip fractures and 133 nonvertebral fractures were confirmed over 7.5 ± 2.0 years of follow-up. The age-adjusted hazard ratio for a 1.0-unit femoral neck BMD T-score decrease in women was 1.88 for hip fracture and 1.52 for nonvertebral fracture. Men had a similar hazard ratio of 5.71 for hip fracture, and 2.17 for nonvertebral fracture. The FRAX score correlated with fracture risk in the diabetic subjects. For a given T-score and age, or for a given FRAX score, subjects with type 2 diabetes mellitus had a higher fracture risk than those without type 2 diabetes. For similar fracture risk, diabetics had a higher T-score than subjects without diabetes. The study concluded that femoral neck BMD T-score and FRAX score were associated with hip and nonvertebral fracture risk in older adults with type 2 diabetes mellitus but that fracture risk was higher in diabetics than nondiabetics for a given T-score and age or for a given FRAX score.

These findings indicate that adults with type 2 diabetes mellitus, like those treated with glucocorticoid therapy, have increased fracture risk beyond that predicted by their femoral neck BMD T-score. In addition, adults with type 2 diabetes mellitus with the same fracture risk as nondiabetics have higher femoral neck BMD T-scores. These data imply that bone quality is decreased in adults with type 2 diabetes mellitus, perhaps because of accumulation of advanced glycation end products or other causes. Adult diabetics should be treated for osteoporosis more aggressively than adults without diabetes who have similar T-scores or FRAX scores.

B. L. Clarke, MD

References

1. Schwartz AV, Sellmeyer DE, Strotmeyer ES, et al; Health ABC Study. Diabetes and bone loss at the hip in older black and white adults. *J Bone Miner Res.* 2005;20: 596-603.
2. Strotmeyer ES, Cauley JA, Schwartz AV, et al. Nontraumatic fracture risk with diabetes mellitus and impaired fasting glucose in older white and black adults: the health, aging, and body composition study. *Arch Intern Med.* 2005;165:1612-1617.
3. de Liefde II, van der Klift M, de Laet CE, van Daele PL, Hofman A, Pols HA. Bone mineral density and fracture risk in type-2 diabetes mellitus: the Rotterdam Study. *Osteoporos Int.* 2005;16:1713-1720.
4. Johnell O, Kanis JA, Oden A, et al. Predictive value of BMD for hip and other fractures. *J Bone Miner Res.* 2005;20:1185-1194.
5. Hillier TA, Cauley JA, Rizzo JH, et al. WHO absolute fracture risk models (FRAX): do clinical risk factors improve fracture prediction in older women without osteoporosis? *J Bone Miner Res.* 2011;26:1774-1782.
6. Trémollieres FA, Pouillès JM, Drewniak N, Laparra J, Ribot CA, Dargent-Molina P. Fracture risk prediction using BMD and clinical risk factors in early postmenopausal women: sensitivity of the WHO FRAX tool. *J Bone Miner Res.* 2010;25:1002-1009.

Fracture Risk in Women With Breast Cancer: A Population-Based Study
Melton LJ III, Hartmann LC, Achenbach SJ, et al (Mayo Clinic, Rochester, MN)
J Bone Miner Res 2012 [Epub ahead of print]

A positive association has been reported between greater bone density and higher breast cancer risk, suggesting that these women could be at reduced risk of fracture. To estimate fracture risk among unselected community women with breast cancer, and to systematically assess associations with various risk factors including breast cancer treatments, we conducted a population-based historical cohort study of 608 Olmsted County, MN women with invasive breast cancer first diagnosed in 1990-99 (mean age, 61.6 ± 14.8 years), who were followed for 5776 person-years. Altogether, 568 fractures were observed in 270 women (98 per 1000 person-years). Overall fracture risk was elevated 1.8-fold; but the absolute increase in risk was only 9%, and 56% of the women did not experience a fracture during follow-up. Excluding pathologic fractures (15%) and those found incidentally (24%), to allow for ascertainment bias, the standardized incidence ratio was 1.2 (95% CI, 0.99-1.3) for total fracture risk and 0.9 (95% CI, 0.7-1.2) for osteoporotic fracture risk alone. Various breast cancer treatments were associated with an increased risk of fracture, but those associations were strongest for pathologic fractures, which were relatively more common among the women who were premenopausal when their breast cancer was diagnosed. Moreover, underlying clinical characteristics prompting different treatments may have been partially responsible for the associated fracture outcomes (indication bias). These data thus demonstrate that breast cancer patients in general are not at greatly increased risk of fracture but neither are they protected from fractures despite any determinants that breast cancer and high bone density may have in common.

▶ Previous studies have reported that women with higher bone mineral density (BMD) have increased breast cancer risk.[1] The assumption has been that exposure to higher levels of endogenous or exogenous estrogen both increases BMD during adult life and simultaneously causes increased likelihood that women will eventually develop breast cancer.[2] In spite of the increased risk of breast cancer, the presence of higher BMD should protect against fracture risk.[3] Other studies have found that prior hip or distal forearm fracture is associated with lower risk of breast cancer, presumably in women who had lower BMD.[4-6]

This study found that women with breast cancer are not at significantly increased risk of fracture, despite therapies used to treat breast cancer, but also that women who have breast cancer are not protected against fracture risk. The study was a population-based study of 608 women with invasive breast cancer diagnosed initially during the decade of the 1990s, of mean age 62 years, who were followed up with for fractures over 5776 person-years. During this interval, 568 fractures occurred in 270 of the women, for a fracture rate of 98 per 1000 person-years. The overall fracture risk was increased by 1.8-fold, with absolute fracture risk increased by 9%, with fractures occurring in 44% of subjects over the follow-up interval. Pathologic fractures accounted for 15% of the total and incidentally found fractures for 24%. If these 36% of the fractures were excluded, the standardized incidence ratio for total fractures was 1.2 and that for osteoporotic fractures 0.9. Breast cancer treatments were associated with increased fracture risk, but the associations were strongest for pathologic fractures, which occurred most commonly among women who were premenopausal when diagnosed. Fracture outcomes may have been partly dependent on the fact that treatments were selected based on clinical characteristics of the subjects. The study concluded that women with breast cancer do not appear to have significantly increased risk of fracture but also that they are not protected from risk of fracture, even though they may have characteristics that both increase BMD and the risk of breast cancer.

The significance of these findings is that while high BMD may protect against fractures in general, this characteristic may also increase the risk of other adverse outcomes. Women with higher BMD have been reported to have a higher risk of breast cancer. This study found that women with invasive breast cancer did not have a higher risk of overall fractures or osteoporotic fractures, despite therapies that might be expected to increase the risk of fracture. However, these women had the expected rate of fracture, indicating that higher BMD did not protect them from fracture.

B. L. Clarke, MD

References

1. Tremollieres F, Ribot C. Bone mineral density and prediction of non-osteoporotic disease. *Maturitas*. 2010;65:348-351.
2. Yager JD, Davidson NE. Estrogen carcinogenesis in breast cancer. *N Engl J Med*. 2006;354:270-282.
3. Riggs BL, Khosla S, Melton LJ 3rd. Sex steroids and the construction and conservation of the adult skeleton. *Endocr Rev*. 2002;23:279-302.
4. Olsson H, Hägglund G. Reduced cancer morbidity and mortality in a prospective cohort of women with distal forearm fractures. *Am J Epidemiol*. 1992;136: 422-427.
5. Persson I, Adami HO, McLaughlin JK, Naessén T, Fraumeni JF Jr. Reduced risk of breast and endometrial cancer among women with hip fractures (Sweden). *Cancer Causes Control*. 1994;5:523-528.
6. Newcomb PA, Trentham-Dietz A, Egan KM, et al. Fracture history and risk of breast and endometrial cancer. *Am J Epidemiol*. 2001;153:1078-1081.

Fracture Risk in Men With Prostate Cancer: A Population-Based Study

Melton LJ III, Lieber MM, Atkinson EJ, et al (Mayo Clinic, Rochester, MN)
J Bone Miner Res 26:1808-1815, 2011

Fractures are increased among men with prostate cancer, especially those on androgen-deprivation therapy (ADT), but few data are available on men with localized prostate cancer. The purpose of this investigation was to estimate fracture risk among unselected community men with prostate cancer and systematically assess associations with ADT and other risk factors for fracture. In a population-based retrospective cohort study, 742 Olmsted County, MN, men with prostate cancer first diagnosed in 1990–1999 (mean age 68.2 ± 8.9 years) were followed for 6821 person-years. We estimated cumulative fracture incidence, assessed relative risk by standardized incidence ratios, and evaluated risk factors in time-to-fracture regression models. All together, 482 fractures were observed in 258 men (71 per 1000 person-years). Overall fracture risk was elevated 1.9-fold, with an absolute increase in risk of 9%. Relative to rates among community men generally, fracture risk was increased even among men not on ADT but was elevated a further 1.7-fold among ADT-treated compared with untreated men with prostate cancer. The increased risk following various forms of ADT was accounted for mainly by associations with pathologic fractures (14% of all fractures). Among men not on ADT (62% of the cohort), more traditional osteoporosis risk factors were implicated. In both groups, underlying clinical characteristics prompting different treatments (indication bias) may have been partially responsible for the associations seen with specific therapies. To the extent that advanced-stage disease and pathologic fractures account for the excess risk, the effectiveness of fracture prevention among men with prostate cancer may be limited.

▶ Men with the highest bone mass have a higher risk of prostate cancer.[1,2] Men with prostate cancer are known to have increased fractures due to metastatic disease, hypogonadism due to androgen deprivation therapy or surgical orchiectomy and other age-related causes.[3] Very little information regarding fracture risk is available in men with localized prostate cancer. Surgical orchiectomy or androgen deprivation therapy both lower serum testosterone and estradiol levels sufficiently that significant bone loss may occur, leading to increased fracture risk. Androgen deprivation therapy is usually given by steroidal antiandrogens, nonsteroidal antiandrogens, or gonadotropin-releasing hormone agonists.[4]

This population-based retrospective cohort study evaluated 742 men with prostate cancer first diagnosed in 1999 and followed up with them for 6821 person-years. Cumulative fracture incidence was estimated, with relative risk assessed by standardized incidence ratios and risk factors identified in time-to-fracture regression models. The study reported 482 fractures in 258 men, for a fracture rate of 71 per 1000 person-years. The overall fracture risk was increased by 1.9-fold over age-matched controls, with an absolute relative risk of 9.0%. Relative to fracture rates in community-dwelling men, fracture risk was increased among men with prostate cancer not on androgen deprivation therapy, but was increased further by 1.7-fold among men treated with androgen deprivation therapy compared with untreated men with prostate cancer. The increased risk after various forms of androgen deprivation therapy was mostly associated with pathologic fractures rather than systemic bone loss, whereas for men not on androgen deprivation therapy, fractures were associated with typical risk factors for osteoporosis. Underlying clinical characteristics may have prompted different treatments, and these may have been partially responsible for the associations seen with specific therapies. Because advanced-stage disease and pathologic fractures account for most of the excess fracture risk in men with prostate cancer, effectiveness of fracture prevention among men with prostate cancer may be limited.

The finding of a 1.9-fold increased fracture risk in unselected men with prostate cancer was consistent with results from a large case-control study in Denmark[5] but not with a case-control study from Canada that showed no increased risk of fractures of the hip, spine, and forearm combined.[6] The findings of the current study imply that fracture risk in men with prostate cancer is mostly due to metastatic disease and pathologic fractures rather than treatment-related bone loss, because pathologic fractures accounted for more than half the difference between observed and expected fractures. The increased fracture risk was seen mainly in the axial skeleton, but many vertebral fractures were discovered only by x-ray. If it is true that excess risk of fractures in prostate cancer is due to advanced-stage disease and pathologic fractures, therapy to prevent fractures may be less successful than therapy to prevent typical osteoporotic fractures.

B. L. Clarke, MD

References

1. Zhang Y, Kiel DP, Ellison RC, et al. Bone mass and the risk of prostate cancer: the Framingham study. *Am J Med.* 2002;113:734-739.
2. Farhat GN, Taioli E, Cauley JA, et al. The association of bone mineral density with prostate cancer risk in the Osteoporotic Fractures in Men (MrOS) Study. *Cancer Epidemiol Biomarkers Prev.* 2009;18:148-154.

3. Ahlborg HG, Nguyen ND, Center JR, Eisman JA, Nguyen TV. Incidence and risk factors for low trauma fractures in men with prostate cancer. *Bone*. 2008;43: 556-560.
4. Higano CS. Management of bone loss in men with prostate cancer. *J Urol*. 2003; 170:S59-S63.
5. Abrahamsen B, Nielsen MF, Eskildsen P, Andersen JT, Walter S, Brixen K. Fracture risk in Danish men with prostate cancer: a nationwide register study. *BJU Int*. 2007;100:749-754.
6. Lau YK, Lee E, Prior HJ, Lix LM, Metge CJ, Leslie WD. Fracture risk in androgen deprivation therapy: a Canadian population based analysis. *Can J Urol*. 2009;16: 4908-4914.

Levels of Serotonin, Sclerostin, Bone Turnover Markers as well as Bone Density and Microarchitecture in Patients With High-Bone-Mass Phenotype Due to a Mutation in Lrp5

Frost M, Andersen T, Gossiel F, et al (Odense Univ Hosp, Denmark; Univ of Sheffield, UK; et al)
J Bone Miner Res 26:1721-1728, 2011

Patients with an activation mutation of the *Lrp5* gene exhibit high bone mass (HBM). Limited information is available regarding compartment-specific changes in bone. The relationship between the phenotype and serum serotonin is not well documented. To evaluate bone, serotonin, and bone turnover markers (BTM) in *Lrp5*-HBM patients, we studied 19 *Lrp5*-HBM patients (T253I) and 19 age- and sex-matched controls. DXA and HR-pQCT were used to assess BMD and bone structure. Serum serotonin, sclerostin, dickkopf-related protein 1 (DKK1), and BTM were evaluated. Z-scores for the forearm, total hip, lumbar spine, forearm, and whole body were significantly increased (mean ± SD) between 4.94 ± 1.45 and 7.52 ± 1.99 in cases versus −0.19 ± 1.19 to 0.58 ± 0.84 in controls. Tibial and radial cortical areas, thicknesses, and BMD were significantly higher in cases. In cases, BMD at the lumbar spine and forearm and cortical thickness were positively associated and trabecular area negatively associated with age ($r = 0.49, 0.57, 0.74$, and $−0.61$, respectively, $p < .05$). Serotonin was lowest in cases (69.5 [29.9−110.4] ng/mL versus 119.4 [62.3−231.0] ng/mL, $p < .001$) and inversely associated with tibial cortical density ($r = −0.49$, $p < .05$) and directly with osteocalcin (OC), bone-specific alkaline phosphatase (B-ALP), and procollagen type 1 amino-terminal propeptide (PINP) ($r = 0.52−0.65$, $p < .05$) in controls only. OC and S-CTX were lower and sclerostin higher in cases, whereas B-ALP, PINP, tartrate-resistant acid phosphatase (TRAP), and dickkopf-related protein 1 (DKK1) were similar in cases and controls. In conclusion, increased bone mass in *Lrp5*-HBM patients seems to be caused primarily by changes in trabecular and cortical bone mass and structure. The phenotype appeared to progress with age, but BTM did not suggest increased bone formation.

▶ Patients with activating mutations of the lipoprotein receptor−related protein 5 (Lrp5) gene have increased bone mineral density (BMD), resulting in a high bone mass phenotype,[1,2] whereas those with inactivating mutations have decreased BMD, leading to the osteoporosis-pseudoglioma syndrome.[3] The high bone mass phenotype develops as a result of enhanced signaling by the canonical Wnt pathway in osteoblasts, which causes increased osteoblast function, due to lack of inactivating signals from Wnt antagonists such as sclerostin[4] and dickkopf-related protein 1 (Dkk1).[5,6] More recently it has been suggested that regulation of bone formation by Lrp5 is not due to direct effects of Lrp5 on bone, but rather through changes in tryptophan hydroxylase 1 (Tph1), an enzyme that synthesizes serotonin in the enterochromaffin cells in the duodenum.[7] Gut-derived serotonin decreases bone mass via the Htr1b receptor in osteoblasts. Patients with high bone mass phenotype have been reported to have reduced serum serotonin levels, and those with osteoporosis-pseudoglioma syndrome, increased serum serotonin levels.[7]

This study evaluated BMD, bone microarchitecture, bone turnover markers, and serotonin and sclerostin levels in 19 mostly female patients from 4 families with Lrp5 T253I mutations causing the high bone mass phenotype and 19 age- and sex-matched controls. Subjects with the high bone mass phenotype had markedly increased BMD at all skeletal sites compared with controls. BMD at the lumbar spine and forearm and cortical thickness correlated with age, whereas trabecular area correlated inversely with age in cases with high bone mass phenotype. Serotonin was lowest in the cases, and negatively correlated with tibial cortical density. Serotonin positively correlated with serum osteocalcin, bone-specific alkaline phosphatase, and P1NP in controls only. Serum osteocalcin and CTx-telopeptide were lower and sclerostin higher in cases, whereas bone-specific alkaline phosphatase, P1NP, tartrate-resistant acid phosphatase, and Dkk1 were similar between cases and controls. The study concluded that high bone mass phenotype in patients with Lrp5-activating mutations appeared to be caused by changes in both trabecular and cortical bone mass and structure, that the phenotype appeared to progress with age, and that markers of bone turnover did not suggest increased bone formation.

These results clarify the physiology of the high bone mass phenotype further. Four novel findings are described, including that increased bone mass is due to significantly increased cortical thickness as well as increased trabecular volumetric BMD, number, and thickness. In addition, lumbar spine and forearm BMD as well as cortical thickness increase with aging. Further, serum serotonin is inversely related to cortical thickness and positively associated with markers of bone turnover in controls. Finally, serum osteocalcin and CTx-telopeptide are lower in cases of high bone mass, whereas serum sclerostin is higher. Further research will be required to fully characterize the significance of these findings in patients with the high bone mass phenotype.

B. L. Clarke, MD

References

1. Boyden LM, Mao J, Belsky J, et al. High bone density due to a mutation in LDL-receptor-related protein 5. *N Engl J Med.* 2002;346:1513-1521.
2. Van Wesenbeeck L, Cleiren E, Gram J, et al. Six novel missense mutations in the LDL receptor-related protein 5 (LRP5) gene in different conditions with an increased bone density. *Am J Hum Genet.* 2003;72:763-771.

3. Gong Y, Slee RB, Fukai N, et al. LDL receptor-related protein 5 (LRP5) affects bone accrual and eye development. *Cell.* 2001;107:513-523.
4. Balemans W, Piters E, Cleiren E, et al. The binding between sclerostin and LRP5 is altered by DKK1 and by high-bone mass LRP5 mutations. *Calcif Tissue Int.* 2008; 82:445-453.
5. Ai M, Holmen SL, Van Hul W, Williams BO, Warman ML. Reduced affinity to and inhibition by DKK1 form a common mechanism by which high bone mass-associated missense mutations in LRP5 affect canonical Wnt signaling. *Mol Cell Biol.* 2005;25:4946-4955.
6. Balemans W, Devogelaer JP, Cleiren E, Piters E, Caussin E, Van Hul W. Novel LRP5 missense mutation in a patient with a high bone mass phenotype results in decreased DKK1-mediated inhibition of Wnt signaling. *J Bone Miner Res.* 2007;22:708-716.
7. Yadav VK, Ryu JH, Suda N, et al. Lrp5 controls bone formation by inhibiting serotonin synthesis in the duodenum. *Cell.* 2008;135:825-837.

Change in Undercarboxylated Osteocalcin Is Associated with Changes in Body Weight, Fat Mass, and Adiponectin: Parathyroid Hormone (1-84) or Alendronate Therapy in Postmenopausal Women with Osteoporosis (the PaTH Study)

Schafer AL, Sellmeyer DE, Schwartz AV, et al (Univ of California, San Francisco; et al)
J Clin Endocrinol Metab 96:E1982-E1989, 2011

Context.—The undercarboxylated form of the osteoblast-secreted protein osteocalcin has favorable effects on fat and glucose metabolism in mice. In human subjects, cross-sectional studies suggest a relevant association.

Objective.—We investigated whether changes in undercarboxylated osteocalcin (ucOC) during osteoporosis treatment are associated with changes in metabolic parameters.

Design, Setting, Participants, and Interventions.—We measured ucOC in sera from a subset of osteoporotic postmenopausal women who were treated with PTH(1-84) or alendronate (n = 64 and n = 33, respectively) during the Parathyroid Hormone and Alendronate study.

Main Outcome Measures.—We measured serum adiponectin, leptin, and insulin and analyzed existing data on body weight, fat mass, and serum glucose concentration. Three-month changes in ucOC levels were evaluated as predictors of 12-month changes in indices of fat and glucose metabolism.

Results.—ucOC levels increased with PTH(1-84) and decreased with alendronate administration ($P \le 0.01$ for both treatment groups). Three-month change in ucOC was inversely associated with 12-month changes in body weight (standardized $\beta = -0.25$, $P = 0.04$) and fat mass ($\beta = -0.23$, $P = 0.06$), after adjustment for the treatment group. Three-month change in ucOC was positively associated with a 12-month change in adiponectin ($\beta = 0.30, P = 0.01$), independent of change in fat mass. There were no interactions between treatment and change in ucOC on changes in weight, fat mass, or adiponectin.

Conclusions.—PTH(1-84) increases and alendronate decreases ucOC levels. Changes in ucOC induced by PTH(1-84) and alendronate are associated with changes in metabolic indices. These associations are consistent with observations from animal models and support a role for ucOC in the skeletal regulation of energy metabolism in humans.

▶ Animal studies have shown that the osteoblast secretory product osteocalcin influences fat and glucose metabolism and functions like a hormone. Osteocalcin is normally released during bone formation into the circulation, thereby serving as a marker of bone formation. It is also incorporated into bone matrix near the osteoblast, to be released later during bone resorption. Homozygous osteocalcin knockout mice have increased fat mass, decreased beta-cell proliferation, decreased insulin secretion, and insulin resistance, whereas mice with increased undercarboxylated osteocalcin have small fat pads, increased beta-cell proliferation, increased insulin sensitivity, and increased serum adiponectin levels, an insulin-sensitizing adipokine.[1] Administration of recombinant undercarboxylated osteocalcin to wild-type mice decreased fat mass, increased adiponectin expression, improved glucose metabolism, and decreased weight gain and glucose intolerance when mice were fed a high-fat diet.[2] Human cross-sectional studies have shown an association between osteocalcin, glucose metabolism, and fat mass.[3-5] Human interventional studies have not yet been done because undercarboxylated osteocalcin is not available for human administration.

This study assessed serum osteocalcin levels in postmenopausal osteoporotic women treated with human parathyroid hormone 1-84 (hPTH 1-84) or alendronate as part of the PaTH clinical trial.[6] hPTH 1-84 is an anabolic agent that stimulates osteoblasts to form new bone and thereby increases bone mineral density. The study showed that hPTH 1-84 increased, and alendronate decreased, serum undercarboxylated osteocalcin over 3 months of treatment. These changes correlated with 12-month decreases in body weight and fat mass and increases in adiponectin, independent of fat mass change. No interactions were seen between treatment and change in serum osteocalcin level, or changes in weight, fat mass, or adiponectin. Given that the changes in undercarboxylated osteocalcin induced by hPTH 1-84 and alendronate are associated with changes in metabolic parameters, the study supports a role for undercarboxylated osteocalcin in regulation of energy metabolism in humans.

These findings add to the human evidence that undercarboxylated osteocalcin plays a role in regulation of fat and glucose metabolism. This study provides the first human longitudinal evidence that changes in undercarboxylated osteocalcin regulate body weight, fat mass, and adiponectin levels. The opposite effects of hPTH 1-84 and alendronate on bone formation magnified the differences seen in undercarboxylated osteocalcin during the study. Subjects with greater increases in undercarboxylated osteocalcin during hPTH 1-84 treatment had greater decreases in body weight and fat mass and greater increases in the insulin-sensitizing adipokine adiponectin. These associations correspond with results from animal studies and may support a role for undercarboxylated osteocalcin in skeletal regulation of human energy metabolism.

B. L. Clarke, MD

References

1. Lee NK, Sowa H, Hinoi E, et al. Endocrine regulation of energy metabolism by the skeleton. *Cell.* 2007;130:456-469.
2. Ferron M, Hinoi E, Karsenty G, Ducy P. Osteocalcin differentially regulates beta cell and adipocyte gene expression and affects the development of metabolic diseases in wild-type mice. *Proc Natl Acad Sci U S A.* 2008;105:5266-5270.
3. Pittas AG, Harriss SS, Eliades M, Stark P, Dawson-Hughes B. Association between serum osteocalcin and markers of metabolic phenotype. *J Clin Endocrinol Metab.* 2009;94:827-832.
4. Kanazawa I, Yamaguchi T, Yamauchi M, et al. Serum undercarboxylated osteocalcin was inversely associated with plasma glucose level and fat mass in type 2 diabetes mellitus. *Osteoporos Int.* 2011;22:187-194.
5. Kanazawa I, Yamaguchi T, Yamamoto M, et al. Serum osteocalcin level is associated with glucose metabolism and atherosclerosis parameters in type 2 diabetes mellitus. *J Clin Endocrinol Metab.* 2009;94:45-49.
6. Black DM, Greenspan SL, Ensrud KE, et al. The effects of parathyroid hormone and alendronate alone or in combination in postmenopausal osteoporosis. *N Engl J Med.* 2003;349:1207-1215.

Metabolic Bone Disease

A Single Infusion of Zoledronic Acid Produces Sustained Remissions in Paget Disease: Data to 6.5 Years

Reid IR, Lyles K, Su G, et al (Univ of Auckland, New Zealand; Duke Univ, Durham, NC; Novartis Pharmaceuticals Corporation, East Hanover, NJ; et al)

J Bone Miner Res 26:2261-2270, 2011

Two trials have shown that a single 5-mg infusion of zoledronic acid achieves much higher response rates in Paget disease of bone than risedronate. The duration of this effect is unknown. We have conducted an open follow-up of responders from the two trials (152 originally treated with zoledronic acid, 115 with risedronate) out to 6.5 years without further intervention. Endpoints were times to relapse (ie, return of serum total alkaline phosphatase activity to within 20% of the pretreatment value) or loss of response (response=normalization of alkaline phosphatase or 75% or greater reduction in its excess). Bone turnover markers were lower in the zoledronic acid group throughout follow-up, with mean alkaline phosphatase (ALP) remaining within the reference range in these patients, whereas the mean in the risedronate group was above normal from 1 year. Relapse rates were substantially greater in the risedronate group (23 of 115, 20%) than in those treated with zoledronic acid (1 of 152, 0.7%, $p < .001$), and loss of response occurred in 19 (12.5%) zoledronic acid patients compared with 71 (62%) risedronate patients ($p < .0001$). Risk ratios for relapse and loss of response in zoledronic acid patients were 0.02 [95% confidence interval (CI) 0.00–0.18] and 0.12 (95% CI 0.07–0.19), respectively. Changes from baseline in quality of life, assessed using SF-36 scores, were more positive in the zoledronic acid group across the follow-up period ($p = .01$). Bone markers at 6 months were predictive of response duration. These data demonstrate an unprecedented duration of remission of Paget disease following treatment with zoledronic acid, accompanied by an improved quality of life.

▶ Paget disease of bone is a localized disorder that causes markedly increased turnover in 1 or more specific bones, resulting in bone pain, deformity in the skull and long bones, premature arthritis, deafness, and pathologic fractures.[1] Increased bone turnover results in formation of disorganized woven bone and loss of normal microarchitecture. Partial control of Paget disease of bone has been possible in recent decades due to potent antiresorptive medications, initially with calcitonin and more recently with oral or intravenous bisphosphonates. Of the bisphosphonates, zoledronic acid is the most potent agent approved for treatment of Paget disease. Two clinical trials have demonstrated that a single infusion of zoledronic acid, 5 mg, on one occasion gives much higher response rates than risedronate.[2,3] These trials showed that 96% of subjects responded at 6 months after a single 5-mg infusion, with normal serum alkaline phosphatase levels achieved in 89% at 6 months and improved quality of life.[4]

This study evaluated the duration of effect of a single dose of zoledronic acid given for treatment of Paget disease. A total of 152 subjects who had previously responded to zoledronic acid and 115 subjects who had responded to risedronate, in the 2 previous clinical trials comparing zoledronic acid with risedronate, were contacted to assess success of previous treatment up to 6.5 years after initial intervention, with no further intervention given. End points assessed were time to relapse, defined as time required for serum total alkaline phosphatase to return to within 20% of the pretreatment value, and loss of response to treatment. Response was defined as normalization of serum total alkaline phosphatase or 75% or greater reduction in its excess value above the normal range. Serum total alkaline phosphatase and other markers of bone turnover were lower in the zoledronic acid group throughout 6.5 years of follow-up, with mean serum total alkaline phosphatase remaining within the normal range in these subjects. Mean serum total alkaline phosphatase level increased above normal in the risedronate group after 1 year. The relapse rate was 20% in the risedronate group and 0.7% in the zoledronic acid group, and loss of response occurred in 12.5% of the zoledronic acid group and 62% of the risedronate group. Markers of bone turnover at 6 months were predictive of the duration of response. Changes in quality of life across the follow-up period were more positive in the zoledronic acid group. The study concluded that a single infusion of zoledronic acid induced an unprecedented duration of remission of Paget disease of bone, associated with increased quality of life.

These findings are striking because of the prolonged duration of effect of a single infusion of zoledronic acid on Paget disease of bone. None of the other approved agents for treatment of Paget disease of bone have nearly as prolonged an effect on this disorder. A similar prolonged effect, although not for as long, has been reported for zoledronic acid in postmenopausal osteoporosis.[5,6] This prolonged duration of effect was not because subjects entering the trials had a milder form of disease; study subjects at baseline had serum total alkaline phosphatase values 4 to 6 times the upper end of the reference range, indicating moderate to severe disease. The markers of bone turnover in this study do not yet show a return toward baseline, indicating that zoledronic acid will likely continue to have treatment effect for some time to come. How long the effect might last is not yet clear. Significant efficacy, long-term safety, convenience, and relatively low cost make zoledronic acid a very useful drug for treatment of Paget disease of bone.

B. L. Clarke, MD

References

1. Silverman SL. Paget disease of bone: therapeutic options. *J Clin Rheumatol.* 2008; 14:299-305.
2. Reid IR, Miller P, Lyles K, et al. Comparison of a single infusion of zoledronic acid with risedronate for Paget's disease. *N Engl J Med.* 2005;353:898-908.
3. Hosking D, Lyles K, Brown JP, et al. Long-term control of bone turnover in Paget's disease with zoledronic acid and risedronate. *J Bone Miner Res.* 2007;22:142-148.
4. Langston AL, Campbell MK, Fraser WD, et al. Clinical determinants of quality of life in Paget's disease of bone. *Calcif Tissue Int.* 2007;80:1-9.
5. Grey A, Bolland MJ, Wattie D, Horne A, Gamble G, Reid IR. The antiresorptive effects of a single dose of zoledronate persist for two years: a randomized, placebo-controlled trial in osteopenic postmenopausal women. *J Clin Endocrinol Metab.* 2009;94:538-544.
6. Bolland MJ, Grey AB, Horne AM, et al. Effects of intravenous zoledronate on bone turnover and BMD persist for at least 24 months. *J Bone Miner Res.* 2008;23: 1304-1308.

Circulating Sclerostin in Disorders of Parathyroid Gland Function

Costa AG, Cremers S, Rubin MR, et al (Columbia Univ, NY; et al)
J Clin Endocrinol Metab 96:3804-3810, 2011

Context.—Sclerostin, a protein encoded by the *SOST* gene in osteocytes and an antagonist of the *Wnt* signaling pathway, is down-regulated by PTH administration. Disorders of parathyroid function are useful clinical settings to study this relationship.

Objective.—The objective of the study was to evaluate sclerostin in two different disorders of parathyroid function, primary hyperparathyroidism and hypoparathyroidism, and to analyze the relationship between sclerostin and PTH, bone markers, and bone mineral density.

Design.—This is a cross-sectional study.

Setting.—The study was conducted at a clinical research center.

Patients.—Twenty hypoparathyroid and 20 hyperparathyroid patients were studied and compared to a reference control group.

Results.—Serum sclerostin was significantly higher in hypoparathyroid subjects than in hyperparathyroid subjects ($P < 0.0001$) and controls ($P < 0.0001$). PTH was negatively associated with sclerostin, achieving statistical significance in hypoparathyroidism ($r = -0.545$; $P = 0.02$). The bone turnover markers, cross-linked C-telopeptide of type I collagen (CTX) and amino-terminal propeptide of type I collagen (P1NP), were differently associated with sclerostin according to the parathyroid disorder. In primary hyperparathyroidism, bone turnover markers were associated negatively with sclerostin (for P1NP, r = −0.490; *P* = 0.03). In hypoparathyroidism, bone turnover markers were associated positively with sclerostin (for CTX, r = +0.571; *P* = 0.01). Although there was no significant correlation between bone mineral density and sclerostin in either parathyroid disorder, there was a significant positive relationship between sclerostin and bone mineral content in hypoparathyroidism.

Conclusions.—The results are consistent with the hypothesis that PTH is a regulator of sclerostin in human disorders of parathyroid function. In addition, the results suggest that bone mineral content may be another factor that influences sclerostin.

▶ Sclerostin is the glycoprotein product of the osteocyte SOST gene that inhibits canonical Wnt and BMP signaling pathways in osteoblasts and osteoblast lineage cells.[1,2] Binding of sclerostin to the LRP5/LRP6 receptor complex leads to inhibition of β-catenin, which is a major activator of anabolic genes in the osteoblast nucleus.[3] Sclerostin has also been shown to inhibit BMP7 secretion by mouse osteocytes.[4] Inhibition of these signaling pathways results in decreased synthesis of new bone by these bone-forming cells. Sclerostin is thought to function primarily as an endogenous inhibitor of new bone formation to prevent overproduction of bone. Mutations in the SOST gene cause exuberant bone production, as seen in the human diseases sclerosteosis and van Buchem disease.[5,6]

Teriparatide (recombinant human parathyroid hormone 1-34 [PTH 1-34]) was approved for the treatment of osteoporosis because it was shown to effectively stimulate new bone formation, in part by decreasing osteocyte production of sclerostin.[7] The decrease in sclerostin production caused by teriparatide suggests that disorders of parathyroid gland function might also affect sclerostin synthesis and secretion by osteocytes. In general, hyperparathyroidism might decrease sclerostin production, and hypoparathyroidism might upregulate its production.

This cross-sectional study evaluated circulating sclerostin levels in 20 patients with primary hyperparathyroidism and 20 with hypoparathyroidism and compared results with a healthy reference control group. Patients with primary hyperparathyroidism had decreased sclerostin levels, and those with hypoparathyroidism had increased sclerostin levels. PTH levels were negatively correlated with sclerostin. Correlation of serum CTx-telopeptide and P1NP, markers of bone resorption and formation, respectively, with sclerostin depended on the disorder. In primary hyperparathyroidism, these markers correlated negatively with sclerostin, but, in hypoparathyroidism, the correlation was positive for unclear reasons. Although there was not a correlation between bone mineral density and sclerostin in either disorder, sclerostin and bone mineral content were positively correlated in hypoparathyroidism. The study concluded that PTH regulates sclerostin in disorders of parathyroid function and that bone mineral content may also regulate sclerostin production by osteocytes.

These findings extend previous observations that circulating sclerostin likely has clinical relevance, even though this glycoprotein primarily acts at the tissue level in the bone microenvironment. Serum osteocalcin has been detected in both women and men[8] and a correlation demonstrated between bone marrow plasma and serum concentrations.[9] This study confirms that PTH downregulates sclerostin production when increased and upregulates production when decreased. The positive correlation of sclerostin with bone mineral content may be due to greater numbers of osteocytes present with increased bone mineral content.

B. L. Clarke, MD

References

1. van Bezooijen RL, Roelen BA, Visser A, et al. Sclerostin is an osteocyte-expressed negative regulator of bone formation, but not a classical BMP antagonist. *J Exp Med.* 2004;199:805-814.
2. Poole KE, van Bezooijen RL, Loveridge N, et al. Sclerostin is a delayed secreted product of osteocytes that inhibits bone formation. *FASEB J.* 2005;19:1842-1844.
3. Semënov M, Tamai K, He X. SOST is a ligand for LRP5/LRP6 and a Wnt signaling inhibitor. *J Biol Chem.* 2005;280:26770-26775.
4. Krause C, Korchynskyi O, de Rooij K, et al. Distinct modes of inhibition by sclerostin on bone morphogenetic protein and Wnt signaling pathways. *J Biol Chem.* 2010;285:41614-41626.
5. Balemans W, Ebeling M, Patel N, et al. Increased bone density in sclerosteosis is due to the deficiency of a novel secreted protein (SOST). *Hum Mol Genet.* 2001;10:537-543.
6. Wergedal JE, Veskovic K, Hellan M, et al. Patients with van Buchem disease, an osteosclerotic genetic disease, have elevated bone formation markers, higher bone density, and greater derived polar moment of inertia than normal. *J Clin Endocrinol Metab.* 2003;88:5778-5783.
7. Keller H, Kneissel M. SOST is a target gene for PTH in bone. *Bone.* 2005;37:148-158.
8. Mödder UI, Clowes JA, Hoey K, et al. Regulation of circulating sclerostin levels by sex steroids in women and in men. *J Bone Miner Res.* 2011;26:27-34.
9. Drake MT, Srinivasan B, Mödder UI, et al. Effects of parathyroid hormone treatment on circulating sclerostin levels in postmenopausal women. *J Clin Endocrinol Metab.* 2010;95:5056-5062.

PTH(1–84) Administration Reverses Abnormal Bone-Remodeling Dynamics and Structure in Hypoparathyroidism

Rubin MR, Dempster DW, Sliney J Jr, et al (Columbia Univ, NY; Helen Hayes Hosp, West Haverstraw, NY)

J Bone Miner Res 26:2727-2736, 2011

Hypoparathyroidism is associated with abnormal structural and dynamic skeletal properties. We hypothesized that parathyroid hormone(1–84) [PTH(1–84)] treatment would restore skeletal properties toward normal in hypoparathyroidism. Sixty-four subjects with hypoparathyroidism were treated with PTH(1–84) for 2 years. All subjects underwent histomorphometric assessment with percutaneous iliac crest bone biopsies. Biopsies were performed at baseline and at 1 or 2 years. Another group of subjects had a single biopsy at 3 months, having received tetracycline before beginning PTH(1–84) and prior to the biopsy (quadruple-label protocol).

Measurement of biochemical bone turnover markers was performed. Structural changes after PTH(1−84) included reduced trabecular width (144 ± 34 μm to 128 ± 34 μm, $p = 0.03$) and increases in trabecular number (1.74 ± 0.34/mm to 2.07 ± 0.50/mm, $p = 0.02$) at 2 years. Cortical porosity increased at 2 years (7.4% ± 3.2% to 9.2% ± 2.4%, $p = 0.03$). Histomorphometrically measured dynamic parameters, including mineralizing surface, increased significantly at 3 months, peaking at 1 year (0.7% ± 0.6% to 7.1% ± 6.0%, $p = 0.001$) and persisting at 2 years. Biochemical measurements of bone turnover increased significantly, peaking at 5 to 9 months of therapy and persisting for 24 months. It is concluded that PTH(1−84) treatment of hypoparathyroidism is associated with increases in histomorphometric and biochemical indices of skeletal dynamics. Structural changes are consistent with an increased remodeling rate in both trabecular and cortical compartments with tunneling resorption in the former. These changes suggest that PTH(1-84) improves abnormal skeletal properties in hypoparathyroidism and restores bone metabolism toward normal euparathyroid levels.

▶ Untreated hypoparathyroidism is characterized by low serum calcium level, high serum phosphorus level, normal renal function, and inappropriately low or absent serum parathyroid hormone (PTH) level. Urinary calcium level is relatively high for the decreased level of serum calcium, and serum 1,25-dihydroxyvitmain D level is low to normal or mildly decreased. This disorder most commonly results from thyroidectomy or parathyroidectomy but may occur due to autoimmune disorders or other rare conditions.[1-3] Low serum PTH levels lead to decreased bone remodeling, which leads to increased bone mineral density (BMD) compared with age-matched and sex-matched controls.[4] Bone from patients with hypoparathyroid may be more dense than normal, but it has abnormal structural and dynamic skeletal properties. Bone histomorphometry performed on iliac crest bone biopsies from patients with hypoparathyroidism has demonstrated greater trabecular bone volume, trabecular width, and cortical width, but dynamic parameters, including mineralizing surface and bone formation rate, were markedly decreased.[5] Three-dimensional micro-CT confirmed the trabecular changes seen on 2-dimensional histomorphometry.[6]

Treatment of patients with hypoparathyroidism with daily PTH 1-84 helps improve serum calcium and phosphorus levels toward normal, reduces the need for high-dose calcium and vitamin D supplementation, and alters BMD. Daily PTH 1-84 has been shown to increase lumbar spine BMD and to decrease one-third distal radius BMD. This study evaluated changes in bone histomorphometry owing to PTH 1-84 treatment in 64 subjects treated for 24 months. Labeled biopsies were taken at baseline and at 1 or 2 years. A subset of subjects underwent labeling before starting treatment and again 3 months after starting therapy, before undergoing biopsy. At 2 years, trabecular width decreased and trabecular number increased, whereas cortical porosity increased. Dynamic parameters, including mineralizing surface, increased significantly by 3 months, peaked at 1 year, and then remained stable until decreasing at 2 years. Levels of markers of bone turnover increased early after starting treatment, peaked by 5 to

9 months, and then remained stable until decreasing at 2 years. The study concluded that the structural changes seen were due to increased remodeling in both trabecular and cortical bone compartments, with tunneling resorption in trabecular bone invoked to explain the increase in trabecular number, and that PTH 1-84 improves abnormal skeletal properties in hypoparathyroidism and restores bone metabolism toward normal.

These results suggest that treatment of patients with hypoparathyroidism with daily PTH 1-84 restores bone metabolism and structure toward normal. The time course of changes in bone turnover markers suggests relatively rapid effects on bone turnover that peak by 5 to 9 months and then persist before decreasing toward the end of 24 months of treatment. Changes in bone histomorphometry follow a similar time course. Structural changes were evident by 1 year, with reduced trabecular thickness and increased trabecular number and cortical porosity. These findings indicate an initial rapid response to PTH 1-84, followed by slow tempering over time.

B. L. Clarke, MD

References

1. Bilezikian JP, Khan A, Potts JT Jr, et al. Hypoparathyroidism in the adult: epidemiology, diagnosis, pathophysiology, target-organ involvement, treatment, and challenges for future research. *J Bone Miner Res.* 2011;26:2317-2337.
2. Ahonen P, Myllärniemi S, Sipilä I, Perheentupa J. Clinical variation of autoimmune polyendocrinopathy-candidiasis-ectodermal dystrophy (APECED) in a series of 68 patients. *N Engl J Med.* 1990;322:1829-1836.
3. Mayer A, Ploix C, Orgiazzi J, et al. Calcium-sensing receptor autoantibodies are relevant markers of acquired hypoparathyroidism. *J Clin Endocrinol Metab.* 2004;89: 4484-4488.
4. Abugassa S, Nordenström J, Eriksson S, Sjödén G. Bone mineral density in patients with chronic hypoparathyroidism. *J Clin Endocrinol Metab.* 1993;76:1617-1621.
5. Rubin MR, Dempster DW, Zhou H, et al. Dynamic and structural properties of the skeleton in hypoparathyroidism. *J Bone Miner Res.* 2008;23:2018-2024.
6. Rubin MR, Dempster DW, Kohler T, et al. Three dimensional cancellous bone structure in hypoparathyroidism. *Bone.* 2010;46:190-195.

Mineral and Vitamin D Metabolism

Diets Higher in Dairy Foods and Dietary Protein Support Bone Health During Diet- and Exercise-Induced Weight Loss in Overweight and Obese Premenopausal Women

Josse AR, Atkinson SA, Tarnopolsky MA, et al (McMaster Univ, Hamilton, Ontario, Canada)

J Clin Endocrinol Metab 97:251-260, 2012

Context.—Consolidation and maintenance of peak bone mass in young adulthood may be compromised by inactivity, low dietary calcium, and diet-induced weight loss.

Objective.—We aimed to determine whether higher intakes of dairy foods, dietary calcium, and protein during diet- and exercise-induced weight loss affected markers of bone health.

Participants.—Participants included premenopausal overweight and obese women.

Design/Intervention.—Ninety participants were randomized into three groups (n = 30 per group): high protein and high dairy (HPHD), adequate protein and medium dairy (APMD), and adequate protein and low dairy (APLD), differing in dietary protein (30, 15, or 15% of energy, respectively), dairy foods (15, 7.5, or <2% of energy from protein, respectively), and dietary calcium (∼1600, ∼1000, or <500 mg/d, respectively).

Outcome Measures.—Serum and urine bone turnover biomarkers, serum osteoprotegerin (OPG), receptor activator of nuclear factor-κB ligand (RANKL), PTH, 25-hydroxyvitamin D, leptin, and adiponectin measured at 0 and 16 wk.

Results.—All groups lost equivalent body weight ($P < 0.05$). N-telopeptide, C-telopeptide (CTX), urinary deoxypyridinoline, and osteocalcin increased in APLD ($P < 0.01$), whereas in HPHD, osteocalcin and procollagen 1 amino-terminal propeptide (P1NP) increased ($P < 0.05$), and all resorption markers remained unchanged. P1NP to CTX and OPG to RANKL ratios increased in HPHD ($P < 0.005$), and P1NP to CTX ratio decreased in APLD ($P < 0.05$). PTH decreased in HPHD and APMD *vs.* APLD ($P < 0.005$), and 25-hydroxyvitamin D increased in HPHD ($P < 0.05$), remained unchanged in APMD, and decreased in APLD ($P < 0.05$). Leptin decreased and adiponectin increased in APMD and HPHD only ($P < 0.001$).

Conclusions.—Hypoenergetic diets higher in dairy foods, dietary calcium, and protein with daily exercise, favorably affected important bone health biomarkers *vs.* diets with less of these bone-supporting nutrients.

▶ Adult bone mass is accrued in the teenage years and between the second and third decade of life. Establishing peak bone mass and maintaining it throughout life is important to prevent osteoporosis. Greater bone mass is achieved with higher body weight persons. However, weight loss after restriction of calories can adversely affect bone health. Remedies to restrict or improve bone loss during weight loss programs would be a great benefit. Diet, supplements, calcium, and vitamin D are some factors that have been recommended to achieve the goal of minimizing bone loss.[1-5] Josse and associates investigated a diet high in dairy foods and protein in supporting bone health in premenopausal women during diet- and exercise-induced weight loss. While weight loss was comparable between the groups, bone health was superior in the high dairy group based on assessment with bone formation and desorption markers. Long-term studies are needed to confirm that bone mineral density would corroborate the apparent benefits based on bone markers.

A. W. Meikle, MD

References

1. Josse AR, Atkinson SA, Tarnopolsky MA, Phillips SM. Diets higher in dairy foods and dietary protein support bone health during diet- and exercise-induced weight loss in overweight and obese premenopausal women. *J Clin Endocrinol Metab.* 2012;97:251-260.

2. Hirota T, Hirota K. Diet for lifestyle-related diseases to maintain bone health. *Clin Calcium.* 2011;21:730-736.
3. Thorpe MP, Jacobson EH, Layman DK, He X, Kris-Etherton PM, Evans EM. A diet high in protein, dairy, and calcium attenuates bone loss over twelve months of weight loss and maintenance relative to a conventional high-carbohydrate diet in adults. *J Nutr.* 2008;138:1096-1100.
4. Huth PJ, DiRienzo DB, Miller GD. Major scientific advances with dairy foods in nutrition and health. *J Dairy Sci.* 2006;89:1207-1221.
5. Bowen J, Noakes M, Clifton P. High dairy-protein versus high mixed-protein energy restricted diets - the effect on bone turnover and calcium excretion in overweight adults. *Asia Pac J Clin Nutr.* 2003;12:S52.

Is Vitamin D a Determinant of Muscle Mass and Strength?

Marantes I, Achenbach SJ, Atkinson EJ, et al (Mayo Clinic, Rochester, MN)
J Bone Miner Res 26:2860-2871, 2011

There remains little consensus on the link between vitamin D levels and muscle mass or strength. We therefore investigated the association of serum 25-hydroxyvitamin D (25(OH)D), 1,25-dihydroxyvitamin D (1,25(OH)$_2$D), and parathyroid hormone (PTH) levels with skeletal muscle mass and strength. We studied 311 men (mean age, 56 years; range, 23−91 years) and 356 women (mean age, 57 years; range, 21−97 years) representing an age-stratified, random sample of community adults. Multivariate linear regression models were used to examine the association of skeletal muscle mass (by total body dual-energy X-ray absorptiometry) and strength (handgrip force and isometric knee extension moment) with each of 25(OH)D, 1,25(OH)$_2$D, and PTH quartiles, adjusted for age, physical activity, fat mass, and season. We found no consistent association between 25(OH)D or PTH and any of our measurements of muscle mass or strength, in either men or women. However, in subjects younger than 65 years, there was a statistically significant association between low 1,25(OH)$_2$D levels and low skeletal mass in both men and women and low isometric knee extension moment in women, after adjustment for potential confounders. Modestly low 25(OH)D or high PTH levels may not contribute significantly to sarcopenia or muscle weakness in community adults. The link between low 25(OH)D and increased fall risk reported by others may be due to factors that affect neuromuscular function rather than muscle strength. The association between low 1,25(OH)$_2$D and low skeletal mass and low knee extension moment, particularly in younger people, needs further exploration.

▶ Vitamin D deficiency has been associated with osteoporosis and fall risk. Studies have shown a moderate correlation between low vitamin D levels and decreased postural stability and poor functional performance that could lead to falls.[1,2] It is not yet clear how vitamin D levels might affect fall risk directly. The vitamin D receptor was previously reported to be found in human skeletal muscle,[3] but a more recent study has disputed this finding.[4] Genotypic variations in the vitamin D receptor have been associated with differences in muscle strength.[5,6]

One potential mechanism by which vitamin D might prevent falls is by improving muscle mass and strength.

This study correlated skeletal muscle mass and strength with serum 25-hydroxyvitamin D, 1,25-dihydroxyvitamin D, and parathyroid hormone (PTH) levels in an age-stratified population-based sample of 311 men age 23—91 years and 356 women age 21—97 years living in the community. Skeletal muscle mass was assessed by total body dual-energy X-ray absorptiometry and muscle strength by handgrip force and isometric knee extension moment. Vitamin D deficiency was present in 42% of study subjects. The overall results showed no consistent association between muscle mass or strength and quartiles of either form of vitamin D or PTH after adjustment for age, physical activity, fat mass, and season. However, subjects younger than 65 years showed a significant correlation between low serum 1,25-dihydroxyvitamin D level and low skeletal muscle mass in men and women, and low isometric knee extension moment in women, after adjustment for potential confounders. The study showed no association between mildly decreased serum 25-hydrxoyvitamin D and increased PTH levels and muscle weakness. The study concluded that the previously reported association between low serum 25-hydroxyvitamin D and fall risk may be due to factors other than muscle strength, and that the association between low serum 1,25-dihydroxyvitamin D and low skeletal muscle mass and decreased knee extension requires further investigation.

These findings failed to confirm an association between serum 25-hydroxyvitamin D and muscle mass or strength in an adult community—dwelling, population-based sample of men and women. However, an association was found between low serum 1,25-dihydroxyvitamin D and decreased skeletal muscle mass in men and women and decreased knee strength in women, although a clear threshold below which muscle mass or strength was lower was not identified. One other study has reported a modest association between low serum 1,25-dihydroxyvitamin D levels and low muscle strength,[7] but others have not.[8,9] Further investigation will be necessary to clarify the relative contributions of 25-hydroxyvitamin D and 1,25-dihydroxyvitmain D levels to muscle mass, muscle strength, and fall risk.

B. L. Clarke, MD

References

1. Bischoff-Ferrari HA, Dawson-Hughes B, Staehelin HB, et al. Fall prevention with supplemental and active forms of vitamin D: a meta-analysis of randomised controlled trials. *BMJ.* 2009;330:b3692.
2. Bischoff-Ferrari HA, Dietrich T, Orav EJ, et al. Higher 25-hydroxyvitamin D concentrations are associated with better lower-extremity function in both active and inactive persons aged ≥60 y. *Am J Clin Nutr.* 2004;80:752-758.
3. Bischoff HA, Borchers M, Gudat F, et al. In situ detection of 1,25-dihydroxyvitamin D3 receptor in human skeletal muscle tissue. *Histochem J.* 2001;33:19-24.
4. Wang Y, DeLuca HF. Is the vitamin D receptor found in muscle? *Endocrinology.* 2011;152:354-363.
5. Windelinckx A, De Mars G, Beunen G, et al. Polymorphisms in the vitamin D receptor gene are associated with muscle strength in men and women. *Osteoporos Int.* 2007;18:1235-1242.
6. Grundberg E, Brändstrom H, Ribom EL, Ljunggren O, Mallmin H, Kindmark A. Genetic variation in the human vitamin D receptor is associated with muscle

strength, fat mass and body weight in Swedish women. *Eur J Endocrinol.* 2004; 150:323-328.
7. Houston DK, Cesari M, Ferrucci L, et al. Association between vitamin D status and physical performance: the InCHIANTI study. *J Gerontol A Biol Sci Med Sci.* 2007;62:440-446.
8. Boonen S, Lysens R, Verbecke G, et al. Relationship between age-associated endocrine deficiencies and muscle function in elderly women: a cross-sectional study. *Age Ageing.* 1998;27:449-454.
9. Mowé M, Haug E, Bøhmer T. Low serum calcidiol concentration in older adults with reduced muscular function. *J Am Geriatr Soc.* 1999;47:220-226.

High Doses of Vitamin D to Reduce Exacerbations in Chronic Obstructive Pulmonary Disease: A Randomized Trial
Lehouck A, Mathieu C, Carremans C, et al (Univ Hosps Leuven, Belgium)
Ann Intern Med 156:105-114, 2012

Background.—Low serum 25-hydroxyvitamin D (25-[OH]D) levels have been associated with lower FEV_1, impaired immunologic control, and increased airway inflammation. Because many patients with chronic obstructive pulmonary disease (COPD) have vitamin D deficiency, effects of vitamin D supplementation may extend beyond preventing osteoporosis.

Objective.—To explore whether supplementation with high doses of vitamin D could reduce the incidence of COPD exacerbations.

Design.—Randomized, single-center, double-blind, placebo-controlled trial. (ClinicalTrials.gov registration number: NCT00666367)

Setting.—University Hospitals Leuven, Leuven, Belgium.

Patients.—182 patients with moderate to very severe COPD and a history of recent exacerbations.

Intervention.—100 000 IU of vitamin D supplementation or placebo every 4 weeks for 1 year.

Measurements.—The primary outcome was time to first exacerbation. Secondary outcomes were exacerbation rate, time to first hospitalization, time to second exacerbation, FEV_1, quality of life, and death.

Results.—Mean serum 25-(OH)D levels increased significantly in the vitamin D group compared with the placebo group (mean between-group difference, 30 ng/mL [95% CI, 27 to 33 ng/mL]; $P < 0.001$). The median time to first exacerbation did not significantly differ between the groups (hazard ratio, 1.1 [CI, 0.82 to 1.56]; $P = 0.41$), nor did exacerbation rates, FEV_1, hospitalization, quality of life, and death. However, a post hoc analysis in 30 participants with severe vitamin D deficiency (serum 25-[OH]D levels <10 ng/mL) at baseline showed a significant reduction in exacerbations in the vitamin D group (rate ratio, 0.57 [CI, 0.33 to 0.98]; $P = 0.042$).

Limitation.—This was a single-center study with a small sample size.

Conclusion.—High-dose vitamin D supplementation in a sample of patients with COPD did not reduce the incidence of exacerbations. In participants with severe vitamin D deficiency at baseline, supplementation may reduce exacerbations.

▶ Epidemiologic studies have associated vitamin D deficiency with many different disorders, including autoimmune diseases, cancer, cardiovascular disease, and infections, including influenza and tuberculosis.[1-4] In spite of the mounting evidence linking vitamin D deficiency to multiple disorders, relatively few therapeutic trials with vitamin D to treat diseases associated with vitamin D deficiency have been completed. Therapeutic trials with vitamin D to prevent osteoporosis and fractures have shown modest benefit, whereas recent trials in multiple sclerosis,[5] diabetes,[6] influenza,[7] and tuberculosis[8] have shown no benefit. One possible reason for the disappointing results published to date may be that the vitamin D doses used were too small. Low serum 25-hydroxyvitamin D levels have been associated with low forced expiratory volume (FEV_1), impaired immunologic control, and increased airway inflammation, as seen in chronic obstructive pulmonary disease (COPD). A previous study showed that 60% to 75% of severe COPD patients had serum 25-hydroxyvitmamin D levels less than 20 ng/mL.[9]

This study evaluated the effect of high-dose vitamin D supplementation on COPD outcomes, including time to first exacerbation, exacerbation rate, time to first hospitalization, time to second exacerbation, FEV_1, quality of life, and death. Subjects were given oral vitamin D 100 000 IU or placebo once a month for 12 months. Mean serum 25-hydroxyvitamin D levels increased from 20 ng/mL at baseline to 52 ng/mL by 4 months in treated subjects during the trial. Disappointingly, the study showed no improvement in median time to first exacerbation, exacerbation rate, hospitalization, quality of life, or death. Post-hoc analysis of 30 subjects with severe baseline vitamin D deficiency, defined as serum 25-hydroxyvitamin D level less than 10 ng/mL, showed a significant reduction in exacerbations in the vitamin D-treated group. The study concluded that high-dose vitamin D supplementation for 1 year did not reduce acute exacerbations, improve lung function, or change other outcomes in a small number of COPD patients compared with placebo. Post-hoc analysis showed that vitamin D supplementation may be beneficial in patients with severe vitamin D deficiency.

These findings join those from other negative studies discussed above and argue that high-dose vitamin D supplementation may not be beneficial except in the most severely deficient patients. The findings are consistent with recent observations from the Lung Health Study, which showed that vitamin D levels did not correlate with rate of decline in FEV_1 in a subset of patients.[10] The lack of demonstrated benefit in these studies could be due to inadequate power, insufficient vitamin D dose, or insensitive endpoints. This study recruited a population prone to severe exacerbations and used high-dose vitamin D to maximize the likelihood of showing benefit, but the small sample size may have minimized this. Future studies will be required to demonstrate whether vitamin D supplementation is able to improve clinical outcomes in populations with diseases associated with vitamin D deficiency.

B. L. Clarke, MD

References

1. Kriegel MA, Manson JE, Costenbader KH. Does vitamin D affect risk of developing autoimmune disease?: a systematic review. *Semin Arthritis Rheum.* 2011; 40:512-531.
2. Krishnan AV, Trump DL, Johnson CS, Feldman D. The role of vitamin D in cancer prevention and treatment. *Endocrinol Metab Clin North Am.* 2010;39: 401-418.
3. Wang TJ, Pencina MJ, Booth SL, et al. Vitamin D deficiency and risk of cardiovascular disease. *Circulation.* 2008;117:503-511.
4. Nnoaham KE, Clarke A. Low serum vitamin D levels and tuberculosis: a systematic review and meta-analysis. *Int J Epidemiol.* 2008;37:113-119.
5. Burton JM, Kimball S, Vieth R, et al. A phase I/II dose-escalation trial of vitamin D3 and calcium in multiple sclerosis. *Neurology.* 2010;74:1852-1859.
6. von Hurst PR, Stonehouse W, Coad J. Vitamin D supplementation reduces insulin resistance in South Asian women living in New Zealand who are insulin resistant and vitamin D deficient - a randomised, placebo-controlled trial. *Br J Nutr.* 2010; 103:549-555.
7. Urashima M, Segawa T, Okazaki M, Kurihara M, Wada Y, Ida H. Randomized trial of vitamin D supplementation to prevent seasonal influenza A in schoolchildren. *Am J Clin Nutr.* 2010;91:1255-1260.
8. Wejse C, Gomes VF, Rabna P, et al. Vitamin D as supplementary treatment for tuberculosis: a double-blind, randomized, placebo-controlled trial. *Am J Respir Crit Care Med.* 2009;179:843-850.
9. Janssens W, Bouillon R, Claes B, et al. Vitamin D deficiency is highly prevalent in COPD and correlates with variants in the vitamin D-binding gene. *Thorax.* 2010; 65:215-220.
10. Kunisaki KM, Niewoehner DE, Singh RJ, Connett JE. Vitamin D status and longitudinal lung function decline in the Lung Health Study. *Eur Respir J.* 2011;37: 238-243.

6 Adrenal Cortex

Introduction

This year's selections highlight interesting observations on adrenal diseases with potential application to their diagnosis and treatment. We have focused on imaging of adrenal lesions, diagnosis and treatment of malignant tumors, the continuing saga on the best procedures to diagnose primary aldosteronism, unusual etiologies of Addison's disease and adrenal and testicular repercussions of congenital adrenal hyperplasia.

Positron Emission Tomography has been useful in distinguishing malignant adrenal lesions with high metabolic activity from benign lesions, but false positive results are being reported by Canter et al in a patient with a benign adrenal adenoma and by Alencar et al in macronodular adrenal hyperplasia. Treatment of advanced adrenal cortical carcinoma (ACC) is most challenging, but a number of reports suggest the possibility of temporary reprieve from the inexorable progression of the disease. Li et al have found that CT-guided microwave ablation of primary and metastatic ACC is a minimally invasive and effective method for treatment of these lesions. The resection of metastases in patients with stage IV ACC is controversial, but den Winkel et al conducted a retrospective study of pulmonary metastasectomies in these patients and concluded the procedure has the potential for producing long-term survival in a highly selected group of patients, particularly younger patients. Casamassima et al report on the experience of the University of Florence with stereotactic radiotherapy for metastatic disease and conclude the treatment is safe and effective with a control rate of 90% at 2 years.

The emergence of ACC in patients with otherwise benign neoplastic disease such as Carney complex was reported almost simultaneously by Anselmo et al in an Azorean family and Moran et al in a patient with this disease. The interesting aspect of these observations was the concomitant presence of ACC and primary pigmented micronodular hyperplasia raising the question of the potential for the hyperplasia to promote a malignant transformation.

Mitotane is standard treatment for ACC, but when combined with other chemotherapeutic drugs it may, by induction of CYP3A4, increase the clearance of these drugs as summarized by Kroiss et al and negate their therapeutic action. There are many tools for distinguishing benign from malignant adrenal tumors. Arlt et al suggest that when using urine steroid metabolomics it is possible to identify steroid precursors that are uniquely increased in ACC. Barreau et al suggest another approach is detection of chromosomal alterations and genomic profiles unique for malignant lesions.

The diagnosis of the type of primary aldosteronism, adenoma versus hyperplasia, continues to be challenging. To improve the performance of adrenal venous sampling (AVS), Rossi et al suggest intraprocedural cortisol measurement in order to confirm the catheter position within the adrenal vein; Burton et al propose ^{11}C-metomidate as a sensitive and specific non-invasive alternative to AVS, and Mulatero et al propose using urine 18OHF, urine 18oxoF and serum 18OHB for the differential diagnosis.

Departing from the more traditional causes of primary adrenal insufficiency (PAI), there are genetic biochemical defects leading to hypoadrenalism. Choi et al investigated the effects of DAX-1 mutations in patients with adrenal hypoplasia congenital, and Parajes et al report 2 brothers with PAI caused by a partial mutation of the gene encoding for P450 side chain cleavage enzyme. Optimal replacement with glucocorticoids and mineralocorticoids in PAI is difficult to achieve. This is because of the circadian nature of cortisol secretion. Patients are frequently overtreated and a possible consequence is decreased bone mineral density. Koetz et al showed that bone mineral density is not reduced when patients receive glucocorticoid replacement in lower doses, an important consideration in the treatment of patients with adrenal insufficiency. An improved method for hydrocortisone replacement is proposed by Johannson et al using a novel once-a-day dual-release formulation.

Finally, it is worth noting the development of testicular adrenal rest tumors in patients with congenital adrenal hyperplasia (CAH). Delfino et al report a high prevalence of testicular adrenal rest cell tumors in 18 patients with CAH. Nermoen et al had similar findings, as well as adrenal myelolipomas, in over 100 Norwegian patients with this diagnosis.

David E. Schteingart, MD

Adrenal Hormone Secretion and Pathology

Intensely Positron Emission Tomography-avid Benign Adrenal Adenoma
Canter D, Simhan J, Wu KN, et al (Fox Chase Cancer Ctr, Philadelphia, PA)
Urology 78:1307-1308, 2011

Both positron emission tomography/computed tomography (CT) and adrenal washout studies are highly accurate in differentiating benign from malignant adrenal lesions. Very few data exist to help guide management when the positron emission tomography and CT adrenal findings contradict each other with regard to the malignant potential. We present a patient with a remote history of breast cancer and a new solitary left adrenal mass. A CT washout study suggested a lipid-poor adenoma; however, positron emission tomography/CT demonstrated intense fluorodeoxyglucose uptake, suggesting malignancy. The pathologic evaluation after laparo-scopic adrenalectomy revealed a benign adrenal adenoma.

▶ The benign or malignant character of adrenal pathology can be discerned by specific imaging techniques well validated over the past 4 decades. For inciden-tally discovered adrenal masses by CT of MRI, lipid content and contrast washout have been found to have high sensitivity and specificity in determining if the lesion is benign or malignant. Benign lesions are lipid rich and have more than 60% contrast washout in 15 minutes. Lipid-poor lesions may still be benign, but additional information is required to establish their character. Positron emis-sion tomography (PET) has been used with increasing frequency to determine if an adrenal lesion is malignant. With 18F-fluorodeoxyglucose (18F-FDG) PET/CT, increased uptake is usually associated with high metabolic activity and high probability of malignancy. However, there is a 5% probability of false-posi-tive results, with high uptake in histologically benign lesions. The authors report on a case of a lipid-poor adrenal cortical adenoma with excellent washout but intense uptake of 18F-FDG. This led to an adrenalectomy with removal of a benign adrenal cortical adenoma. This article gives a word of caution in inter-preting PET/CT findings in light of other discrepant imaging data and particularly in making decisions regarding surgical resection of these lesions. Follow-up imaging over a period of time might have clarified the likely nature of the adrenal tumor.

D. E. Schteingart, MD

CT-Guided Percutaneous Microwave Ablation of Adrenal Malignant Carcinoma: Preliminary Results
Li X, Fan W, Zhang L, et al (Sun Yat Sen Univ, Guangzhou, China)
Cancer 117:5182-5188, 2011

Background.—Microwave ablation has recently been developed as a safe and effective treatment for a variety of tumors. The authors evalu-ated the safety and efficacy of computed tomography (CT)-guided percu-taneous microwave ablation of adrenal malignant tumors.

Methods.—Nine patients between 41 and 83 years of age (average age, 54 years) with adrenal carcinoma (a total of 10 lesions) received CT-guided percutaneous water-cooled microwave ablation. The 9 cases included 1 primary adrenocortical carcinoma and 8 metastatic carcinomas (4 from lung cancer, 2 from hepatocellular carcinoma, 1 from intrahepatic cholangiocarcinoma, and 1 from left tibial osteosarcoma). Of the 8 meta-static cases, 7 were unilateral, and 1 was bilateral. All cases were patholog-ically confirmed by aspiration biopsy or postsurgical biopsy. The tumor diameters ranged from 2.1 cm to 6.1 cm (average, 3.8 cm). The average number of ablation sites was 1.5 sites (1-3 sites), and the average accumu-lated ablation time was 7.7 minutes (4-15 minutes). The procedures were performed using a cooled-shaft antenna.

Results.—The patients were followed for 3-37 months, with an average of 11.3 months. Nine of 10 lesions were completely necrotized after first treatment. The other lesion was completely necrotized after 2 treatments. One of the patients experienced hypertensive crisis during treatment. No patient experienced recurrent tumor at the treated site, and this lack of recurrence indicated effective local control. All patients had progression of metastatic disease at extra-adrenal sites.

Conclusions.—CT-guided percutaneous water-cooled microwave ablation is a minimally invasive and effective method for the treatment of adrenal carcinoma.

▶ Adrenal cortical carcinoma (ACC) is a rare type of cancer with an incidence of 1 or 2 cases per million people per year, and it carries a poor prognosis. While patients discovered in stages I or II have a better than 50% 5-year survival rate, 40% to 70% are diagnosed in advance stages with local extension and distant metastases. For patients in stage IV with multiple pulmonary or hepatic metastases, systemic cytotoxic chemotherapy or targeted molecular therapy is recommended. Surgical resection of the primary tumor offers the best chance of prolonged tumor-free survival. There remains the question whether repeat resection of recurrences or surgical excision of single metastatic lesions has survival advantages. Over the years, we have resected single hepatic lesions and pulmonary lesions when present in limited numbers. Alternatives to surgical resection have been proposed with the use of external radiation therapy, brachytherapy, radiofrequency ablation, CT-guided percutaneous microwave ablation, and stereotactic radiotherapy. In addition to resection of primary ACC metastases, there is interest in ablating single metastatic lesions to the adrenal gland in some patients with other solid tumors as a way of controlling the disease. These authors from China report on 9 patients with adrenal malignancies (1 ACC, 8 metastatic from various primaries) of less than 6 cm who underwent CT-guided percutaneous microwave ablation. This heat-related treatment caused complete tumor necrosis after the first application. Tumors less than 5 cm had the best response. The procedure appeared safe with minimal complications. Although the treated lesions did not recur, patients had progression of their disease in extra-adrenal sites. The question is whether local control of the disease has an overall therapeutic advantage in terms of overall life expectancy, symptomatology, or quality of life.

D. E. Schteingart, MD

Drug interactions with mitotane by induction of CYP3A4 metabolism in the clinical management of adrenocortical carcinoma
Kroiss M, Quinkler M, Lutz WK, et al (Univ of Würzburg, Germany; Charité Univ Medicine Berlin, Germany)
Clin Endocrinol 75:585-591, 2011

Mitotane [1-(2-chlorophenyl)-1-(4-chlorophenyl)-2,2-dichloroethane, (*o,p'*-DDD)] is the only drug approved for the treatment for adrenocortical carcinoma (ACC) and has also been used for various forms of glucocorti-coid excess. Through still largely unknown mechanisms, mitotane inhibits adrenal steroid synthesis and adrenocortical cell proliferation. Mitotane increases hepatic metabolism of cortisol, and an increased replacement dose of glucocorticoids is standard of care during mitotane treatment. Recently, sunitinib, a multityrosine kinase inhibitor (TKI), has been found to be rapidly metabolized by CYP3A4 during mitotane treatment, indicating clinically relevant drug interactions with mitotane. We here summarize the current evidence concerning mitotane-induced changes in hepatic monooxygenase expression, list drugs potentially affected by mitotane-related CYP3A4 induction and suggest alternatives. For example, using standard doses of macrolide antibiotics is unlikely to reach sufficient plasma levels, making fluoroquinolones in many cases a superior choice. Similarly, statins such as simvastatin are metabolized by CYP3A4, whereas others like pravastatin are not. Importantly, in the past, several clinical trials using cytotoxic drugs but also targeted therapies in ACC yielded disappointing results. This lack of antineoplastic activity may be explained in part by insufficient drug exposure owing to enhanced drug metabolism induced by mitotane. Thus, induction of CYP3A4 by mitotane needs to be considered in the design of future clinical trials in ACC.

▶ Mitotane has been used in the treatment of patients with metastatic adrenal cortical carcinoma, either as monotherapy or in combination with other chemo-therapeutic drugs. It has adrenalytic antitumor effects and also inhibits cortisol production. When used in combination with other cytotoxic drugs, mitotane may add its adrenalytic effect to them or enhance their action by inhibiting the multidrug resistance gene (MDR) and increasing their retention within the target cells. Mitotane causes significant toxicity in therapeutically effective doses, but the adverse effects are dose dependent and maximal at doses above 6 g daily. Treatment with mitotane inhibits hormone production and eventually causes necrosis of the contralateral adrenal gland resulting in adrenal insufficiency. Mitotane has significant peripheral extra-adrenal effects. It increases binding of cortisol to corticosteroid binding globulin, and hydrocortisone substitution to cover for adrenal insufficiency requires supraphysiologic doses of 25 to 35 mg daily. Synthetic glucocorticoids, such as prednisone and dexamethasone, are less desirable because their metabolism may also be enhanced by mitotane, making it difficult to determine the optimal replacement dose. Mitotane increases cholesterol by induction of HMG-Co A reductase and causes gynecomastia in more than 50% of men by induction of sex hormone binding globulin (SHBG). Mitotane may interfere with the activity of coadministered drugs by important drug—drug interaction. This is nicely documented in a review article by Kroiss et al. Mitotane induces CYP3A4, and a variety of drugs, including the multityro-sine kinase inhibitor sunitinib, may be rapidly metabolized in the presence of mitotane with loss of its pharmacologic activity.

The authors claim the mechanism of action of mitotane is largely unknown, but unfortunately they ignore a large body of literature over the last several decades[1-7] providing convincing evidence on how mitotane induces its adrenalytic effect. It involves transformation to an acyl chloride via P450-mediated hydroxylation and covalent binding to specific bionucleophiles. The target appears to be a mitochondrial steroid hydroxylase P450c11 involved in xenobiotic metabolism. The adrenalytic effect also involves oxidative damage with formation of free radicals and induction of lipid peroxidation.

D. E. Schteingart, MD

References

1. Schteingart DE. Adjuvant mitotane therapy of adrenal cancer-use and controversy. Editorial. *N Engl J Med.* 2007;356:2415-2418.
2. Pineiro-Sanchez ML, Vaz ADN, Counsell RE, Schteingart DE, Sinsheimer JE. Adrenal metabolism of mitotane: Role of cytochrome P-450. Abstract. *FASEB J.* 1994;8:45.
3. Martz F, Straw JA. The in vitro metabolism of 1-(o-chlorophenyl)-1-(p-chlorophenyl)-2,2-dichloroethane (o, p'-DDD) by dog adrenal mitochondria and metabolite covalent binding to mitochondrial macromolecules: a possible mechanism for the adrenocorticolytic effect. *Drug Metab Dispos.* 1977;5:482-486.
4. Cai W, Counsell RE, Djanegara T, Schteingart DE, Sinsheimer JE, Wotring LL. Metabolic activation and binding of mitotane in adrenal cortex homogenates. *J Pharm Sci.* 1995;84:134-138.
5. Cai W, Benitez R, Counsell RE, et al. Bovine adrenal cortex transformations of mitotane [1-(2-chlorophenyl)-1-(4-chlorophenyl)-2,2-dichorethane; o,p'-DDD] and its p, p'- and m,p'- isomers. *Biochem Pharmacol.* 1995;49:1483-1489.
6. Sinsheimer JE, Freeman CJ. Mitotane (1-(o-chlorophenyl)-1-(p-chlorophenyl)-2,2-dichloroethane) metabolism in perfusion studies with dog adrenal glands. *Drug Metab Dispos.* 1987;15:267-269.
7. Lund BO, Lund J. Novel involvement of a mitochondrial steroid hydroxylase (P450c11) in xenobiotic metabolism. *J Biol Chem.* 1995;270:20895-20897.

---

^{18}F-FDG-PET/CT Imaging of ACTH-Independent Macronodular Adrenocortical Hyperplasia (AIMAH) Demonstrating Increased ^{18}F-FDG Uptake

Asmar Alencar G, Villares Fragoso MCB, Itaya Yamaga LY, et al (Hospital das Clínicas da Faculdade de Medicina da Universidade de São Paulo, Brazil; Hospital Israelita Albert Einstein, São Paulo, Brazil)
J Clin Endocrinol Metab 96:3300-3301, 2011

Background.—Integrated 2-[fluorine 18] fluoro-2-deoxy-D glucose (^{18}F-FDG) positron emission tomography/computed tomography (PET/CT) may permit the discrimination of benign from malignant adrenal masses. However, at least 5% of the adrenal abnormalities identified using this imaging modality are false-positive for malignancy. A benign adrenal disease was found to produce an intense ^{18}F-FDG uptake on PET/CT.

Case Reports.—Three women, 49, 51, and 60, demonstrated the clinical features of hypercortisolism and were diagnosed with adrenocorticotropic hormone (ACTH)-n-independent Cushing's syndrome. The women were not related. Their symptoms and signs included an abnormal overnight 1-mg dexamethasone suppression test, elevated

24-hour urinary cortisol levels, and undetectable plasma ACTH levels. Bilateral macronodular adrenal masses were noted on unenhanced CT. ^{18}F-FDG-PET/CT revealed the ^{18}F-FDG uptake in these masses was visibly higher than in the liver, with levels usually associated with malignant tumors and metastases. Bilateral adrenalectomy was performed in each woman, with pathologic evaluation indicating ACTH-independent macronodular adrenocortical hyperplasia (AIMAH).

Conclusions.—AIMAH is a benign adrenal disease. Based on the findings in this study, it should be considered in the differential diagnosis of adrenal lesions with increased ^{18}F-FDG activity, which includes carcinoma and metastases.

▶ Positron emission tomography (PET) has been used with increasing frequency to determine if an adrenal lesion is malignant. With ^{18}F-fluorodeoxyglucose (^{18}F-FDG) PET/computed tomography (CT), increased uptake is usually associated with high metabolic activity and high probability of malignancy. However, there is a 5% probability of false-positive results, that is, high uptake in histologically benign lesions. Alencar et al from Brazil report on high FDG uptake in a patient with Cushing syndrome secondary to adrenocorticotropic hormone—independent macronodular adrenocortical hyperplasia. With many solid tumors that are not functional, increased FDG uptake probably correlates well with the characteristic increased metabolic activity of malignant growth. The adrenal gland may be an exception, especially with functioning lesions that actively secrete steroids, a feature that may require a metabolically active process. PET/CT scans are useful in the identification of extra-adrenal lesions in patients with a history of acinar cell carcinoma.

D. E. Schteingart, MD

Metastatic Adrenocortical Carcinoma: Results of 56 Pulmonary Metastasectomies in 24 Patients
op den Winkel J, Pfannschmidt J, Muley T, et al (Thoraxklinik am Universitatsklinikum Heidelberg, Germany; Univ of Würzburg, Germany)
Ann Thorac Surg 92:1965-1970, 2011

Background.—Surgical resection is an important form of treatment for metastatic disease in patients with adrenocortical carcinoma (ACC). However, data about the results of this treatment are sparse. We reviewed our experience with the resection of pulmonary lesions metastatic from ACC as a means of evaluating such results.

Methods.—A retrospective review of the database at a German national registry for ACC identified 24 patients (9 men and 15 women; median age, 41 years) who underwent pulmonary metastasectomy for primary ACC during the study period of 1989 through 2009. Only patients who met the criteria for potentially curative surgery, defined as the presumed feasibility of resecting all visualized tumorous lesions, were included.

Results.—No perioperative deaths occurred in 56 pulmonary metastasectomies done on the patients in the study. The overall cumulative rate of 5-year survival, calculated from the time of first pulmonary surgery, was 24.5%, and the median survival was 50.2 months. Age younger than 41 years at the time of first pulmonary metastasectomy and repeated pulmonary metastasectomy were associated with longer survival in a univariate analysis. In accord with this, we observed a median survival of 31.9 months in patients 41 years of age or older as compared with a median survival of 59.3 months in younger patients ($p = 0.004$). In patients with repeated pulmonary metastasectomies, median survival after the first resection was significantly longer, at 59.3 months than in patients who had only one pulmonary resection, whose median survival was 31.9 months ($p = 0.001$).

Conclusions.—We conclude that surgical resection of pulmonary metastases for ACC should be regarded as safe, with the potential for producing long-term survival in a highly selected group of patients. Younger patients may benefit more than older ones from such resection, and the recurrence of pulmonary metastases should not preclude repeated surgical resections of these lesions.

▶ Adrenal cortical carcinoma (ACC) is a rare type of cancer with an incidence of 1 or 2 cases per 1 million people per year and with poor prognosis. Although patients discovered in stages I or II have a better than 50% 5-year survival rate, 40% to 70% are diagnosed in advance stages with local extension and distant metastases. For patients in stage IV with multiple pulmonary or hepatic metastases, systemic cytotoxic chemotherapy or targeted molecular therapies are recommended. Surgical resection of the primary tumor offers the best chance of prolonged tumor-free survival. There remains the question whether repeat resection of recurrences or surgical excision of single metastatic lesions has survival advantages. Over the years we have resected single hepatic lesions and pulmonary lesions when present in limited numbers. These authors report on a retrospective review of 56 pulmonary metastasectomies in 24 patients with metastatic ACC. The overall cumulative rate of 5-year survival was 24.5% and median survival was 50.2 months. Survival was longer in patients aged 41 years or less at the time of the first procedure and in patients who underwent repeated resections. In 20 of 24 patients, hilar and mediastinal lymph node resection was done during the pulmonary resection. The conclusion is that resection of pulmonary metastases is safe and results in longer-term survival. However, it is uncertain why resection of metastatic lesions extends life expectancy. Metastatic adrenal cortical carcinoma is a systemic disease, and it is unclear to what extent resection of metastases forestalls progression of the disease. This retrospective, multi-institutional report may have focused on selected patients, and how the findings can be extended to an unselected population of patients with ACC remains to be determined. Given the low incidence of ACC, it will be difficult to conduct a prospective randomized study of surgical resection of pulmonary or hepatic metastases. Until then, this report offers encouragement to consider resection of minimal pulmonary metastatic lesions in patients with advanced ACC but with a limited number of metastases.

D. E. Schteingart, MD

Urine Steroid Metabolomics as a Biomarker Tool for Detecting Malignancy in Adrenal Tumors
Arlt W, Biehl M, Taylor AE, et al (Univ of Birmingham, UK; Univ of Groningen, The Netherlands; et al)
J Clin Endocrinol Metab 96:3775-3784, 2011

Context.—Adrenal tumors have a prevalence of around 2% in the general population. Adrenocortical carcinoma (ACC) is rare but accounts for 2−11% of incidentally discovered adrenal masses. Differentiating ACC from adrenocortical adenoma (ACA) represents a diagnostic challenge in patients with adrenal incidentalomas, with tumor size, imaging, and even histology all providing unsatisfactory predictive values.

Objective.—Here we developed a novel steroid metabolomic approach, mass spectrometry-based steroid profiling followed by machine learning analysis, and examined its diagnostic value for the detection of adrenal malignancy.

Design.—Quantification of 32 distinct adrenal derived steroids was carried out by gas chromatography/mass spectrometry in 24-h urine samples from 102 ACA patients (age range 19−84 yr) and 45 ACC patients (20−80 yr). Underlying diagnosis was ascertained by histology and metastasis in ACC and by clinical follow-up [median duration 52 (range 26−201) months] without evidence of metastasis in ACA. Steroid excretion data were subjected to generalized matrix learning vector quantization (GMLVQ) to identify the most discriminative steroids.

Results.—Steroid profiling revealed a pattern of predominantly immature, early-stage steroidogenesis in ACC. GMLVQ analysis identified a subset of nine steroids that performed best in differentiating ACA from ACC. Receiver-operating characteristics analysis of GMLVQ results demonstrated sensitivity = specificity = 90%(area under the curve = 0.97) employing all 32 steroids and sensitivity = specificity = 88% (area under the curve = 0.96) when using only the nine most differentiating markers.

Conclusions.—Urine steroid metabolomics is a novel, highly sensitive, and specific biomarker tool for discriminating benign from malignant adrenal tumors, with obvious promise for the diagnostic work-up of patients with adrenal incidentalomas.

▶ Adrenal cortical carcinomas (ACC) are rare, highly malignant tumors that account for only 0.2% of deaths due to cancer. Their incidence has been estimated at 2 per 1 million people annually. About half of these tumors produce hormonal and metabolic syndromes that lead to their discovery. The other half are silent and discovered with metastasis or when the primary tumor becomes large enough to produce abdominal symptoms. Cushing syndrome is the most common clinical presentation in adult patients with hormonally functioning tumors and may seriously complicate their clinical course. Although virilization frequently accompanies Cushing syndrome, the predominant clinical manifestations may be those of androgen excess, with only subtle evidence of hypercortisolism. Hormonal findings in patients with clinical manifestations of Cushing syndrome include high urinary-free cortisol, serum cortisol and dehydroepiandrosterone sulfate at baseline, and failure to suppress with a high (8 mg) dose of dexamethasone. Corticotropin levels are usually suppressed.

For several decades it has been known that the steroid profile in serum or urine can help distinguish benign from malignant adrenal cortical tumors because of the presence of intermediary precursors in the steroid biosynthesis pathway or their metabolites in patients with malignant neoplasms. Specifically, serum levels of progesterone, pregnenolone, 17-hydroxyprogesterone, 17-hydroxypregnenolone, and dehydroepiandrosterone measured by gas chromatography/mass spectroscopy (MS/GC) are increased in ACC. Levels of 11-deoxycortisol were thought to be less specific a measurement because they are increased in both benign and malignant tumors. The main limitation for measuring these steroid profiles has been the complexity of the methodology involved. Using MS/GC, the authors quantified 32 distinct adrenal-derived steroids in the 24-hour urine of 102 patients with adrenal cortical adenomas (ACA) and 45 patients with ACC. Of those with ACA, 32% had evidence of hormone excess, while 73% of those with ACC had evidence of hormone excess. The hormone profile of the 2 groups differed in that patients with ACC had increased excretion of hormone precursors as it had been previously reported. Of interest is that some of those with apparently nonfunctioning tumors also had excretion of steroid precursors. The most discriminating precursor was 11-deoxycortisol and its tetrahydro derivative, tetrahydro-11-deoxycortisol (THS), which was elevated in patients with ACC but not in ACA. This differs from earlier observations that THS was not as specific a discriminating biomarker. The study largely confirms old literature but offers a method for accurate measurement of what is being proposed as a highly sensitive and specific biomarker tool for detecting malignancy in adrenal tumors.

D. E. Schteingart, MD

Bone Mineral Density Is Not Significantly Reduced in Adult Patients on Low-Dose Glucocorticoid Replacement Therapy
Koetz KR, Ventz M, Diederich S, et al (Charité Univ Medicine Berlin, Germany; Endokrinologikum, Berlin, Germany)
J Clin Endocrinol Metab 97:85-92, 2012

Context.—Patients with primary adrenal insufficiency (PAI) and patients with congenital adrenal hyperplasia (CAH) receive glucocorticoid replacement therapy, which might cause osteoporosis.

Objectives.—Questions addressed by this study were: 1) Is bone mineral density (BMD) reduced in PAI and CAH on lower glucocorticoid doses than previously reported? 2) Is BMD in PAI influenced by the type of glucocorticoid used? and 3) Does DHEA treatment affect BMD in PAI women?

Design and Patients.—We conducted a prospective, cross-sectional study including 81 PAI patients and 41 CAH patients.

Main Outcome Measures.—BMD was measured by dual-energy x-ray absorptiometry. Serum levels of bone turnover markers, minerals, vitamins, hormones, and urinary crosslinks were measured.

Results.—PAI and CAH patients received average daily hydrocortisone doses of 12.0 ± 2.7 mg/m^2 (range, 4.9–19.1) and 15.5 ± 7.8 mg/m^2 (range, 5.7–33.7), respectively. BMD varied within the normal reference range (-2 to $+2$) in both cohorts. However, lower Z-scores for femoral neck and Ward's region were found in CAH compared to PAI women, but not in men. Prednisolone treatment showed significant lower osteocalcin levels and lower Z-scores for lumbar spine and femoral neck compared to PAI patients on hydrocortisone. PAI women treated with DHEA had significantly lower urinary collagen crosslinks and bone alkaline phosphatase, and significantly higher Z-scores in lumbar spine and femoral Ward's region compared to non-DHEA-treated women.

Conclusions.—Adult PAI and CAH patients on low glucocorticoid doses showed normal BMD within the normal reference range. The use of longer acting prednisolone resulted in significantly lower BMD in PAI. In addition, DHEA treatment may have a beneficial effect on bone in Addison's women.

▶ Osteopenia or osteoporosis is a frequent complication of long-term corticosteroid therapy or severe Cushing syndrome. The mechanism for the decrease in bone mass is complex and involves the loss of bone matrix because of the protein catabolic effect of glucocorticoids (GC), interference with intestinal calcium absorption because of the inhibitory effect of GC on vitamin D intestinal action, and direct effects of GC on osteoblasts and osteocytes, possibly inducing apoptosis.[1] These effects are clearly encountered in patients on chronic pharmacological doses of corticosteroids but are not definitive in patients on replacement doses. Patients with primary adrenal insufficiency (PAI) are usually replaced with physiological doses of hydrocortisone or prednisone, and patients with congenital adrenal hyperplasia (CAH) are replaced with doses of prednisone sufficient to suppress excessive androgen production and compensate for limited cortisol secretion. There have been reports that many of these patients develop osteoporosis after several years of corticosteroid treatment, but it is likely that this depends on the dose of steroid received. The authors conducted a prospective cross-sectional study of 81 patients with PAI and 41 patients with CAH. They measured bone mineral density (BMD) by dual-energy x-ray densitometry (DEXA) and biomarkers of bone turnover, including osteocalcin, β-crosslaps, and bone resorption marker collagen crosslink *N*-telopeptide. Their results were interesting and important. Patients treated with low glucocorticoid doses showed normal BMD compared with patients who received higher doses, even within the "physiological" replacement range. The message is that we use too generous a dose of GC replacement in PAI, and that patients probably need no more than 12 to 20 mg of hydrocortisone for adequate replacement. Normal cortisol production rates by isotopic dilution are 12 to 22 mg per day.

Patients with CAH, who frequently receive borderline high doses of GC for suppression of adrenal androgens, are more likely to develop lower osteocalcin levels and Z scores for lumbar spine and femoral neck than those with PAI on hydrocortisone. Replacement with prednisolone, a GC with more prolonged half-life than hydrocortisone, is also associated with higher risk of decreased BMD. Men with PAI and CAH on corticosteroid replacement appear to be more protected than women with these conditions because of their androgen production. Similarly, the administration of dehydroepiandrosterone, an adrenal androgen, seems to have a bone protective effect in women with PAI on GC replacement therapy.

D. E. Schteingart, MD

Reference

1. Xia X, Kar R, Gluhak-Heinrich J, et al. Glucocorticoid-induced autophagy in osteocytes. *J Bone Miner Res.* 2010;25:2479-2488.

Stereotactic radiotherapy for adrenal gland metastases: University of Florence experience
Casamassima F, Livi L, Masciullo S, et al (Univ of Florence, Italy)
Int J Radiat Oncol Biol Phys 82:919-923, 2012

Purpose.—To evaluate a retrospective single-institution outcome after hypofractionated stereotactic body radiotherapy (SBRT) for adrenal metastases.

Methods and Materials.—Between February 2002 and December 2009, we treated 48 patients with SBRT for adrenal metastases. The median age of the patient population was 62.7 years (range, 43–77 years). In the majority of patients, the prescription dose was 36 Gy in 3 fractions (70% isodose, 17.14 Gy per fraction at the isocenter). Eight patients were treated with single-fraction stereotactic radiosurgery and forty patients with multifraction stereotactic radiotherapy.

Results.—Overall, the series of patients was followed up for a median of 16.2 months (range, 3–63 months). At the time of analysis, 20 patients were alive and 28 patients were dead. The 1- and 2-year actuarial overall survival rates were 39.7% and 14.5%, respectively. We recorded 48 distant failures and 2 local failures, with a median interval to local failure of 4.9 months. The actuarial 1-year disease control rate was 9%; the actuarial 1- and 2-year local control rate was 90%.

Conclusion.—Our retrospective study indicated that SBRT for the treatment of adrenal metastases represents a safe and effective option with a control rate of 90% at 2 years.

▶ There is interest in ablating single metastatic lesions to the adrenal glands in some patients with primary extra-adrenal solid tumors as a way of controlling the disease. Alternatives to surgical resection have been proposed with the use of external radiation therapy, brachytherapy, radiofrequency ablation, CT-guided percutaneous microwave ablation, and stereotactic radiotherapy. In a retrospective study from Italy, these authors from Italy have evaluated the results of stereotactic radiosurgery in 48 patients with adrenal metastases. Although the procedure was safe and lesions became stable in 60% of treated patients during a follow-up median period of 16.2 months, patients had progression of their disease. The 1-year actuarial overall survival rate was 39.7% and the 2-year survival rate was 14.5%. The rationale for treating adrenal metastatic lesions in the manner described is the possibility that by reducing the tumor burden, the disease can be better controlled. This, unfortunately, remains to be proven.

D. E. Schteingart, MD

Clinical and Pathophysiological Implications of Chromosomal Alterations in Adrenocortical Tumors: An Integrated Genomic Approach

Barreau O, de Reynies A, Wilmot-Roussel H, et al (Institut Cochin, Paris, France; Ligue Nationale Contre Le Cancer, Paris, France; et al)
J Clin Endocrinol Metab 97:E301-E311, 2012

Purpose.—Diagnosing malignancy of adrenocortical tumors (ACT) and predicting prognosis in carcinomas are often challenging. Transcriptome markers have recently emerged, providing promising clinical relevance and improved pathophysiological knowledge. Whether tumoral chromosomal alterations provide similar information is not known. The aim was to evaluate the diagnostic and prognostic value of chromosomal alterations in ACT and to identify genes associated with benign and malignant tumorigenesis.

Experimental Design.—Chromosomal alterations of 86 adenomas and 52 carcinomas were identified by comparative genomic hybridization arrays and/or quantitative PCR.

Results.—A larger proportion of the genome is altered in carcinomas compared with adenomas (44 *vs.* 10%, $P = 2.10^{-10}$). In adenomas, the 9q34 region, which includes the steroidogenic factor 1 locus, is commonly gained and associated with an overexpression of steroidogenic factor 1 (*SF-1*). In carcinomas, recurrent gains include chromosomes 5, 7, 12, 16, 19, and 20 and recurrent losses chromosomes 13 and 22. Filtering the genes from these regions according to their expression profile identified genes potentially relevant to adrenocortical tumorigenesis. A diagnostic tool was built by combining DNA copy number estimates at six loci (5q, 7p, 11p, 13q, 16q, and 22q). This tool discriminates carcinomas from adenomas in an independent validation cohort (sensitivity 100%, specificity 83%). In carcinomas, the number of chromosomal alterations was not associated with survival (Cox $P = 0.84$). A prognostic tool based on tumor DNA was designed with a clustering strategy and validated in an independent cohort.

Conclusions.—Chromosomal alterations in ACT discriminate carcinomas from adenomas and contain prognostic information. Chromosomal alterations alter the expression of genes important for tumorigenesis.

▶ Clonality studies of adrenal cortical tumors using X-chromosome inactivation analysis indicate monoclonal expansion of a single cell as the origin of adrenal carcinomas (ACC). There are multiple chromosomal alterations in ACC.[1] Chromosomal gains are observed in chromosomes 5, 12, and 19, and most losses occur in chromosomes 1 p, 17 p and 11. Mutations in key genes involved in adrenal cortical cell proliferation may lead to tumor development. Cases of adrenal cancer have been described in families with a hereditary cancer syndrome who exhibit mutations in tumor-suppressor genes. One such condition is the Li-Fraumeni syndrome, a rare autosomal-dominant syndrome caused by germline mutations in the TP53 tumor-suppressor gene and associated with high susceptibility to a variety of malignancies, including sarcoma, breast cancer, brain tumors, lung cancer, laryngeal carcinoma, leukemia, and ACC. However, adrenal cancer occurs infrequently in this syndrome. The deleterious genotype in these cases is expressed through several generations in both children and adults. Studies on the genetics of these familial syndromes helped identify mutations in sporadic cases. Somatic mutations of the tumor-suppressor gene TP53 are associated with one-third of ACC with p53 protein nuclear accumulation and a worse prognosis. Studies of specific genes and pangenomic analysis show that the IGF-II gene is the most commonly expressed, being detected in 85% of cases of ACC. Transcriptome studies have identified an IGF-II cluster of genes (containing mainly growth factors and growth factor receptor genes) significantly overexpressed in ACC. Perturbation of the IGF-II locus appears to be a dominant event in ACC. In contrast, a cluster of steroidogenic genes (CYP11A, CYP11B, HSD3B1) is more expressed in adenomas. Transcriptome analysis also suggests that the Wnt signaling pathway is activated in ACC. About one-third of adrenal cortical tumors harbor somatic-activating mutations of the β-catenin gene. In the absence of the Wnt signal, β-catenin is captured within a destructive complex and eventually degraded. In contrast, activation of Wnt signaling allows β-catenin to accumulate and enter the nucleus, where it activates genes that instruct the cell to proliferate and remain in an undifferentiated state. Using transcriptome profiling, a set of genes identified with Wnt dysregulation was identified in ACC. Another potential mechanism of tumorigenesis involves upregulation of telomerase, a multisubunit ribonucleoprotein complex that adds telomere repeats to the ends of linear chromosomes, a process critical for normal tissue progenitor cell function and cancer development. Telomerase is found to be upregulated in 90% of human cancers, where it serves to stabilize telomeres and allows unlimited cell division. In the presence of p53, senescence is activated as an antioncogenic mechanism. With the loss of p53 seen in adrenal cancer, telomere maintenance mechanisms are active and lead to tumor development. As proposed in other malignant solid tumors, activated adrenal cortical cancer stem cells may provide a mechanism for perpetuating progenitor cells that ultimately contribute to the persistent proliferation of mature cancer cells.

Microarray analysis of adrenal tumors and normal adrenals has also shown upregulation of Jagged1 and Notch pathways in a majority of adrenal cortical carcinomas. These pathways could be important contributors to adrenal tumorigenesis and targets for pharmacologic inhibition of cell proliferation. FOXM1, a proliferation-specific transcription factor of the Forkhead family, was also shown to be overexpressed in malignant versus benign tumors or normal tissues. Thus, FOXM1 may be a good marker for malignant adrenocortical tumors and may play a role in tumorigenesis.

A variety of other genetic defects have been described in ACC, but it is uncertain what role they play in the initiation and progression of the neoplastic process. As with the TP53 gene, allelic loss at the Rb gene locus on chromosome 13q has been described in ACC. Other genetic markers examined have included the H19 and the p57kip2 genes. These genes have been mapped to chromosome 11p15.513 and appear to be important for fetal growth and development. The levels of expression of the H19 are very high in human fetal adrenal glands, but they subsequently decrease by 50% in adults. The gene product for p57kip2, a member of the p21cip1 cyclin-dependent kinase family, appears to regulate cell proliferation, exit from the cell cycle, and maintenance of differentiated cells. Loss of activity of the p57kip2 gene product has been detected in virilizing adenomas and ACC, suggesting that this gene product plays a role in the normal maintenance of adrenal cortical differentiation and function. H19 and p57kip2 gene expression is adrenocorticotropic hormone dependent, and regulation of the p57kip2 gene appears to be related to the cyclic adenosine monophosphate—dependent protein kinase pathway. The gene product for p57kip2 is usually found to be high in most normal human tissues. A markedly reduced expression of the H19 gene has been found in both nonfunctioning and functioning ACC, especially in tumors that produce cortisol and aldosterone. Reduced expression of the p57kip2 has been found in Beckwith-Wiedemann syndrome, a congenital overgrowth disorder characterized by high risk of development of childhood tumors, including ACC. In general, genetic changes increase as the tumor increases its malignancy grade.

Some of the genetic changes described are uncovered in the late stages of the disease, and it is likely that a better understanding of early events may lead to a more effective control of the process of tumorigenesis. The recent identification of specific genetic defects in adrenal cortical carcinomas is likely to be important in understanding the process of tumorigenesis as well as the diagnosis, prognosis, and targeted therapy of adrenal cancer.

For the last several years, several molecular/genetic studies have attempted to classify adrenal tumors, correlate the genomic profile with tumor progression, and determine prognosis. In last year's issue of the YEAR BOOK we commented on several articles attempting to define biomarkers for ACC. The effort continues. Barreau et al report on chromosomal alterations of 86 adrenal adenomas (AA) and 52 ACC by comparative genomic hybridization arrays or quantitative polymerase chain reaction. Not surprisingly, carcinomas exhibited more alterations than adenomas with chromosomal deletions and gains and gene over- and underexpression that allowed for separation of the 2 types of tumors. ACC had specific chromosomal gains (5, 7, 12, 16, 19, 20) and losses (13 and 22) with corresponding overexpression of some oncogenes. In AA, overexpression was noted of steroidogenic enzyme genes such as steroidogenic factor 1 (SF-1). However, SF-1 is also expressed in ACC, and high expression has poor prognostic value.[2] ACC genomes clustered in 2 groups with apparently different clinical outcomes, suggesting the gene profile may be useful in categorizing ACC according to their biological characteristics. Giordano et al[3] have recently reported on similar findings. Using Affymetrix Human Genome U133 plus 2.0 oligonucleotide arrays, they generated transcriptional profiles for 10 normal adrenal cortices (NC), 22 adrenocortical adenomas (ACA), and 33 ACCs. Like in Barreaus' study, cluster analysis of the ACCs found 2 subtypes that reflected tumor proliferation, as measured by mitotic counts and cell cycle genes. Kaplan-Meier analysis of these ACC clusters showed a significant difference in survival ($P < .020$).

Genomic studies are still in their infancy, but they open new pathways for better understanding the process of tumorigenesis, its clinical consequence, and possibilities for targeted therapies.

D. E. Schteingart, MD

References

1. Schteingart DE. Neoplasms of the adrenal cortex, Cancer Medicine, 8th edition, 88:1269–1274. In: Holland JF, Frei E, editors. People's Medical Publishing House-USA, Shelton, CT; 2010;75:933-939.
2. Sbiera S, Schmull S, Assie G, et al. High Diagnostic and prognostic value of steroidogenic factor-1 expression in adrenal tumors. *J Clin Endocrinol Metab.* 2010;95:E161-E171.
3. Giordano TJ, Kuick R, Else T, et al. Molecular classification and prognostication of adrenocortical tumors by transcriptome profiling. *Clin Cancer Res.* 2009;15: 668-676.

Autoimmunity and Addison's Disease

Functional effects of DAX-1 mutations identified in patients with X-linked adrenal hypoplasia congenita
Choi J-H, Park J-Y, Kim G-H, et al (Univ of Ulsan College of Medicine, Seoul, South Korea; et al)
Metab Clin Exp 60:1545-1550, 2011

X-linked adrenal hypoplasia congenita with hypogonadotropic hypogonadism and adrenal insufficiency is a rare disorder caused by mutations of DAX-1. In this study, we investigated the functional defects of DAX-1 caused by mutations identified in 3 unrelated Korean patients with adrenal hypoplasia congenita. The DAX-1 gene was directly sequenced using genomic DNA isolated from peripheral blood leukocytes. The functional defects of DAX-1 caused by mutations were evaluated using an in vitro promoter assay. After mutagenesis of DAX-1 complementary DNA in the pcDNA3.1 vector, steroidogenic factor 1 and the promoter region of steroidogenic acute regulatory protein (StAR) genes in pGL4.10[luc2] were transiently cotransfected into human embryonic kidney 293 cells, followed by luminometry measurements of the luciferase activity of StAR.

Mutation analysis of 3 patients revealed p.L386delfsX2, p.W105X, and p.Q252X mutations of the DAX-1 gene. The mutant DAX-1 proteins showed lower repressive activity on the StAR gene promoter when compared with normal DAX-1. Nonsense and frameshift mutations of the DAX-1 gene partially eliminated the ability of DAX-1 to repress the transcription of StAR in an in vitro assay.

▶ The most common etiology of primary adrenal insufficiency (PAI) in the United States is autoimmune adrenalitis, which occurs in 65% of cases either by itself or as part of familial autoimmune pluriglandular syndrome. In these cases, the adrenal cortex is atrophied, but the medulla is intact and functional. Infectious etiologies such as tuberculosis, systemic mycosis, and acute sepsis usually destroy the whole gland, including the medulla. In some patients, the etiology is an infiltrative process such as lymphoma, amyloidosis, or metastatic neoplasm. The most common primaries metastasizing to the adrenal are from lung (60%), renal cell, melanoma, breast, prostate, and pancreas. Adrenal infarction or hemorrhage can lead to acute adrenal insufficiency, usually in patients under physical stress who are on anticoagulants. Patients with classical forms of congenital adrenal hyperplasia may present with acute adrenal insufficiency in the neonatal or infancy period and with severe dehydration and shock. Surgical adrenalectomy for Cushing syndrome or treatment of adrenal cancer with adrenolytic therapy such as mitotane also results in permanent adrenal insufficiency. Finally, rare mutations in early steroidogenic enzymes result in adrenal hypoplasia and PAI in early childhood. DAX-1 is an orphan nuclear receptor that encodes a 470-aminoacid protein and serves to activate target genes involved in hypothalamic—adrenal—gonadal axis development and function. DAX-1 is a general repressor of steroid biosynthesis through repression of steroidogenic factor-1 (SF-1)—mediated transactivation of many genes in the steroid biosynthetic pathway.

The authors report on the functional effects of DAX-1 mutations in 3 Korean children who developed PAI in the neonatal period. The 3 patients also had hypogonadotropic hypogonadism, a condition associated with DAX-1 mutations. The sequencing of DAX-1 in the 3 patients showed that the mutations encountered diminished repressive activity compared to normal DAX-1 and abolished the repression activity of both steroidogenic acute regulatory protein (StAR) and *SF-1* gene promoter activation.

D. E. Schteingart, MD

A Novel Entity of Clinically Isolated Adrenal Insufficiency Caused by a Partially Inactivating Mutation of the Gene Encoding for P450 Side Chain Cleavage Enzyme (CYP11A1)
Parajes S, Kamrath C, Rose IT, et al (Univ of Birmingham, UK; Justus-Liebig-Univ, Giessen, Germany; et al)
J Clin Endocrinol Metab 96:E1798-E1806, 2011

Context.—Cytochrome P450 side-chain cleavage enzyme (CYP11A1) facilitates the first and rate-limiting step of steroidogenesis. Only nine patients with CYP11A1 deficiency have been described. All patients presented with adrenal insufficiency (AI) and disorder of sex development in 46,XY individuals.

Objective.—Our objective was to define the pathogenic consequences of a novel *CYP11A1* mutation (p.R451 W) found in two brothers with isolated adrenal insufficiency.

Patients.—The two brothers (46,XY) presented with AI and normal male genital development. The older boy first presented with signs and symptoms suggestive of AI at the age of 2.8 yr but was only diagnosed at the age of 4.1 yr during an adrenal crisis. The younger brother was diagnosed with AI at the age of 2.5 yr while being clinically asymptomatic. Both boys had entirely normal appearance of their external genitalia.

Results.—The novel p.R451W mutation and five published missense *CYP11A1* mutations were characterized employing two *in vitro* approaches using the natural substrate cholesterol and the intermediate 22R-hydroxycholesterol, respectively. Pregnenolone generation was measured by highly specific liquid chromatography tandem mass spectrometry. p.R451 W had 30% of wild-type activity consistent with the clinical phenotype in our patients. Two previously published mutations (p.L222P and p.A359V) had 2- to 3-fold higher *in vitro* activities than originally reported, correlating better with the associated phenotypes.

Conclusions.—We provide the first evidence that partial CYP11A1 deficiency has to be considered as a differential diagnosis in clinically isolated adrenal insufficiency. Our assays demonstrate a tighter genotype-phenotype correlation in CYP11A1 deficiency than previous *in vitro* studies.

▶ Primary adrenocortical insufficiency (PAI) is manifested by a common clinical and biochemical presentation, despite a variety of possible etiologies, leading to the destruction of the adrenal cortex. Typical biochemical findings are low cortisol and aldosterone levels, high corticotropin and renin, and absent adrenal cortical response to synthetic corticotropin stimulation. The most common etiology in the United States is autoimmune adrenalitis, which occurs in 65% of cases either by itself or as part of autoimmune pluriglandular syndrome. The adrenal cortex is atrophied, but the medulla is intact and functional. Infectious etiologies such as tuberculosis, systemic mycosis, and acute sepsis usually destroy the whole gland, including the medulla. In some patients, the etiology is an infiltrative process such as lymphoma, amyloidosis, and metastatic neoplasms. The most common primaries metastasizing to the adrenal are from lung (60%), renal cell, melanoma, breast, prostate, and pancreas. Adrenal infarction or hemorrhage can lead to acute adrenal insufficiency, usually in patients under physical stress who are on anticoagulants. Patients with classical forms of congenital adrenal hyperplasia may present with acute adrenal insufficiency in the neonate or infancy period. Surgical adrenalectomy for Cushing syndrome or treatment of adrenal cancer with adrenolytic therapy such as mitotane also results in permanent adrenal insufficiency. Finally, rare mutations in early steroidogenic enzymes result in adrenal hypoplasia and PAI in early childhood. An example of this condition is presented by these authors. They describe

2 brothers diagnosed with PAI secondary to a novel, partially inactivating mutation of the gene encoding for P450 side chain cleavage enzyme (CYP11A1).
This enzyme catalyzes the conversion of cholesterol to pregnenolone, and its
total deficiency results in lack of development of the external genitalia in addition to deficiency of cortisol, aldosterone, and sex hormone secretion. Because
in the cases reported, the enzyme inactivation was partial, and the patients had
normal-appearing external genitalia. The molecular genetic analysis of the
CYP11A1 gene showed a homozygous novel C to T transition at nucleotide
9298. These cases are important because the identification of the genetic defect
gives a more precise understanding of the phenotype and allows for the
screening and detection of other affected family members and their early diagnosis and treatment. The bottom line is that establishing the etiology of PAI is
important for proper patient management.

D. E. Schteingart, MD

**Improved Cortisol Exposure-Time Profile and Outcome in Patients with
Adrenal Insufficiency: A Prospective Randomized Trial of a Novel
Hydrocortisone Dual-Release Formulation**
Johannsson G, Nilsson AG, Bergthorsdottir R, et al (Univ of Gothenburg,
Sweden; et al)
J Clin Endocrinol Metab 97:473-481, 2012

Context.—Patients with treated adrenal insufficiency (AI) have increased
morbidity and mortality rate. Our goal was to improve outcome by developing a once-daily (OD) oral hydrocortisone dual-release tablet with
a more physiological exposure-time cortisol profile.

Objective.—The aim was to compare pharmacokinetics and metabolic
outcome between OD and the same daily dose of thrice-daily (TID) dose
of conventional hydrocortisone tablets.

Design and Setting.—We conducted an open, randomized, two-period,
12-wk crossover multicenter trial with a 24-wk extension at five university
hospital centers.

Patients.—The trial enrolled 64 adults with primary AI; 11 had concomitant diabetes mellitus (DM).

Intervention.—The same daily dose of hydrocortisone was administered
as OD dual-release or TID.

Main Outcome Measure.—We evaluated cortisol pharmacokinetics.

Results.—Compared with conventional TID, OD provided a sustained
serum cortisol profile 0–4 h after the morning intake and reduced the late
afternoon and the 24-h cortisol exposure. The mean weight (difference =
-0.7 kg, $P = 0.005$), systolic blood pressure (difference $= -5.5$ mm Hg, $P =$
0.0001) and diastolic blood pressure (difference: -2.3 mmHg; $P = 0.03$), and
glycated hemoglobin (absolute difference $= -0.1\%$, $P = 0.0006$) were all
reduced after OD compared with TID at 12 wk. Compared with TID,
a reduction in glycated hemoglobin by 0.6% was observed in patients with
concomitant DM during OD $(P = 0.004)$.

Conclusion.—The OD dual-release tablet provided a more circadian-based serum cortisol profile. Reduced body weight, reduced blood pressure, and improved glucose metabolism were observed during OD treatment. In particular, glucose metabolism improved in patients with concomitant DM.

▶ Primary adrenal insufficiency (PAI) is characterized by partial or complete deficiency of cortisol, aldosterone, and sex hormone secretion. For decades, patients have been treated with substitution therapy with glucocorticoids and mineralocorticoids and occasionally adrenal androgens. The most commonly used glucocorticoid is hydrocortisone in doses of 20 to 30 mg/d, and the usually used mineralocorticoid is fludrocortisone in doses of 0.05 to 0.2 mg/d. Replacement with fludrocortisone is rather simple; most patients require a single daily dose. Aldosterone levels fluctuate with posture, but in replacing aldosterone, this is not an important consideration. Adjustments are made based on blood pressure, serum electrolytes, and plasma renin levels. In contrast, determining the optimal dose of hydrocortisone is challenging. Cortisol is secreted according to a circadian rhythm, with peak values between 6 and 8 AM, and the cortisol exposure-time profile seems to be a critical factor in establishing optimal replacement. Other factors include cortisol binding to corticosteroid-binding globulin, the level of circulating free cortisol, and its peripheral metabolism and clearance. Lack of optimal replacement therapy with hydrocortisone has serious consequence. Patients with PAI have more than double the standardized mortality rate, and mortality is increased 7-fold in patients with adrenal insufficiency and hypopituitarism. Likely reasons are supraphysiologic maintenance doses, poor diurnal glucocorticoid exposure-time profile, and inadequate coverage during situations of stress. The optimal maintenance dose of hydrocortisone during nonstress conditions can be established by measuring a 24-hour urinary free cortisol. The level should be in the middle of the reference range for the assay. The following case illustrates the utility of 24-hour urinary free cortisol measurements in determining the optimal replacement dose. A 60-year-old woman underwent transsphenoidal pituitary surgery for Cushing disease, developed adrenal insufficiency postoperatively, and was placed on hydrocortisone, 25 mg/d. She developed clinical features of Cushing syndrome, and urine free cortisol was high (250 µg/d [normal 20–90 µg/d]). The dose was gradually reduced to 12.5 mg/d, her clinical features resolved, and her urine free cortisol decreased to 50 µg/d.

In an important article on hydrocortisone replacement in patients with PAI, Johannsson et al report on the use of a novel, once-daily, dual-release hydrocortisone tablet to improve cortisol exposure-time profile. This tablet releases two-thirds of the dose during the first 4 hours and the rest over the following 20 hours, recapitulating a normal circadian rhythm. They conducted an open, randomized, 2-period, 12-week crossover multicenter trial, comparing in 64 patients with PAI the once daily, 30-mg dual release hydrocortisone tablet with a standard hydrocortisone dosing of 30 mg administered in unequally divided doses (15-10-5). As shown in Fig 2 in the original article, patients receiving the once-a-day tablet had a smoother and more physiologic cortisol profile than those on the standard treatment. In addition, these patients had significant clinical improvement with decrease in body weight, blood pressure, hemoglobin A1c and quality-of-life testing.

For decades, we have been treating patients with PAI without serious attention to dose or manner of administration of replacement steroids. Some patients have received prednisone instead of hydrocortisone to minimize the doses patients need to take daily. Even when using hydrocortisone, patients occasionally receive supraphysiologic, equally divided doses without consideration of the importance of preserving a normal circadian rhythm. The study by Johannsson et al should make physicians aware of the complexity of treating patients who have adrenal insufficiency.

D. E. Schteingart, MD

Congenital Adrenal Hyperplasia

High frequency of adrenal myelolipomas and testicular adrenal rest tumours in adult Norwegian patients with classical congenital adrenal hyperplasia because of 21-hydroxylase deficiency

Nermoen I, Rørvik J, Holmedal SH, et al (Univ of Oslo, Norway; Univ of Bergen, Norway; Akershus Univ Hosp, Lørenskog, Norway; et al)
Clin Endocrinol 75:753-759, 2011

Background.—Increased frequencies of adrenal tumours and testicular adrenal rest tumours (TART) have been reported in patients with 21-hydroxylase deficiency (21OHD).

Objective.—Patients, methods and design From a cross-sectional population-based study of 101 adult Norwegian patients with 21OHD, sixty-two participated in this study (23 men, 39 women; age range 18–75); thirty-two were salt wasting (SW) and 30 simple virilizing (SV); they were assessed with adrenal computed tomography (CT), testicular ultrasound and hormone measurement in the morning after overnight medication fast.

Results.—Nine adrenal tumours were detected in seven (11%) patients (bilateral in 2); four were myelolipomas and one a phaeochromocytoma. Seventeen (27%) had normal adrenal size, whereas 36 (58%) had persisting hyperplasia, and seven (11%) adrenal hypoplasia. Abnormal adrenals were more common in SW than in SV. TART occurred exclusively in SW and was present in seven (57%) of these men. Testicular volumes were small compared with normative data. Morning ACTH and 17-hydroxy-progesterone levels correlated positively with adrenal dimensions and frequency of TART.

Conclusion.—In this unselected population of patients with classical 21OHD, we found high frequencies of adrenal tumours, particularly mye-lolipomas, and of hyperplasia and hypoplasia, and TART in SW. It is important that physicians are aware that benign adrenal and testicular tumours occur frequently in 21OHD. Furthermore, these findings may reflect inappropriate glucocorticoid therapy, making a case for the advancement of novel physiological treatment modalities.

▶ Patients with classical forms of congenital adrenal hyperplasia (CAH) usually present in childhood with primary adrenal insufficiency and virilization. The most common type results from 21-hydroxylase deficiency. With severe enzyme deficiency, patients develop the salt-wasting (SW) type with mineralocorticoid deficiency, while with lesser degrees of deficiency, only cortisol synthesis is impaired and the phenotype is predominantly simple virilization (SV). Standard treatment consists of corticotropin (ACTH) and adrenal cortical suppression with corticosteroids to replace deficient cortisol secretion and suppress excessive androgen production. The dose of corticosteroid required for optimal suppression frequently exceeds normal physiological replacement. In contrast to women with CAH, men are suppressed less vigorously, since virilization is less of a clinical problem. However, adrenal androgens can suppress pituitary gonadotropins and inhibit testicular function, including spermatogenesis, causing oligospermia and infertility. Incomplete suppression of plasma ACTH levels in these patients results in persistent adrenal cortical hyperplasia and stimulation of gonadal adrenal rests. We had commented on an article by Delfino et al[1] on testicular adrenal rest cell tumors in patients with CAH. This article from Sweden and Norway focuses on the same issue. The authors studied 62 patients (23 men, 39 women) with 21-hydroxylase deficiency with adrenal CT and, in men, testicular ultrasound. There were more adrenal tumors in men than in women, and myelolipomas were found only in men. Adrenal hyperplasia was found in half of the men and women, and these findings coincided with higher ACTH and 17-hydroxyprogesterone levels, suggesting incomplete suppression. One-third of the men had testicular adrenal rest cell tumors, and these were more prevalent in patients with the SW type, the more severe form of CAH. This article warns against testicular biopsies in these patients. The tumors often shrink or disappear with more effective corticosteroid suppression. It is clear that better ways of suppressing ACTH levels and the abnormal steroidogenic pathway need to be found without inducing Cushing syndrome.

D. E. Schteingart, MD

Reference

1. Delfino M, Elia J, Imbrogno N, et al. Testicular adrenal rest tumors in patients with congenital adrenal hyperplasia: prevalence and sonographic, hormonal, and seminal characteristics. *J Ultrasound Med.* 2012;31:383-388.

Testicular Adrenal Rest Tumors in Patients With Congenital Adrenal Hyperplasia: Prevalence and Sonographic, Hormonal, and Seminal Characteristics

Delfino M, Elia J, Imbrogno N, et al (Univ of Rome "Sapienza," Italy)
J Ultrasound Med 31:383-388, 2012

Objective.—Testicular adrenal rest tumors have been described in patients with congenital adrenal hyperplasia (CAH). The aim of this work was to (1) evaluate the prevalence of testicular adrenal rest tumors in patients with CAH; (2) study the hormonal profile; (3) define the sonographic features; (4) assess the seminal profile; and (5) initiate a longitudinal study on the possible role of corticotropin (ACTH) plasma levels in the induction and persistence of testicular adrenal rest tumors.

Methods.—Eighteen patients affected by CAH, aged 21 to 41 years, were studied. These were all patients referred to our endocrinology unit for the first time to undergo a clinical evaluation. All of the patients were taking long-term cortisone acetate and fludrocortisone replacement therapy. The study included (1) a physical examination, (2) testis sonography, (3) a hormonal profile, (4) semen analysis.

Results.—Sonography showed testicular adrenal rest tumors in 11 patients (61.1%); of these, 9 cases (50.0%) were bilateral, and 2 (11.1%) were unilateral. The diameter ranged from 4 to 38 mm. In 9 patients, the lesions were hypoechoic, whereas in 2, they were hyperechoic. High plasma ACTH levels were detected in all of the patients with tumors despite long-term therapy. Semen analysis found 2 cases of azoospermia and 6 cases of oligoasthenoteratozoospermia; the 3 remaining patients were normospermic. The preliminary longitudinal study has shown 3 patients with a disappearance or reduction of the tumors after 6 months of modified treatment.

Conclusions.—This study confirms the high prevalence of testicular adrenal rest tumors in patients with CAH and the major role played in its pathogenesis by high plasma ACTH levels.

▶ Patients with classical forms of congenital adrenal hyperplasia (CAH) are usually treated with glucocorticoids to replace deficient cortisol secretion and suppress plasma corticotropin (ACTH) levels and excessive androgen production. In contrast to women with CAH, men are suppressed less vigorously because virilization is not usually a clinical problem. However, adrenal androgens can suppress pituitary gonadotropins and inhibit testicular function, including spermatogenesis, causing oligospermia and infertility. Incomplete suppression of plasma ACTH levels in these patients results in adrenal cortical hyperplasia and stimulation of gonadal adrenal rests. There are reports in these patients of adrenal myelolipomas and testicular adrenal rest cell tumors. Delfino et al reported on the prevalence of testicular adrenal rest cell tumors in 18 adult men with CAH on long-term replacement therapy with cortisone acetate and fludrocortisone. They all had high plasma ACTH levels. Testicular sonography showed adrenal rest cell tumors ranging in size from 4 to 38 mm in 61% of the patients, and semen analysis showed disturbed spermatogenesis in 72%. Of interest is that better suppression of ACTH levels caused disappearance of these tumors. The importance of this study is that it calls attention to the gonadal consequence of incomplete ACTH suppression in men with CAH. The challenge is being able to suppress ACTH without inducing Cushing syndrome.

D. E. Schteingart, MD

Cushing's Disease: Diagnosis and Treatment

A Large Family with Carney Complex Caused by the S147G PRKAR1A Mutation Shows a Unique Spectrum of Disease Including Adrenocortical Cancer

Anselmo J, Medeiros S, Carneiro V, et al (Hospital Divino Espírito Santo, São Miguel, Azores, Portugal; et al)
J Clin Endocrinol Metab 97:351-359, 2012

Context.—Most tumors in Carney complex (CNC) are benign, including primary pigmented nodular adrenocortical disease (PPNAD), the main endocrine tumor in CNC. Adrenocortical cancer (AC) has never been observed in the syndrome. Herein, we describe a large Azorean family with CNC caused by a point mutation in the *PRKAR1A* gene coding for type 1-α (RIα) regulatory subunit of the cAMP-dependent protein kinase A, in which the index patient presented with AC.

Objective.—We studied the genotype-phenotype correlation in CNC.

Design and Setting.—We reported on case series and *in vitro* testing of the *PRKAR1A* mutation in a tertiary care referral center.

Patients.—Twenty-two members of a family were investigated for Cushing syndrome and other CNC components; their DNA was sequenced for *PRKAR1A* mutations.

Results.—Cushing syndrome due to PPNAD occurred in four patients, including the proposita who presented with AC and three who had Cushing syndrome and/or PPNAD. Lentigines were found in six additional patients who did not have PPNAD. A base substitution (c.439A>G/p.S147G) in *PRKAR1A* was identified in the proposita, in the three others with PPNAD, in the proposita's twin daughters who had lentigines but no evidence of hypercortisolism, and in five other family members, including one without lentigines or evidence of hypercortisolism. Unlike in other RIα defects, loss of heterozygosity was not observed in AC. The S147G mutation was compared to other expressed *PRKAR1A* mutations; it led to decreased cAMP and catalytic subunit binding by RIα and increased protein kinase A activity *in vitro*.

Conclusions.—In a large family with CNC, one amino acid substitution caused a spectrum of adrenal disease that ranged from lack of manifestations to cancer. PPNAD and AC were the only manifestations of CNC in these patients, in addition to lentigines. These data have implications for counseling patients with CNC and are significant in documenting the first case of AC in the context of PPNAD.

▶ Carney complex is a genetic syndrome with autosomal dominant transmission. Patients present with multiple tumors, usually benign, in addition to cutaneous pigmented lesions. Typical manifestations include pituitary adenomas with acromegaly, Sertoli cell calcifying testicular tumors, cardiac myxomas, and melanotic schwannomas. The cutaneous lesions include lentigines, frequently around the mouth, blue nevi, and subcutaneous myxomas. The adrenal glands are frequently involved, presenting with Cushing syndrome (CS) secondary to corticotropin (ACTH)-independent primary pigmented micronodular adrenocortical hyperplasia (PPNAD). The pathology consists of normal-weight glands with multiple darkly-pigmented functioning nodules less than 10 mm in size, internodular atrophy, and brown intracellular pigment (lipofuscin). When patients present with CS, cortisol levels may be normal or high with loss of normal circadian rhythm, but ACTH is suppressed.

The genetics of Carney complex has been well worked out. Two genetic loci have been described: one at 17q24 and the other at 2p16. In the genetic locus 17q24, there are mutations at the protein kinase A-R1 alpha subunit (*PRKAR1A*). The function of protein kinase A is to serve as a tumor suppressor gene by regulating cell proliferation and growth. Nearly 120 mutations have been described in patients with Carney, but not all of these genetic mutations are associated with specific phenotypes.

Most of the reports in the literature on PPNAD fail to describe adrenal malignancies as part of the syndrome. This has changed with this study describing a family from the Portuguese Azores with Carney complex, where the index case presented with a combination of PPNAD and adrenal cortical carcinoma (ACC). Both pathologies coexisted in the same gland.

The patient had severe CS, but it is not clear how much the PPNAD and the ACC contributed to the hypercortisolemia. An important question in this case is whether the development of ACC was a random event in this patient with PPNAD or if the genetic mutation predisposed the adrenal cortex to malignant transformation. It is likely that the coexistence of PPNAD and ACC is a rare event in Carney complex, and counseling about the risk of ACC in these patients and their families is premature. This case is described as a first report of the coexistence of PPNAD and ACC in Carney complex, but keep reading. A second report appeared almost simultaneously showing another case with a similar finding.[1]

D. E. Schteingart, MD

Reference

1. Morin E, Mete O, Wasserman JD, et al. Carney complex with adrenal cortical carcinoma. *J Clin Endocrinol Metab*. 2012;97:E202-E206.

Carney Complex with Adrenal Cortical Carcinoma

Morin E, Mete O, Wasserman JD, et al (Univ Health Network, Toronto, Ontario, Canada; Hosp for Sick Children, Toronto, Ontario, Canada)
J Clin Endocrinol Metab 97:E202-E206, 2012

Context.—Carney complex is a genetically heterogenous multiple neoplasia syndrome. Adrenal cortical carcinoma is a rare malignancy with a poor prognosis that is not recognized to be associated with this syndrome.

Objective.—We report a 22-yr-old female presenting with Carney complex who developed adrenal carcinoma. The response to adjunctive therapy is also described.

Methods.—We performed a detailed pathology review of the adrenal tumor to examine morphologic changes, Ki-67 labeling, and p53 expression. We also performed genetic testing of candidate genes and describe the response to radiation and kinase inhibition therapy.

Results.—The patient presented with an 8.5-cm adrenal mass with a MIB-1 labeling index of 20% and unequivocal angioinvasion classified as a T3NXM0 carcinoma. The nontumorous adrenal cortex revealed characteristic features of primary pigmented nodular adrenocortical disease. Genetic analysis revealed a novel PRKAR1 frame shift mutation resulting in a premature stop codon and a heterozygous p53 polymorphic substitution previously noted in other solid carcinomas. Disease recurrence in the liver showed partial response to combined stereotactic radiotherapy and sorafenib multikinase inhibition.

Conclusion.—This represents an initial characterization of a malignancy among patients with Carney complex. Our findings have implications for disease surveillance and management of individuals with this genetic syndrome.

▶ Carney complex is a genetic syndrome with autosomal dominant transmission. Patients present with multiple tumors, usually benign, in addition to cutaneous pigmented lesions. Two genetic loci have been described, one at 17q24 and the other at 2p16. In the genetic locus 17q24 there are mutations at the protein kinase A-R1 alpha subunit (PRKAR1A). The function of protein kinase A is to serve as a tumor suppressor gene by regulating cell proliferation and growth. The authors report on a case of Carney complex that presented with Cushing syndrome and an 8.5-cm right adrenal mass. The pathology was consistent with adrenocortical carcinoma (ACC), but the nontumorous adrenal cortex had evidence of primary pigmented nodular adrenal disease (PPNAD) lesions. Genetic analysis showed a novel PRKAR1 frame shift mutation, resulting in a premature stop codon and a heterozygous p53 polymorphic substitution. This second case of ACC developing on the background of PPNAD raises the question of the influence of the genetic mutation type on the process of adrenal tumorigenesis. As further cases are recognized, it will be possible to link the genetic profile with the risk of developing ACC in these patients.

D. E. Schteingart, MD

Primary Aldosteronism

Intraprocedural Cortisol Measurement Increases Adrenal Vein Sampling Success Rate in Primary Aldosteronism

Rossi E, Regolisti G, Perazzoli F, et al (Santa Maria Nuova Hosp, Reggio Emilia, Italy; Univ of Parma, Italy; et al)
Am J Hypertens 24:1280-1285, 2011

Background.—Adrenal venous sampling (AVS) is the gold standard for the identification of unilateral primary aldosteronism (PA), but is technically difficult. The aim of our study was to assess whether intraprocedural cortisol measurement (IPCM) increases AVS success rate.

Methods.—Twenty-five consecutive PA patients underwent cosyntropin-stimulated AVS. Cortisol was measured immediately in a first set of samples drawn from adrenal veins and inferior vena cava. The selectivity criterion was an adrenal vein-to-inferior vena cava cortisol ratio ≥ 5. If bilateral selectivity was not achieved in a first set of samples, a second set was obtained during the same radiological session. PA was judged as unilateral if the gradient of cortisol-corrected aldosterone between dominant and nondominant side was >3.5. Twenty-five consecutive PA patients who had previously been submitted to AVS without IPCM served as historical controls. Lateralizing patients who underwent unilateral adrenalectomy were followed for 2 years after surgery.

Results.—Bilateral selectivity using IPCM was achieved in 19/25 patients in the first set of samples, and in an additional four cases in the second set (92% vs. 76%; $P = 0.06$). The final rate of bilateral selectivity was higher than that obtained in the historical series (23/25 vs. 16/25, $P = 0.04$), whereas bilateral selectivity in the first set of samples was not different from that achieved in the historical series. Nineteen lateralizing patients (13 of the present series, six of the historical series) were submitted to adrenalectomy, resulting in reversal of PA.

Conclusions.—IPCM increases the success rate of AVS.

▶ Determination of the primary aldosteronism (PA) subtype—aldosterone-producing adenoma (APA) versus bilateral adrenal hyperplasia (BAH)—requires adrenal venous sampling. When properly performed, this test is the gold standard to determine which therapeutic approach is most indicated for any given patient. This is important because patients with PA secondary to an APA can be cured with unilateral laparoscopic adrenalectomy, but patients with BAH may not benefit from surgery. This invasive test is not always easy to perform, and the success of the test depends on the experience of the interventional radiologist involved. A major difficulty has been certainty about the placement of the catheters, especially in the right adrenal vein that connects directly to the inferior vena cava, sometimes in a common opening with the hepatic vein. To confirm the position of the catheter, cortisol is measured simultaneously with aldosterone, and an adrenal vein to inferior vena cava ratio of greater than 5 indicates the catheter is properly positioned. The challenge is the timeliness of the cortisol measurement, because if one waits until the measurements have been completed and the catheters are not in place, there is no opportunity for correction. Auchus et al[1] in 2009 had already proposed intraprocedural measurement of cortisol to optimize catheter positioning. A similar study is now reported by these authors, comparing 25 patients with PA undergoing adrenal venous sampling (AVS) with intraprocedural cortisol measurements with 25 patients who had undergone AVS without the cortisol monitoring. They found that cortisol monitoring led to more successful bilateral catheterization and more accurate results. The major concern in both reports is the logistics of performing cortisol measurements during the AVS procedure. Patients need to keep the catheters or their sheaths in place for several hours; the measurement of cortisol is not instantaneous, and if there is a need to reposition the catheters, several more hours are required before the procedure can be completed. The procedure turns out to be not only uncomfortable for the patient, but it is also expensive, given the length of time the radiology unit will be used.

The concept of confirming the catheter position during the procedure is important, but it will require development of a faster method for measuring cortisol, preferably in the same room by the procedure table. What is reassuring is that radiologists who are experienced in adrenal vein catheterization can confirm the catheter position by contrast imaging and make adjustments when the catheters are not in the right place.

D. E. Schteingart, MD

Reference

1. Auchus RJ, Michaelis C, Wians FH Jr, et al. Rapid cortisol assays improve the success rate of adrenal vein sampling for primary aldosteronism. *Ann Surg.* 2009;249:318-321.

Evaluation of the Sensitivity and Specificity of ^{11}C-Metomidate Positron Emission Tomography (PET)-CT for Lateralizing Aldosterone Secretion by Conn's Adenomas

Burton TJ, Mackenzie IS, Balan K, et al (Univ of Cambridge, UK; Addenbrooke's Hosp, Cambridge UK)

J Clin Endocrinol Metab 97:100-109, 2012

Context.—Identification of unilateral aldosterone-producing (Conn's) adenomas has traditionally required lateralization by the invasive and technically difficult procedure of adrenal vein sampling (AVS). ^{11}C-metomidate, a potent inhibitor of adrenal steroidogenic enzymes, is a positron emission tomography (PET) radiotracer that is selectively accumulated by Conn's adenomas.

Objective.—The objective of the study was to compare the sensitivity and specificity of ^{11}C-metomidate PET-computed tomography (CT) against the current gold standard of AVS.

Design.—The design of the study was within-patient comparison of diagnostic techniques.

Setting.—The study was conducted at a single center-university teaching hospital.

Patients.—Thirty-nine patients with primary hyperaldosteronism (PHA) and five with nonfunctioning adenomas (incidentalomas) participated in the study.

Intervention(s).—The first six PHA patients were studied on three occasions to determine whether steroid pretreatment reduced ^{11}C-metomidate uptake by normal adrenal. Subsequent patients received dexamethasone for 3 d prior to injection of ^{11}C-metomidate 150–500 MBq.

Main Outcome Measure(s).—Maximum standardized uptake values (SUV_{max}) over regions of interest determined from 35–45 min after injection were measured.

Results.—Dexamethasone increased tumor to normal adrenal SUV_{max} ratio by $25.6 \pm 5.0\%$ ($P < 0.01$). PET-CT visualized subcentimeter adenomas and distinguished hot from cold adenomas within a gland. In 25 patients with PHA and AVS lateralization to the side of an adenoma, SUV_{max} over tumor (mean ± SEM) of 21.7 ± 1.6 was greater than over normal adrenal, 13.8 ± 0.6 ($P = 0.00003$); this difference was absent in 10 patients without lateralization on AVS ($P = 0.28$) and in four of five incidentalomas. On receiver-operator characteristics analysis, an SUV_{max} ratio of 1.25:1 provided a specificity of 87% [95% confidence interval (69, 104)] and sensitivity of 76% (59, 93); in tumors with SUV_{max} greater than 17, the specificity rose to 100%.

Conclusions.—[11]C-metomidate PET-CT is a sensitive and specific noninvasive alternative to AVS in the management of PHA (Fig 2A, B).

▶ Most cases of primary aldosteronism (PA) were initially attributed to an adrenal cortical adenoma (AA), but it is currently believed that 60% of cases of PA are secondary to bilateral adrenocortical hyperplasia (BAH). Biochemically, patients with PA have elevated aldosterone and suppressed renin secretion. A high aldosterone/renin ratio of greater than 40 with a serum aldosterone greater than 15 ng/dL strongly suggest a diagnosis of PA. Confirmatory tests are based on lack of aldosterone suppression with a saline infusion. But the test does not distinguish between adenoma and hyperplasia. Computed tomography of the abdomen may show an adenoma or hyperplasia, but the adenomas are frequently small (< 1 cm), and the radiographic finding may lead to a high proportion of erroneous determination between hyperplasia and adenoma. In some cases, there is a clear adrenal cortical adenoma in 1 adrenal and a completely normal-appearing adrenal on the contralateral side, a situation that may exclude the need for invasive localization, but, in general, determination of the PA subtype, AA versus BAH, requires adrenal venous sampling (AVS). This invasive test is not always easy to perform, but it remains the gold standard for a diagnosis of PA and a decision whether to surgically treat these patients. This is important because patients with PA secondary to AA can be cured with unilateral laparoscopic adrenalectomy, but patients with BAH may not benefit from surgery.

Burton et al report on the use of 11C-metomidate Positron Emission Tomography (PET-CT) for lateralizing aldosterone secretion by AA in 39 patients with

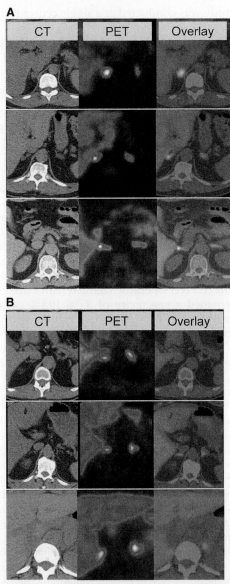

FIGURE 2.—PET-CT images from illustrative patients in each diagnostic group. A, Unilateral PHA and positive lateralization on PET-CT. CT, PET, and overlay images are shown for subjects 1 (*upper panels*), 6 (*middle panels*), and 15 (*lower panels*). All three patients lateralized to the right on AVS. B, Bilateral PHA and no lateralization on PET-CT. CT, PET, and overlay images are shown for subjects 28 (*upper panels*), 31 (*middle panels*), and 29 (*lower panels*). These subjects did not lateralize significantly on AVS and are true negatives in the ROC analysis. (Reprinted from Burton TJ, Mackenzie IS, Balan K, et al. Evaluation of the sensitivity and specificity of ^{11}C-metomidate positron emission tomography (PET) CT for lateralizing aldosterone secretion by Conn's adenomas. *J Clin Endocrinol Metab.* 2012;97:100-109, Copyright 2012, with permission from The Endocrine Society.)

PA and 5 with nonfunctioning, incidentally discovered adrenal cortical tumors. They determined the sensitivity and specificity of the imaging procedure and compared it with the results of adrenal venous sampling and adrenalectomy. Most patients were pretreated with suppressive doses of dexamethasone for 3 days to increase the tumor to normal adrenal maximum standardized uptake values (SUV_{max}). There was a high SUV_{max} ratio between the AA and normal adrenal in patients with lateralizing AVS but no SUV_{max} difference in those without lateralization. Specificity was 87% and sensitivity was 76%, but in tumors with higher SUV_{max}, specificity increased to 100%. The availability of 11C-metomidate PET-CT will determine how easily it will be used instead of AVS. But as shown in Fig 2A, images with positive lateralization results are impressive, especially when compared with that of patients without lateralization (Fig 2B).

D. E. Schteingart, MD

18-Hydroxycorticosterone, 18-Hydroxycortisol, and 18-Oxocortisol in the Diagnosis of Primary Aldosteronism and Its Subtypes
Mulatero P, di Cella SM, Monticone S, et al (Univ of Torino, Italy; et al)
J Clin Endocrinol Metab 97:881-889, 2012

Context.—Diagnosis of primary aldosteronism (PA) is made by screening, confirmation testing, and subtype diagnosis (computed tomography scan and adrenal vein sampling). However, some tests are costly and unavailable in most hospitals.

Objective.—The aim of the study was to evaluate the role of serum 18-hydroxycorticosterone (s18OHB), urinary and serum 18-hydroxycortisol (u- and s18OHF), and urinary and serum 18-oxocortisol (u- and s18oxoF) in the diagnosis of PA and its subtypes, aldosterone-producing adenoma (APA) and bilateral adrenal hyperplasia (BAH).

Patients.—The study included 62 patients with low-renin essential hypertension (EH), 81 patients with PA (20 APA, 61 BAH), 24 patients with glucocorticoid-remediable aldosteronism, 16 patients with adrenal incidentaloma, and 30 normotensives.

Intervention and Main Outcome Measures.—We measured s18OHB, s18OHF, and s18oxoF before and after saline load test (SLT) and 24-h u18OHF and u18oxoF.

Results.—PA patients displayed significantly higher levels of s18OHB, u18OHF, and u18oxoF compared to EH and normal subjects; APA patients displayed s18OHB, u18OHF, and u18oxoF levels significantly higher than BAH patients. Similar results were obtained for s18OHF and s18oxoF. SLT significantly reduced s18OHB, s18OHF, and s18oxoF in all groups, but steroid reduction was much less for APA patients compared to BAH and EH. The s18OHB/aldosterone ratio after SLT more than doubled in EH but remained unchanged in APA patients.

Conclusions.—u18OHF, u18oxoF, and s18OHB measurements in patients with a positive aldosterone/plasma renin activity ratio correlate with confirmatory tests and adrenal vein sampling in PA patients. If verified, these steroid assays would refine the diagnostic workup for PA.

▶ Most cases of primary aldosteronism (PA) were initially attributed to an adrenal cortical adenoma (AA), but it is currently believed that 60% of cases of PA are secondary to bilateral adrenocortical hyperplasia (BAH). Clinically, patients with PA secondary to an AA exhibit hypertension and hypokalemia with metabolic alkalosis, but patients with BAH may have milder clinical manifestations and hypokalemia may not be present. There is uncertainty about the possibility of subclinical PA in patients who present with hypertension and mildly elevated aldosterone levels that cause cardiac and renal fibrosis. Biochemically, patients with PA have elevated aldosterone and suppressed renin secretion. A high aldosterone–renin ratio (ARR) of greater than 40 with a serum aldosterone greater than 15 ng/dL strongly suggests a diagnosis of PA. Studies of the accuracy of the ARR as a diagnostic screening tool showed a highly significant within-patient correlation ($r = 0.69$; $P < .0001$) and reproducibility, and only 7% of the values fell out of the 95% confidence interval for the between-test difference. The accuracy of ARR for pinpointing aldosterone-producing adenoma patients was 80%, and its reproducibility supports its use for screening of primary aldosteronism.[1] Confirmatory tests are based on a lack of aldosterone suppression with a saline infusion. After reclining overnight, patients receive 2 L of 0.9% saline infusion, over 4 hours. Aldosterone is measured before and after infusion. In one report, levels after infusion in patients with PA (2 patients) were 18.6 +/– 12.9 ng/dL, while a comparison group of patients with essential hypertension were 5.7 +/– 1.9 ng/dL ($P < .0001$).[2] The test does not distinguish between adenoma and hyperplasia. CT of the abdomen may show an adenoma or hyperplasia, but the adenomas are frequently small, less than 1 cm, and the radiographic finding may lead to erroneous determination between hyperplasia and adenoma. Determination of the PA subtype, AA versus BAH, requires an additional test, adrenal venous sampling. This invasive test is not always easy to perform, but it remains the gold standard for a diagnosis of PA and a decision whether to surgically treat these patients. This is important because patients with PA secondary to an AA can be cured with unilateral laparoscopic adrenalectomy, but patients with BAH may not benefit from surgery. Medical treatment is recommended for patients with mineralocorticoid antagonists such as spironolactone (50–200 mg/day) or eplerenone (10–30 mg/day).

In response to the difficulties with adrenal venous sampling in the evaluation of patients with PA, several studies have recently been published with possible alternatives. This study examined the role of serum 18-hydroxycorticosterone (18-OHB) and serum and urine 18-hydroxycortisol (18-OHF) and 18-oxocortisol (18-OXOF) in 213 patients (81 patients with PA, 62 patients with low renin essential hypertension, 24 patients with glucocorticoid remediable aldosteronism, 16 patients with adrenal incidentaloma, and 30 patients who were normotensive). 18-OHB is a precursor of aldosterone synthesis in the zona glomerulosa and has long been suggested as a useful measurement in patients suspected of PA because levels are increased in that condition. 18-OHF and 18-OXOF are defined as hybrid steroids because they are synthesized by aldosterone synthase using

11β-hydroxylase as a substrate in the zona fasciculata. As shown in Fig 2 in the original article of this article, urinary levels of 18-OHF and 18-OXOF were elevated in PA and highest in patients with AA. Although there was some overlap between AA and BAH at lower levels, the separation was more definitive at the higher levels. As shown in Fig 4 in the original article, the authors propose an algorithm to incorporate the measurement of these hybrid steroids in the workup of patients with possible PA.

D. E. Schteingart, MD

References

1. Rossi GP, Seccia TM, Palumbo G, et al. Within-patient reproducibility of the aldosterone: renin ratio in primary aldosteronism. *Hypertension.* 2010;55:83-89.
2. Lucarelli G, Arnaldi G, Giacchetti G, et al. Saline infusion test in the diagnosis of primary aldosteronism. *Am J Hypert.* 2000;13:184A-185A.

7 Reproductive Endocrinology

Introduction

This year's selections include many citations related to androgen action, polycystic ovary syndrome, aging, metabolic syndrome, hypogonadism in men and hormonal influences on bone metabolism.

PEDIATRIC REPRODUCTIVE ENDOCRINOLOGY

Ibanez et al (11-191) report that metformin therapy in girls with precocious pubarche improved adverse effects of androgens and improved menstrual function.

FEMALE REPRODUCTIVE ENDOCRINOLOGY

Follicle counts predict live-birth rates associated with assisted reproductive function in women with PCOS (Holte et al, 11-197). Postmenopausal cigarette smoking women have higher circulating androgens, estrogens, 17-hydroxyprogesterone and SHBG, as found by Brand et al (11-189).

BONE HEALTH

Diets high in dairy foods and protein are protective of bone health during exercise-induced weight loss in obesity and overweight premenopausal women, as observed by Josse et al (11-210). Anorexia nervosa results in severe bone loss, which can be reduced in the spine by risdedronate but not by low-dose testosterone (Miller et al, 11-196). Although estradiol declines in aging women, those with higher testosterone concentrations have greater bone mineral density, lean body mass and total fat mass, as observed by Rariy et al (11-202).

POLYCYSTIC OVARY SYNDROME

Follicle counts on sonogram and serum anti-Mülleran hormone concentrations add to the diagnosis of PCOS, according to the findings of Dewailly and associates (11-195). Schmidt et al (11-200) determined that cardiovascular risk factors were more common in women with PCOS than controls, but this did not translate into higher rates of cardiovascular events during post menopause.

Metformin has been successful in treating hyperandrogenemia in women with PCOS, but Banaszwska et al (11-208) provide evidence that simvastatin is perhaps more effective than metformin. Crisosto et al (11-192) reported that improving hyperandrogenism and hyperinsulinemia during pregnancy in women with PCOS might reduce ovarian follicle mass in their daughters.

MALE REPRODUCTIVE FUNCTION

Using liquid chromatography tandem mass spectrometry in a community based population, Bhasin et al (11-204) generated normal reference intervals in healthy men.

HYPOGONADISM AND AGING

Total and free testosterone was the only hormone consistently associated with overall sexual function in middle-aged and older men, as reported by O'Connor et al (11-205). Hypogonadism in aging men is associated with an increased risk of all-cause and cardiovascular disease deaths (Araujo and associates, 11-206). This study was confirmed by Barrett-Connor et al (11-194), who reported that high serum testosterone predicted a reduced risk for cardiovascular events in elderly men.

PEDIATRIC GONADAL FUNCTION

Cryptorchidism risk in Hispanic white boys appears to be encoded by shorter androgen receptor CAG repeat lengths (Davis-Dao, 11-263). Boys with Klinefelter's syndrome exhibit adverse effects on all testicular cell types, but the depletion of cells occurs at different stages of gonadal development (Rey et al, 11-175).

ANDROGENS MECHANISM OF ACTION

Memarzadeh and associates (11-190) concluded that autonomous androgen receptor signaling contributed to the initiation of prostate cancer. Rubinow et al (11-193) provide evidence that testosterone improves insulin sensitivity by showing that acute testosterone deprivation decreases insulin sensitivity. Abiraterone is a 17 lyase inhibitor and blocks the formation of steroid hormones and androgen action in prostate cancer of bone, as reported by Efstathiou and associates (11-278). Taxanes are used to treat prostate cancer, and blocking nuclear androgen receptor accumulation is a possible mechanism for their effects in the cancer, according to Dashan et al (11-185).

A. Wayne Meikle, MD

Androgen Mechanism of Action

Role of autonomous androgen receptor signaling in prostate cancer initiation is dichotomous and depends on the oncogenic signal

Memarzadeh S, Cai H, Janzen DM, et al (Univ of California, Los Angeles; et al)
Proc Natl Acad Sci U S A 108:7962-7967, 2011

The steroid hormone signaling axis is thought to play a central role in initiation and progression of many hormonally regulated epithelial tumors. It is unclear whether all cancer-initiating signals depend on an intact hormone receptor signaling machinery. To ascertain whether cell autonomous androgen receptor (AR) is essential for initiation of prostate intraepithelial neoplasia (PIN), the response of AR-null prostate epithelia to paracrine and cell autonomous oncogenic signals was assessed in vivo by using the prostate regeneration model system. Epithelial-specific loss of AR blocked paracrine FGF10-induced PIN, whereas the add back of exogenous AR restored this response. In contrast, PIN initiated by cell-autonomous, chronicactivated AKT developed independent of epithelial AR signaling. Our findings demonstrate a selective role for AR in the initiation of PIN, dependent on the signaling pathways driving tumor formation. Insights into the role of hormone receptor signaling in the initiation of epithelial tumors may help define this axis as a target for chemoprevention of carcinomas.

▶ Hormone receptor signaling is a target for therapy for several epithelial tumors including those of breast and prostate. Prostate is regulated by hormone, particularly androgens, but it is uncertain whether receptor signaling has a causative role in initiation of prostate cancer.[1,2] Androgen deprivation has been used for years in initial treatment of prostate cancer, but this does not establish a causal relationship. Memarzadeh et al provide evidence for autonomous androgen receptor signaling in the initiation of prostate cancer.[3] The critical issue is whether chemoprevention can be achieved in men at high risk for prostate cancer. In some men, 5α-reductase inhibitors reduce the risk for prostate cancer. Androgen deprivation would not be acceptable to most men. Newer selective agents need to be developed for prostate cancer prevention. It is uncertain when chemoprevention should be initiated for the patients at risk. These questions will require a large study to find an acceptable therapy.

A. W. Meikle, MD

References

1. Chang HH, Chen BY, Wu CY, et al. Hedgehog overexpression leads to the formation of prostate cancer stem cells with metastatic property irrespective of androgen receptor expression in the mouse model. *J Biomed Sci.* 2011;18:6.
2. Takayama K, Tsutsumi S, Katayama S, et al. Integration of cap analysis of gene expression and chromatin immunoprecipitation analysis on array reveals genome-wide androgen receptor signaling in prostate cancer cells. *Oncogene.* 2011;30:619-630.
3. Lawson DA, Zong Y, Memarzadeh S, Xin L, Huang J, Witte ON. Basal epithelial stem cells are efficient targets for prostate cancer initiation. *Proc Natl Acad Sci U S A.* 2010;107:2610-2615.

Taxane-Induced Blockade to Nuclear Accumulation of the Androgen Receptor Predicts Clinical Responses in Metastatic Prostate Cancer

Darshan MS, Loftus MS, Thadani-Mulero M, et al (Weill Cornell Med College of Cornell Univ, NY; et al)

Cancer Res 71:6019-6029, 2011

Prostate cancer progression requires active androgen receptor (AR) signaling which occurs following translocation of AR from the cytoplasm to the nucleus. Chemotherapy with taxanes improves survival in patients with castrate resistant prostate cancer (CRPC). Taxanes induce microtubule stabilization, mitotic arrest, and apoptotic cell death, but recent data suggest that taxanes can also affect AR signaling. Here, we report that taxanes inhibit ligand-induced AR nuclear translocation and downstream transcriptional activation of AR target genes such as prostate-specific antigen. AR nuclear translocation was not inhibited in cells with acquired β-tubulin mutations that prevent taxane-induced microtubule stabilization, confirming a role for microtubules in AR trafficking. Upon ligand activation, AR associated with the minus-end-microtubule motor dynein, thereby trafficking on microtubules to translocate to the nucleus. Analysis of circulating tumor cells (CTC) isolated from the peripheral blood of CRPC patients receiving taxane chemotherapy revealed a significant correlation between AR cytoplasmic sequestration and clinical response to therapy. These results indicate that taxanes act in CRPC patients at least in part by inhibiting AR nuclear transport and signaling. Further, they suggest that monitoring AR subcellular localization in the CTCs of CRPC patients might predict clinical responses to taxane chemotherapy.

▶ Prostate cancer (PC) is the leading cause of cancer in men and the second leading cause of death in men. While androgens are not considered the cause of the PC, they contribute to its growth and progression. Therapies include blockade of androgen signals or androgen withdrawal by surgical or medical castration. In the past 20 years, few cytotoxic chemotherapies have been successful in treating androgen-unresponsive PCs.[1-6] Taxanes have been used with some success in treating those androgen-unresponsive PCs. Darshan et al sought to explore the mechanism for the effect of taxanes on metastatic PC.[1] Despite apparent androgen resistance of these cancers, they observed that taxanes inhibit androgen receptor nuclear transport and hence signaling. These findings are consistent with other modalities that further suppress castrate concentrations of testosterone. Further study is needed to clarify the mechanism of action of taxanes and to develop more effective preparations of this class of agents.

A. W. Meikle, MD

References

1. Darshan MS, Loftus MS, Thadani-Mulero M, et al. Taxane-induced blockade to nuclear accumulation of the androgen receptor predicts clinical responses in metastatic prostate cancer. *Cancer Res.* 2011;71:6019-6029.

2. Dayyani F, Gallick GE, Logothetis CJ, Corn PG. Novel therapies for metastatic castrate-resistant prostate cancer. *J Natl Cancer Inst.* 2011;103:1665-1675.
3. Gomella LG, Gelpi F, Kelly WK. New treatment options for castrate-resistant prostate cancer: a urology perspective. *Can J Urol.* 2011;18:5767-5777.
4. Seruga B, Tannock IF. Chemotherapy-based treatment for castration-resistant prostate cancer. *J Clin Oncol.* 2011;29:3686-3694.
5. Madan RA, Pal SK, Sartor O, Dahut WL. Overcoming chemotherapy resistance in prostate cancer. *Clin Cancer Res.* 2011;17:3892-3902.
6. Petrylak DP. Current clinical trials in castrate-resistant prostate cancer. *Curr Urol Rep.* 2011;12:173-179.

Acute testosterone deprivation reduces insulin sensitivity in men

Rubinow KB, Snyder CN, Amory JK, et al (Univ of Washington School of Medicine, Seattle)
Clin Endocrinol 76:281-288, 2012

Objective.—In men with prostate cancer, androgen deprivation reduces insulin sensitivity; however, the relative roles played by testosterone and estradiol are unknown. To investigate the respective effects of these hormones on insulin sensitivity in men, we employed a model of experimental hypogonadism with or without hormone replacement.

Design.—Placebo-controlled, randomized trial.

Participants.—Twenty-two healthy male volunteers, 18—55 years old.

Methods.—Following screening, subjects received the gonadotrophin-releasing hormone antagonist acyline plus one of the following for 28 days: Group 1, placebo transdermal gel and placebo pills; Group 2, transdermal testosterone gel 10 g/day plus placebo pills; Group 3, transdermal testosterone gel 10 g/day plus the aromatase inhibitor anastrozole 1 mg/day to normalize testosterone while selectively reducing serum estradiol. Fasting insulin, glucose, adipokines and hormones were measured bi-weekly.

Results.—With acyline administration, serum testosterone was reduced by >90% in all subjects in Group 1. In these men, mean fasting insulin concentrations were significantly increased compared with baseline ($P = 0\cdot02$) at 28 days, despite stable body weight and no changes in fasting glucose concentrations. Decreased insulin sensitivity was also apparent in the insulin sensitivity indices homeostasis model of insulin resistance ($P = 0\cdot03$) and quantitative insulin sensitivity check index ($P = 0\cdot04$). In contrast, in Groups 2 and 3, testosterone concentrations remained in the physiologic range, despite significant reduction in mean estradiol in Group 3. In these groups, no significant changes in insulin sensitivity were observed.

Conclusions.—Acute testosterone withdrawal reduces insulin sensitivity in men independent of changes in body weight, whereas estradiol withdrawal has no effect. Testosterone appears to maintain insulin sensitivity in normal men (Figs 2 and 3).

▶ Chronic testosterone administration is used to treat hypogonadism, in body-building, and in male contraception and results in increase in lean body mass

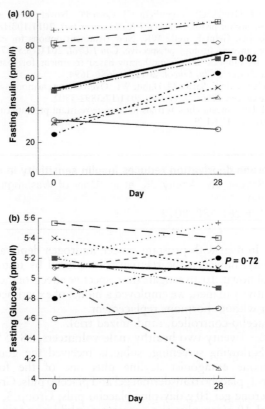

FIGURE 2.—Serum insulin (a) and glucose (b) in eight healthy young men administered the GnRH antagonist acyline and placebo testosterone gel and placebo anastrozole. Note the preservation of normal glucose concentrations by the significantly increased concentrations of serum insulin. The group mean is depicted in solid black. (Reprinted from Rubinow KB, Snyder CN, Amory JK, et al. Acute testosterone deprivation reduces insulin sensitivity in men. *Clin Endocrinol.* 2012;76:281-288, with permission from Blackwell Publishing Ltd.)

and decrease in body fat content. Androgen deprivation therapy in men treated for prostate cancer is associated with risks for type 2 diabetes, decreased sensitivity to insulin, cardiovascular disease, and the metabolic syndrome.[1,2] Testosterone is converted to estradiol and could also influence insulin sensitivity. There is little known about the effect of acute testosterone deprivation on insulin sensitivity in men. Rubinow et al investigated the relative effects of testosterone and estradiol on insulin sensitivity in healthy normal volunteers by suppressing serum testosterone concentrations and then administering testosterone with or without an estrogen synthesis inhibitor.[3,4] Their results suggest that short-term testosterone therapy also improves insulin sensitivity, and this effect is not mediated by estrogen. While leptin and insulin increased with androgen deprivation, adiponectin increased, which seems paradoxical to improved insulin sensitivity. This suggests a more direct effect of testosterone in regulating adiponectin.

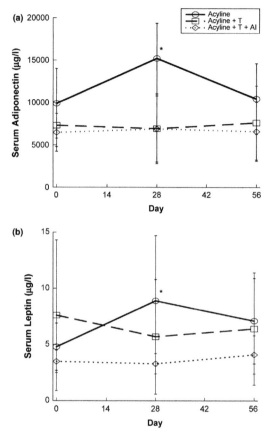

FIGURE 3.—Serum adiponectin (a) and leptin (b) over time in healthy young men administered the GnRH antagonist acyline and placebo (solid line, $n = 8$), acyline and testosterone (broken line, $n = 6$), or acyline, testosterone and the aromatase inhibitor anastrozole (dotted line, $n = 8$). Values are expressed as means ± SD. *$P < 0.05$ compared with baseline. (Reprinted from Rubinow KB, Snyder CN, Amory JK, et al. Acute testosterone deprivation reduces insulin sensitivity in men. *Clin Endocrinol.* 2012;76:281-288, with permission from Blackwell Publishing Ltd.)

Further study is needed to unravel the complex effects of testosterone on insulin responses in men.

A. W. Meikle, MD

References

1. Rubinow KB, Page ST. Testosterone, oestradiol, and insulin sensitivity in men. *Clin Endocrinol (Oxf).* 2012 Feb 22 [Epub ahead of print].
2. Rabiee A, Dwyer AA, Caronia LM, et al. Impact of acute biochemical castration on insulin sensitivity in healthy adult men. *Endocr Res.* 2010;35:71-84.
3. Rosano GM, Sheiban I, Massaro R, et al. Low testosterone levels are associated with coronary artery disease in male patients with angina. *Int J Impot Res.* 2007;19:176-182.

4. Lee CH, Kuo SW, Hung YJ, et al. The effect of testosterone supplement on insulin sensitivity, glucose effectiveness, and acute insulin response after glucose load in male type 2 diabetics. *Endocr Res.* 2005;31:139-148.

Effects of Abiraterone Acetate on Androgen Signaling in Castrate-Resistant Prostate Cancer in Bone

Efstathiou E, Titus M, Tsavachidou D, et al (The Univ of Texas MD Anderson Cancer Ctr, Houston; Roswell Park Cancer Inst, Buffalo, NY; et al)
J Clin Oncol 30:637-643, 2012

Purpose.—Persistent androgen signaling is implicated in castrate-resistant prostate cancer (CRPC) progression. This study aimed to evaluate androgen signaling in bone marrow—infiltrating cancer and testosterone in blood and bone marrow and to correlate with clinical observations.

Patients and Methods.—This was an open-label, observational study of 57 patients with bone-metastatic CRPC who underwent transiliac bone marrow biopsy between October 2007 and March 2010. Patients received oral abiraterone acetate (1 g) once daily and prednisone (5 mg) twice daily. Androgen receptor (AR) and CYP17 expression were assessed by immuno-histochemistry, testosterone concentration by mass spectrometry, AR copy number by polymerase chain reaction, and *TMPRSS2-ERG* status by fluo-rescent in situ hybridization in available tissues.

Results.—Median overall survival was 555 days (95% CI, 440 to 965+ days). Maximal prostate-specific antigen decline ≥ 50% occurred in 28 (50%) of 56 patients. Homogeneous, intense nuclear expression of AR, combined with ≥ 10% CYP17 tumor expression, was correlated with longer time to treatment discontinuation (> 4 months) in 25 patients with tumor-infiltrated bone marrow samples. Pretreatment CYP17 tumor ex-pression ≥ 10% was correlated with increased bone marrow aspirate testosterone. Blood and bone marrow aspirate testosterone concentrations declined to less than picograms-per-milliliter levels and remained sup-pressed at progression.

Conclusion.—The observed pretreatment androgen-signaling signature is consistent with persistent androgen signaling in CRPC bone metastases. This is the first evidence that abiraterone acetate achieves sustained suppression of testosterone in both blood and bone marrow aspirate to less than picograms-per-milliliter levels. Potential admixture of blood with bone marrow aspirate limits our ability to determine the origin of measured testosterone.

▶ Recent studies have suggested that so-called castrate-resistant prostate cancer might be associated with persistent androgen signaling.[1-4] This evidence has sug-gested that these prostate cancers might still be responsive to inhibition of androgen synthesis by inhibiting CYP17 lyase or more potent androgen receptor blockade. Abiraterone acetate is a CYP17 lyase inhibitor, and Efstathiou et al investigated its effects on blood and bone marrow testosterone concentrations in men with castrate-resistant prostate cancer. They observed that abiraterone acetate attained suppression of testosterone and decrease prostate-specific antigen and prolonged survival. Their results suggested that uniform and intense tumor nuclear androgen receptor expression and cytoplasmic CYP17 expression are linked to lack of primary resistance to abiraterone acetate. The drawback of use of abiraterone acetate is that increased backdoor biosynthesis of dihydrotestosterone might account for resistance to the treatment. These results are provocative, but additional studies are needed to determine if complete androgen blockade is the answer to control these cancers.

A. W. Meikle, MD

References

1. Zhang Y, Castaneda S, Dumble M, et al. Reduced expression of the androgen receptor by third generation of antisense shows antitumor activity in models of prostate cancer. *Mol Cancer Ther.* 2011;10:2309-2319.
2. Larsson R, Mongan NP, Johansson M, et al. Clinical trial update and novel therapeutic approaches for metastatic prostate cancer. *Curr Med Chem.* 2011;18: 4440-4453.
3. Ryan CJ, Tindall DJ. Androgen receptor rediscovered: the new biology and targeting the androgen receptor therapeutically. *J Clin Oncol.* 2011;29:3651-3658.
4. Massard C, Fizazi K. Targeting continued androgen receptor signaling in prostate cancer. *Clin Cancer Res.* 2011;17:3876-3883.

Estrogen and Coronary Artery Disease

Cardiovascular Disease and Risk Factors in PCOS Women of Postmenopausal Age: A 21-Year Controlled Follow-Up Study
Schmidt J, Landin-Wilhelmsen K, Brännström M, et al (Univ of Gothenburg, Göteborg, Sweden)
J Clin Endocrinol Metab 96:3794-3803, 2011

Context.—Polycystic ovary syndrome (PCOS) is associated with the metabolic syndrome and, consequently, with a potentially increased risk of cardiovascular disease (CVD) and related mortality later in life. Studies regarding CVD and mortality in PCOS women well into the postmenopausal age are lacking.

Objective.—Our objective was to examine whether postmenopausal PCOS women differ from controls regarding cardiovascular risk factors, myocardial infarction (MI), stroke and mortality.

Design and Setting.—We conducted, at a university hospital, a prospective study of 35 PCOS women (61–79 yr) and 120 age-matched controls. The study was performed 21 yr after the initial study.

Participants.—Twenty-five PCOS women (Rotterdam criteria) and 68 controls participated in all examinations. Data on morbidity were based on 32 of 34 PCOS women and on 95 of 119 controls.

Interventions.—Interventions included reexamination, interviews, and data from the National Board of Health and Welfare and from the Hospital Discharge Registry.

Main Outcome Measures.—Blood pressure, glucose, insulin, triglycerides, total cholesterol, high- and low-density lipoprotein, apolipoprotein A1 and B, fibrinogen, and plasminogen activator inhibitor antigen were studied. Incidences of MI, stroke, hypertension, diabetes, cancer, cause of death, and age at death were recorded.

Results.—PCOS women had a higher prevalence of hypertension ($P = 0.008$) and higher triglyceride levels ($P = 0.012$) than controls. MI, stroke, diabetes, cancer, and mortality prevalence was similar in the two cohorts with similar body mass index.

Conclusions.—The well-described cardiovascular/metabolic risk profile in pre- and perimenopausal PCOS women does not entail an evident increase in cardiovascular events during the postmenopausal period.

▶ Polycystic ovary syndrome (PCOS) is the most common endocrine disorder in women and is characterized by oligomenorrhea, hyperandrogenism, infertility, and polycystic ovaries. The metabolic syndrome is commonly observed in them as is insulin resistance, hyperglycemia, waist/hip ratio, and elevated triglycerides.[1-5] Schmidt et al followed up with women with PCOS for 21 years to assess their risk of cardiovascular disease (CVD) and metabolic risk factors. Despite having risk factors more commonly for CVD than controls, they were not at increased risk for myocardial infarction, stroke, or dying from CVD. The explanation for the failure to observe expected increased risk of CVD was that the PCOS women had higher concentrations of high-density lipoprotein than in later life. Serum testosterone concentrations are lower in men at risk for CVD, and the authors speculate that hyperandrogenism might be protective for CVD in women with PCOS. A limitation of the study was the small sample size, which might preclude detection of more subtle difference between controls and PCOS women.

A. W. Meikle, MD

References

1. Bentley-Lewis R, Seely E, Dunaif A. Ovarian hypertension: polycystic ovary syndrome. *Endocrinol Metab Clin North Am.* 2011;40:433-449. ix-x.
2. de Groot PC, Dekkers OM, Romijn JA, Dieben SW, Helmerhorst FM. PCOS, coronary heart disease, stroke and the influence of obesity: a systematic review and meta-analysis. *Hum Reprod Update.* 2011;17:495-500.
3. Sasaki A, Emi Y, Matsuda M, et al. Increased arterial stiffness in mildly-hypertensive women with polycystic ovary syndrome. *J Obstet Gynaecol Res.* 2011;37:402-411.
4. Lambrinoudaki I. Cardiovascular risk in postmenopausal women with the polycystic ovary syndrome. *Maturitas.* 2011;68:13-16.
5. Tomlinson J, Millward A, Stenhouse E, Pinkney J. Type 2 diabetes and cardiovascular disease in polycystic ovary syndrome: what are the risks and can they be reduced? *Diabet Med.* 2010;27:498-515.

Female Reproductive Function

Antral follicle counts are strongly associated with live-birth rates after assisted reproduction, with superior treatment outcome in women with polycystic ovaries

Holte J, Brodin T, Berglund L, et al (Uppsala Univ, Sweden)
Fertil Steril 96:594-599, 2011

Objective.—To evaluate the association of antral follicle count (AFC) with in vitro fertilization/intracytoplasmic sperm injection (IVF-ICSI) outcome in a large unselected cohort of patients covering the entire range of AFC.

Design.—Prospective observational study.

Setting.—University-affiliated private infertility center.

Patient(s).—2,092 women undergoing 4,308 IVF-ICSI cycles.

Intervention(s).—AFC analyzed for associations with treatment outcome and statistically adjusted for repeated treatments and age.

Main Outcome Measure(s).—Pregnancy rate, live-birth rate, and stimulation outcome parameters.

Result(s).—The AFC was log-normally distributed. Pregnancy rates and live-birth rates were positively associated with AFC in a log-linear way, leveling out above AFC ~ 30. Treatment outcome was superior among women with polycystic ovaries, independent from ovulatory status. The findings were significant also after adjustment for age and number of oocytes retrieved.

Conclusion(s).—Pregnancy and live-birth rates are log-linearly related to AFC. Polycystic ovaries, most often excluded from studies on ovarian reserve, fit as one extreme in the spectrum of AFC; a low count constitutes the other extreme, with the lowest ovarian reserve and poor treatment outcome. The findings remained statistically significant also after adjustment for the number of oocytes retrieved, suggesting this measure of ovarian reserve comprises information on oocyte quality and not only quantity (Fig 1).

▶ Prediction of ovarian reserve has become an important determinant of fertility success. Several factors, including age, adnexal surgery, chemotherapy, smoking, and pelvic radiation are known to affect ovarian reserve. Assessment of ovarian reserve has utilized basal, stimulated gonadotropins, or anti-Müllerian hormone concentrations, ultrasound estimates of ovarian volume, and number of antral follicles.[1,2] Most studies have failed to establish high predictive values of oocyte quantity and quality for pregnancy success.[3,4] Holte et al investigated whether there was an association with live births between ultrasound-determined antral follicle count (AFC) with in vitro fertilization/intracytoplasmic sperm injections. They observed a strong association between ovarian reserve estimated by AFC and assisted reproduction success. This association with the treatment outcome improved until the AFC reached 30 and then reached a plateau. They used individual gonadotropin doses for ovarian stimulation, which might have affected

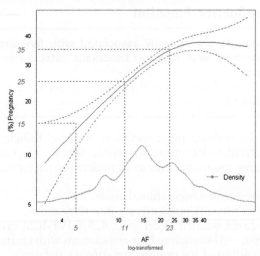

FIGURE 1.—Pregnancy rate (%) per started stimulation (*solid line*) relative to log transformed antral follicle count (AFC), with confidence interval (*dotted lines*). Pregnancy rates increased (log−) linearly and leveled out above the AFC ~30. The corresponding graph for the live-birth rate described the same pattern. AF = antral follicles. Density (*red*) denotes the distribution after log transformation. The AFC numbers given along the x-axis are back-transformed for ease of interpretation. N = 4,308 IVF-ICSI treatment cycles. For interpretation of the references to color in this figure legend, the reader is referred to web version of this article. (Reprinted from Holte J, Brodin T, Berglund L, et al. Antral follicle counts are strongly associated with live-birth rates after assisted reproduction, with superior treatment outcome in women with polycystic ovaries. *Fertil Steril*. 2011;96:594-599, Copyright 2011, with permission from American Society for Reproductive Medicine.)

the results. Their results suggested that ovarian reserve, when expressed as AFC, was a quantitative measure and an age-independent component.

A. W. Meikle, MD

References

1. Coccia ME, Rizzello F. Ovarian reserve. *Ann N Y Acad Sci*. 2008;1127:27-30.
2. Gnoth C, Schuring AN, Friol K, Tigges J, Mallmann P, Godehardt E. Relevance of anti-Mullerian hormone measurement in a routine IVF program. *Hum Reprod*. 2008;23:1359-1365.
3. Broekmans FJ, Kwee J, Hendriks DJ, Mol BW, Lambalk CB. A systematic review of tests predicting ovarian reserve and IVF outcome. *Hum Reprod Update*. 2006; 12:685-718.
4. Bongioanni F, Revelli A, Gennarelli G, Guidetti D, Delle Piane LD, Holte J. Ovarian endometriomas and IVF: a retrospective case-control study. *Reprod Biol Endocrinol*. 2011;9:81.

Cigarette Smoking and Endogenous Sex Hormones in Postmenopausal Women

Brand JS, Chan M-F, Dowsett M, et al (Univ Med Ctr Utrecht, The Netherlands; Univ of Cambridge, UK; et al)

J Clin Endocrinol Metab 96:3184-3192, 2011

Context.—Sex hormones play a key role in women's health, but little is known about lifestyle factors that influence their levels.

Objective.—The objective of the study was to investigate the relationship between cigarette smoking habits and endogenous sex hormone levels in postmenopausal women.

Design and Participants.—This was a cross-sectional study among 2030 postmenopausal women aged 55–81 yr from the Norfolk population of the European Prospective Investigation into Cancer. All women were at least 1 yr postmenopausal and not currently using hormone replacement therapy. General linear models were used to examine the relationship between smoking habits and sex hormone levels.

Results.—Among current smokers, the daily number of cigarettes smoked was associated with increased levels of testosterone (19–37%), free testosterone (19–34%), 17-hydroxprogesterone (17–22%), androstenedione (2–23%), SHBG (6–10%), and estradiol (−2 to 15%). Stratified analysis for body mass index revealed an interaction such that the association with SHBG was restricted to lean women, whereas a smoking-related increase in free estradiol was found only in overweight women. No clear dose-response relationship was observed for estrone, although its levels were highest in heavy smokers. Current smoking habit was associated with a larger difference in sex hormone levels than lifetime cigarette exposure as measured by pack-years. Among former smokers, sex hormones were at levels of never smokers within 1–2 yr of smoking cessation.

Conclusions.—Cigarette smoking is associated with higher circulating levels of androgens, estrogens, 17-hydroxprogesterone, and SHBG in postmenopausal women. The almost immediate lower levels with smoking cessation may indicate that hormone related disease risks could potentially be modified by changing smoking habits.

▶ Elevated serum concentrations of estrogens and androgens are associated with higher risk of breast and endometrial cancer, but these hormones are protective for osteoporosis and fractures. In addition, high circulating estradiol and testosterone levels might contribute to higher risk of type 2 diabetes. Cigarette smoking is a risk for many common chronic diseases and affects the function of the pituitary, adrenals, and ovaries.[1-5] In their cross-sectional study of 2030 postmenopausal women, Brand and associates did not seek to establish a causal relationship between the hormone changes and disease, but they determined the relationship between smoking and sex hormones.[1] The effect of smoking cessation on sex hormone concentrations was also studied. In comparison to nonsmokers, smokers had high serum concentrations of free and total testosterone, 17-OH progesterone, androstenedione, sex hormone—binding globulin, and estradiol. The study does not establish any cause-and-effect relationship between smoking, the sex hormone changes, and disease. It also does not document the mechanism for the altered sex steroid concentrations, but adrenal dysfunction was implicated in the changes.

A. W. Meikle, MD

References

1. Brand JS, Chan MF, Dowsett M, et al. Cigarette smoking and endogenous sex hormones in postmenopausal women. *J Clin Endocrinol Metab.* 2011;96:3184-3192.
2. Goldstein LB, Bushnell CD, Adams RJ, et al. Guidelines for the primary prevention of stroke: a guideline for healthcare professionals from the American Heart Association/American Stroke Association. *Stroke.* 2011;42:517-584.
3. Cochran CJ, Gallicchio L, Miller SR, Zacur H, Flaws JA. Cigarette smoking, androgen levels, and hot flushes in midlife women. *Obstet Gynecol.* 2008;112:1037-1044.
4. Wang PH, Horng HC, Cheng MH, Chao HT, Chao KC. Standard and low-dose hormone therapy for postmenopausal women—focus on the breast. *Taiwan J Obstet Gynecol.* 2007;46:127-134.
5. Goldstein LB, Adams R, Alberts MJ, et al. Primary prevention of ischemic stroke: a guideline from the American Heart Association/American Stroke Association Stroke Council: cosponsored by the Atherosclerotic Peripheral Vascular Disease Interdisciplinary Working Group; Cardiovascular Nursing Council; Clinical Cardiology Council; Nutrition, Physical Activity, and Metabolism Council; and the Quality of Care and Outcomes Research Interdisciplinary Working Group. *Circulation.* 2006;113:e873-e923.

Diagnosis of polycystic ovary syndrome (PCOS): revisiting the threshold values of follicle count on ultrasound and of the serum AMH level for the definition of polycystic ovaries

Dewailly D, Gronier H, Poncelet E, et al (Hôpital Jeanne de Flandre, Lille, France; et al)
Hum Reprod 26:3123-3129, 2011

Background.—Polycystic ovarian morphology (PCOM) at ultrasound is currently used in the diagnosis of polycystic ovary syndrome (PCOS). We hypothesized that the previously proposed threshold value of 12 as an excessive number of follicles per ovary (FN) is no longer appropriate because of current technological developments. In this study, we have revisited the thresholds for FN and for the serum Anti-Müllerian hormone (AMH) level (a possible surrogate for FN) for the definition of PCOM.

Methods.—Clinical, hormonal and ultrasound data were consecutively recorded in 240 patients referred to our department between 2008 and 2010 for exploration of hyperandrogenism (HA), menstrual disorders and/or infertility.

Results.—According to only their symptoms, patients were grouped as: non-PCOS without HA and with ovulatory cycles (group 1, $n = 105$), presumption of PCOS with only HA or only oligo-anovulation (group 2, $n = 73$) and PCOS with HA and oligo-anovulation (group 3, $n = 62$).

By cluster analysis using androgens, LH, FSH, AMH, FN and ovarian volume, group 1 appeared to be constituted of two homogeneous clusters, most likely a non-PCOM non-PCOS subgroup ($n = 66$) and a PCOM, non-PCOS (i.e. asymptomatic) subgroup ($n = 39$). Receiver operating characteristic curve analysis was applied to distinguish the non-PCOM non-PCO members of group 1 and to group 3. For FN and serum AMH respectively, the areas under the curve were 0.949 and 0.973 and the best compromise between sensitivity (81 and 92%) and specificity (92 and 97%) was obtained with a threshold values of 19 follicles and 35 pmol/l (5 ng/ml).

Conclusions.—For the definition of PCOM, the former threshold of >12 for FN is no longer valid. A serum AMH >35 pmol/l (or >5 ng/ml) appears to be more sensitive and specific than a FN >19 and should be therefore included in the current diagnostic classifications for PCOS (Fig 2).

▶ Polycystic ovary syndrome (PCOS) affects about 10% of women of reproductive age and is associated with hyperandrogenism, oligo-anovulation, obesity, insulin resistance, dyslipidemia, and polycystic ovaries. The Rotterdam criteria use pelvic ultrasound scan to define cystic ovaries, whereas the National Institutes of Health criteria do not require pelvic ultrasound scan. Previous studies[1-5] have suggested that excess of less than 10 mm ovarian follicles determined by pelvic ultrasound scan predicted hyperandrogenism as did high concentrations of anti-Müllerian hormone (AMH), which is produced by granulose cells of the ovarian follicles. The issue investigated by Dewailly et al was whether AMH

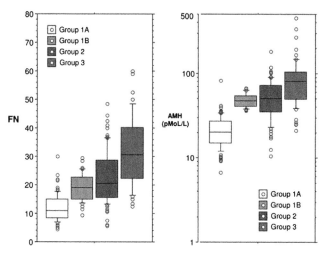

FIGURE 2.—Box-and-whisker plots showing the values of the follicle count (left) and serum AMH level (right, logarithmic scale) in the four subgroups of patients (see text). Horizontal small bars represent the 5–95th percentile range, and the boxes indicate the 25–75th percentile range. The horizontal line in each box corresponds to the median. (Reprinted from Dewailly D, Gronier H, Poncelet E, et al. Diagnosis of polycystic ovary syndrome (PCOS): revisiting the threshold values of follicle count on ultrasound and of the serum AMH level for the definition of polycystic ovaries. *Hum Reprod.* 2011;26:3123-3129, with permission from The Author on behalf of the European Society of Human Reproduction and Embryology.)

could accurately predict polycystic ovary morphology and thus replace pelvic ultrasound scan measurements of ovarian cysts. A serum AMH greater than 5 ng/mL was considered more sensitive than follicle number. Confirmation of these observations will require additional study, but the omission of a pelvic ultrasound scan in the diagnosis of PCOS would be welcomed by many women and clinicians. Obviously, an accurate reproducible assay for AMH is critical for this study.

A. W. Meikle, MD

References

1. Li HW, Anderson RA, Yeung WS, Ho PC, Ng EH. Evaluation of serum antimullerian hormone and inhibin B concentrations in the differential diagnosis of secondary oligoamenorrhea. *Fertil Steril.* 2011;96:774-779.
2. Lin YH, Chiu WC, Wu CH, Tzeng CR, Hsu CS, Hsu MI. Antimüllerian hormone and polycystic ovary syndrome. *Fertil Steril.* 2011;96:230-235.
3. Codner E, Iñiguez G, Hernández IM, et al. Elevated anti-Müllerian hormone (AMH) and inhibin B levels in prepubertal girls with type 1 diabetes mellitus. *Clin Endocrinol (Oxf).* 2011;74:73-78.
4. Dewailly D, Pigny P, Soudan B, et al. Reconciling the definitions of polycystic ovary syndrome: the ovarian follicle number and serum anti-Müllerian hormone concentrations aggregate with the markers of hyperandrogenism. *J Clin Endocrinol Metab.* 2010;95:4399-4405.
5. Tehrani FR, Solaymani-Dodaran M, Hedayati M, Azizi F. Is polycystic ovary syndrome an exception for reproductive aging? *Hum Reprod.* 2010;25:1775-1781.

Hypogonadism and Aging

Are Klinefelter boys hypogonadal?

Rey RA, Gottlieb S, Pasqualini T, et al (Hospital de Niños R. Gutiérrez, Buenos Aires, Argentina)
Acta Paediatr 100:830-838, 2011

Male hypogonadism implies decreased function of one or more testicular cell population, i.e. germ, Leydig and/or Sertoli cells. In the normal prepubertal boy, Sertoli cells are very active, as indicated by high anti-Müllerian hormone (AMH) and inhibin B secretion, whereas the functional activity of Leydig cells is minimal, as evidenced by low testosterone production, and germ cells do not undergo the full spermatogenic process. Klinefelter syndrome is the most frequent cause of hypogonadism in the adult male. In this review, we discuss whether the gonadal failure is already established during infancy and childhood. In Klinefelter syndrome, there is increased germ cells degeneration from mid-foetal life - resulting in a decreased number at birth - which persists during infancy and childhood and becomes dramatic during puberty. Controversial results exist in the literature regarding Leydig cell function in Klinefelter boys: while some authors have found normal to low testosterone levels in infancy and childhood, others have reported normal to high values. Sertoli cell products AMH and inhibin B are normal in prepubertal boys and only decline during mid- to late puberty.

Conclusion.—Klinefelter syndrome is a primary hypogonadism affecting all testicular cell populations. Germ cells are affected from foetal life, and a severe depletion occurs at puberty. Leydig cell function may be normal or mildly affected in foetal and early postnatal life. Sertoli cell function is not impaired until mid- to late puberty, as reflected by normal AMH and inhibin B in Klinefelter boys.

▶ Klinefelter syndrome is characterized as adult with small testes, azoospermia, gynecomastia, and karyotype 47XXY. Rey et al summarize gonadal function in boys with Klinefelter syndrome at various stages of development. During fetal life, Sertoli cells secrete anti-Müllerian hormone, which suppresses Müllerian ducts. Leydig cells secrete testosterone resulting in differentiation of the Wolffian ducts. These boys exhibit a neonatal increase in testosterone that then remains quiescent until puberty. During childhood, testes are of normal size, but germ cell numbers decrease, particularly during mid to late puberty when testicular failure develops. Many boys with Klinefelter syndrome go undiagnosed and present with decreased verbal abilities, motor development, and education problems. Many are shy, quiet, immature, and dependent. Despite apparent developmental sexual deficits, they have male gender identity and sexual orientation. After late puberty, germ cell numbers are markedly decreased and many have low or low normal serum testosterone concentrations. Eunuchoidal features are observed in many associated with hypogonadism.

A. W. Meikle, MD

Endogenous Testosterone and Mortality in Men: A Systematic Review and Meta-Analysis

Araujo AB, Dixon JM, Suarez EA, et al (New England Res Insts, Inc, Watertown, MA; et al)
J Clin Endocrinol Metab 96:3007-3019, 2011

Context.—Low testosterone levels have been associated with outcomes that reduce survival in men.

Objective.—Our objective was to perform a systematic review and meta-analysis of published studies to evaluate the association between endogenous testosterone and mortality.

Data Sources.—Data sources included MEDLINE (1966 to December 2010), EMBASE (1988 to December 2010), and reference lists.

Study Selection.—Eligible studies were published English-language observational studies of men that reported the association between endogenous testosterone and all-cause or cardiovascular disease (CVD) mortality. A two-stage process was used for study selection. 1) Working independently and in duplicate, reviewers screened a subset (10%) of abstracts. Results indicated 96% agreement, and thereafter, abstract screening was conducted in singlicate. 2) All full-text publications were reviewed independently and in duplicate for eligibility.

Data Extraction.—Reviewers working independently and in duplicate determined methodological quality of studies and extracted descriptive, quality, and outcome data.

Data Synthesis.—Of 820 studies identified, 21 were included in the systematic review, and 12 were eligible for meta-analysis [n = 11 studies of all-cause mortality (16,184 subjects); n = 7 studies of CVD mortality (11,831 subjects)]. Subject mean age and testosterone level were 61 yr and 487 ng/dl, respectively, and mean follow-up time was 9.7 yr. Between-study heterogeneity was observed among studies of all-cause ($P < .001$) and CVD mortality ($P = 0.06$), limiting the ability to provide valid summary estimates. Heterogeneity in all-cause mortality (higher relative risks) was observed in studies that included older subjects ($P = 0.020$), reported lower testosterone levels ($P = 0.018$), followed subjects for a shorter time period ($P = 0.010$), and sampled blood throughout the day ($P = 0.030$).

Conclusion.—Low endogenous testosterone levels are associated with increased risk of all-cause and CVD death in community-based studies of men, but considerable between-study heterogeneity, which was related to study and subject characteristics, suggests that effects are driven by differences between cohorts (e.g. in underlying health status).

▶ Serum concentrations of testosterone are subnormal in a high percentage of men with type 2 diabetes, andropause, obesity,[1-6] the metabolic syndrome, and other disorders. Many have clinical symptoms of hypogonadism, and obese men tend to have elevated inflammatory markers and insulin resistance that might be associated with risk of cardiovascular disease. Studies have established a close association between subnormal serum testosterone concentrations.[2] There is also evidence that testosterone therapy in men with testosterone deficiency show improvement in insulin sensitivity and obesity, which might be expected to lower their risk of mortality and cardiovascular disease and mortality. Araujo et al did a systematic review and meta-analysis on endogenous testosterone and mortality in men, and confirmed that all-cause and cardiovascular disease death was higher in men with low testosterone concentrations compared with those with higher values. Long-term studies will be needed to confirm that correcting testosterone deficiency will prolong life in men with low testosterone values.

A. W. Meikle, MD

References

1. Hyde Z, Norman PE, Flicker L, et al. Low free testosterone predicts mortality from cardiovascular disease but not other causes: the Health in Men Study. *J Clin Endocrinol Metab.* 2012;97:179-189.
2. Corona G, Rastrelli G, Monami M, et al. Hypogonadism as a risk factor for cardiovascular mortality in men: a meta-analytic study. *Eur J Endocrinol.* 2011; 165:687-701.
3. Corona G, Rastrelli G, Vignozzi L, Mannucci E, Maggi M. Testosterone, cardiovascular disease and the metabolic syndrome. *Best Pract Res Clin Endocrinol Metab.* 2011;25:337-353.
4. Ruige JB, Mahmoud AM, De Bacquer D, Kaufman JM. Endogenous testosterone and cardiovascular disease in healthy men: a meta-analysis. *Heart.* 2011;97:870-875.

5. Haring R, Völzke H, Steveling A, et al. Low serum testosterone levels are associated with increased risk of mortality in a population-based cohort of men aged 20-79. *Eur Heart J.* 2010;31:1494-1501.
6. Vikan T, Schirmer H, Njolstad I, Svartberg J. Endogenous sex hormones and the prospective association with cardiovascular disease and mortality in men: the Tromsø Study. *Eur J Endocrinol.* 2009;161:435-442.

The Relationships between Sex Hormones and Sexual Function in Middle-Aged and Older European Men

O'Connor DB, the European Male Ageing Study Group (Univ of Leeds, UK; et al)

J Clin Endocrinol Metab 96:E1577-E1587, 2011

Context.—Limited data are available exploring the associations between sex hormones, multiple domains of sexual functioning, and sexual function-related distress in nonpatient samples in Europe.

Objectives.—The aim of the study was to investigate the relationships between serum testosterone (T), estradiol (E2), and dihydrotestosterone (DHT) and sexual function in a multicenter population-based study of aging in men.

Design.—Using stratified random sampling, 2838 men aged 40–79 yr completed the European Male Ageing Study-Sexual Function Questionnaire and provided a blood sample for hormone measurements. T, E2, and DHT were measured using gas chromatography-mass spectrometry.

Setting.—We conducted a community-based population survey in eight European centers.

Main Outcome Measures.—Self-reported sexual function (overall sexual function, sexual function-related distress, erectile dysfunction, masturbation) was measured.

Results.—Total and free T, but not E2 or DHT, was associated with overall sexual function in middle-aged and older men. E2 was the only hormone associated with sexual function-related distress such that higher levels were related to greater distress. Free T levels were associated with masturbation frequency and erectile dysfunction in the fully adjusted models, such that higher T was associated with less dysfunction and greater frequency. Moreover, there was a T threshold for the relationship between total T, sexual function, and erectile dysfunction. At T concentrations of 8 nmol/liter or less, T was associated with worse sexual functioning, whereas at T levels over 8 nmol/liter, the relationship came to a plateau.

Conclusions.—These findings suggest that different hormonal mechanisms may regulate sexual functioning (T) *vs.* the psychological aspects (E2) of male sexual behavior. Moreover, there was a T threshold for overall sexual function such that at levels greater than 8 nmol/liter the relationship between T and sexual function did not become stronger.

▶ Testosterone impacts the maintenance of sexual function in men, and libido and erectile function wane with testosterone deficiency.[1] However, the relationship between sexual dysfunction and serum testosterone concentrations is not very tight. Testosterone replacement therapy does not always correct libido and erectile function in hypogonadal men and might therefore lead to disappointment and frustration for the patient.[2,3] As men age, the influence of aging and hypogonadism blurs, and testosterone therapy might improve libido but fail to correct erectile dysfunction.[4] There is less information about sexual function and symptoms in men and other sex hormones, such as estradiol and dihydrotestosterone (DHT). O'Connor et al included 2838 men aged 40 to 79 in a study of relationship between sex hormones and sexual function. Total and free testosterone but not estradiol or DHT were associated with overall sexual function, and free testosterone was associated with masturbation frequency and erectile dysfunction. While there was scatter in the relationships, there was an established threshold between total testosterone (8 nmol/L = 230 ng/dL) and overall sexual function. The strength of the study was its size, and the main weakness of the study was that it was a cross-sectional study and not interventional.

A. W. Meikle, MD

References

1. Goh VH, Tong TY. The moderating impact of lifestyle factors on sex steroids, sexual activities and aging in Asian men. *Asian J Androl.* 2011;13:596-604.
2. Lackner JE, Rucklinger E, Schatzl G, Lunglmayr G, Kratzik CW. Are there symptom-specific testosterone thresholds in aging men? *BJU Int.* 2011;108:1310-1315.
3. Wu FC, Tajar A, Beynon JM, et al. Identification of late-onset hypogonadism in middle-aged and elderly men. *N Engl J Med.* 2010;363:123-135.
4. Raynaud JP, Tichet J, Born C, et al. Aging Male Questionnaire in normal and complaining men. *J Sex Med.* 2008;5:2703-2712.

High Serum Testosterone Is Associated With Reduced Risk of Cardiovascular Events in Elderly Men: The MrOS (Osteoporotic Fractures in Men) Study in Sweden

Ohlsson C, Barrett-Connor E, Bhasin S, et al (Univ of Gothenburg, Sweden; Univ of California San Diego, La Jolla; Boston School of Medicine and Boston Med Ctr, MA; et al)
J Am Coll Cardiol 58:1674-1681, 2011

Objectives.—We tested the hypothesis that serum total testosterone and sex hormone–binding globulin (SHBG) levels predict cardiovascular (CV) events in community-dwelling elderly men.

Background.—Low serum testosterone is associated with increased adiposity, an adverse metabolic risk profile, and atherosclerosis. However, few prospective studies have demonstrated a protective link between endogenous testosterone and CV events. Polymorphisms in the SHBG gene are associated with risk of type 2 diabetes, but few studies have addressed SHBG as a predictor of CV events.

Methods.—We used gas chromatography/mass spectrometry to analyze baseline levels of testosterone in the prospective population-based MrOS

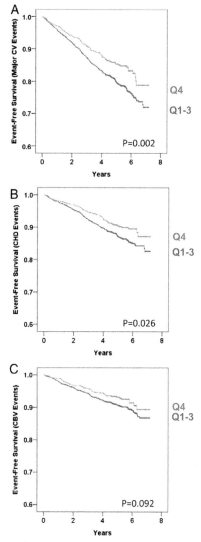

FIGURE 2.—Kaplan-Meier Plots by Testosterone Levels. Kaplan-Meier curves of event-free survival by serum testosterone for major CV events (**A**) CHD events (**B**), and CBV events (**C**). In quartile 4 of serum testosterone (**green lines**) or quartiles 1 to 3 (**blue lines**). p value assessed by logrank test. Abbreviations as in Figure 1 in the original article. For interpretation of the references to color in this figure legend, the reader is referred to web version of this article. (Reprinted from Ohlsson C, Barrett-Connor E, Bhasin S, et al. High serum testosterone is associated with reduced risk of cardiovascular events in elderly men: the MrOS (osteoporotic fractures in men) study in Sweden. *J Am Coll Cardiol.* 2011;58:1674-1681, Copyright 2011, with permission from the American College of Cardiology.)

(Osteoporotic Fractures in Men) Sweden study (2,416 men, age 69 to 81 years). SHBG was measured by immunoradiometric assay. CV clinical outcomes were obtained from central Swedish registers.

Results.—During a median 5-year follow-up, 485 CV events occurred. Both total testosterone and SHBG levels were inversely associated with the risk of CV events (trend over quartiles: $p = 0.009$ and $p = 0.012$, respectively). Men in the highest quartile of testosterone (≥ 550 ng/dl) had a lower risk of CV events compared with men in the 3 lower quartiles (hazard ratio: 0.70, 95% confidence interval: 0.56 to 0.88). This association remained after adjustment for traditional CV risk factors and was not materially changed in analyses excluding men with known CV disease at baseline (hazard ratio: 0.71, 95% confidence interval: 0.53 to 0.95). In models that included both testosterone and SHBG, testosterone but not SHBG predicted CV risk.

Conclusions.—High serum testosterone predicted a reduced 5-year risk of CV events in elderly men (Fig 2).

▶ Low testosterone has recently been associated with increased risk of death and higher risk of type 2 diabetes, but high-dose testosterone produced adverse cardiovascular (CV) events in aging men.[1,2] Thus, conflicting reports on the effects of testosterone on CV risk have been reported.[2-5] Testosterone has metabolic actions in men, such as favorable body composition, improved insulin sensitivity, and improved lipid metabolism. These actions might be expected to reduce CV mortality. Insulin resistance and obesity are associated with low sex hormone binding globulin. Ohlsson et al observed that high serum testosterone was associated with reduced risk of CV events in elderly men during a 5-year follow-up. While total testosterone was associated with CV risk benefit, free testosterone was weakly and not significantly associated with CV risk. There are limitations in the study, such as single measurement of sex steroids and sex hormone—binding globulin and it was not an interventional study. Large interventional trials are needed to confirm their observations.

A. W. Meikle, MD

References

1. Corona G, Rastrelli G, Forti G, Maggi M. Update in testosterone therapy for men. *J Sex Med.* 2011;8:639-654.
2. Lin JW, Lee JK, Wu CK, et al. Metabolic syndrome, testosterone, and cardiovascular mortality in men. *J Sex Med.* 2011;8:2350-2360.
3. Jones TH. Cardiovascular risk during androgen deprivation therapy for prostate cancer. *BMJ.* 2011;342:d3105.
4. Jones TH, Arver S, Behre HM, et al. Testosterone replacement in hypogonadal men with type 2 diabetes and/or metabolic syndrome (the TIMES2 study). *Diabetes Care.* 2011;34:828-837.
5. Basaria S, Coviello AD, Travison TG, et al. Adverse events associated with testosterone administration. *N Engl J Med.* 2010;363:109-122.

Relation between Sex Hormone Concentrations, Peripheral Arterial Disease, and Change in Ankle-Brachial Index: Findings from the Framingham Heart Study
Haring R, Travison TG, Bhasin S, et al (Boston Univ School of Public Health, MA; et al)
J Clin Endocrinol Metab 96:3724-3732, 2011

Objective.—Our objective was to investigate cross-sectional and longitudinal associations of sex hormone concentrations with ankle-brachial index (ABI) and peripheral arterial disease (PAD).

Methods and Results.—We used data from 3034 (1612 women) participants of the Framingham Heart Study. ABI was measured and PAD defined as ABI below 0.90, intermittent claudication, or lower extremity revascularization. Sex hormone concentrations were measured by liquid chromatography-tandem mass spectrometry [total testosterone (T), total estradiol, and estrone], immunofluorometric assay (SHBG), or calculated (free T). Sex-specific multivariable linear and logistic regression models were conducted for each sex hormone separately. Cross-sectional multivariable analyses revealed that men with lower free T and higher estrone (E1) concentrations had a significantly lower ABI [for free T, lowest *vs.* higher quartiles, $\beta = -0.02$, with 95% confidence interval (CI) = -0.04 to -0.001; and for E1, highest *vs.* lower quartiles, $\beta = -0.02$, with 95% CI = -0.04 to -0.002, respectively). Lower total T and SHBG concentrations were also associated with prevalent PAD in age-adjusted [odds ratio (OR) = 2.24, 95% CI = 1.17–4.32; and OR = 2.06; 95% CI = 1.07–3.96, lowest *vs.* highest quartile, respectively), but not in multivariable logistic regression models. Longitudinal multivariable analyses showed an association of lower SHBG with ABI change (decline ≥0.15; n = 69) in men [OR for SHBG quartiles 1, 2, and 3 as compared with quartile 4 were 2.56 (95% CI = 1.01–6.45), 2.28 (95% CI = 0.98–5.32), and 2.93 (95% CI = 1.31–6.52), respectively]. In women, none of the investigated associations yielded statistically significant estimates.

Conclusion.—Our investigation of a middle-aged community-based sample suggests that sex hormone concentrations in men but not in women may be associated with PAD and ABI change.

▶ Peripheral artery disease (PAD) is a risk factor for cardiovascular disease (CVD) and manifests atherosclerosis. A measure of risk for PAD is ankle-brachial index (ABI), which associates highly with CVD and mortality from CVD. In men low serum testosterone has been associated with co-morbidities of CVD including the metabolic syndrome, obesity, diabetes, sex hormone binding globulin, dyslipidemia, hypertension and mortal.[1-7] In women the associations between high testosterone and low sex hormone binding globulin as risk factors for CVD are less well defined. In this Framingham heart study, Haring and associates used ABI as an index of PAD, and reported in a cross sectional study of men and women that men with lower free testosterone and higher estrone had significantly lower age-adjusted concentrations in association with low ABI. In women, sex hormones were not associated with PAD and ABI change. In men it is also uncertain whether the hormonal changes observed pre-exist or art acquired. A limitation of the study was that it was cross sectional and longitudinal cause and effect relationships could not be determine.

A. W. Meikle, MD

References

1. Hyde Z, Norman PE, Flicker L, et al. Low free testosterone predicts mortality from cardiovascular disease but not other causes: the Health in Men Study. *J Clin Endocrinol Metab*. 2012;97:179-189.
2. Corona G, Rastrelli G, Monami M, et al. Hypogonadism as a risk factor for cardiovascular mortality in men: a meta-analytic study. *Eur J Endocrinol*. 2011; 165:687-701.
3. Araujo AB, Dixon JM, Suarez EA, Murad MH, Guey LT, Wittert GA. Clinical review: endogenous testosterone and mortality in men: a systematic review and meta-analysis. *J Clin Endocrinol Metab*. 2011;96:3007-3019.
4. Corona G, Rastrelli G, Vignozzi L, Mannucci E, Maggi M. Testosterone, cardiovascular disease and the metabolic syndrome. *Best Pract Res Clin Endocrinol Metab*. 2011;25:337-353.
5. Ruige JB, Mahmoud AM, De Bacquer D, Kaufman JM. Endogenous testosterone and cardiovascular disease in healthy men: a meta-analysis. *Heart*. 2011;97: 870-875.
6. Haring R, Völzke H, Steveling A, et al. Low serum testosterone levels are associated with increased risk of mortality in a population-based cohort of men aged 20-79. *Eur Heart J*. 2010;31:1494-1501.
7. Vikan T, Schirmer H, Njolstad I, Svartberg J. Endogenous sex hormones and the prospective association with cardiovascular disease and mortality in men: the Tromsø Study. *Eur J Endocrinol*. 2009;161:435-442.

Male Reproductive Function

Are Klinefelter boys hypogonadal?

Rey RA, Gottlieb S, Pasqualini T, et al (Hospital de Niños R. Gutiérrez, Buenos Aires, Argentina; Hospital Italiano, Buenos Aires, Argentina; et al)
Acta Paediatr 100:830-838, 2011

Male hypogonadism implies decreased function of one or more testicular cell population, i.e. germ, Leydig and/or Sertoli cells. In the normal prepubertal boy, Sertoli cells are very active, as indicated by high anti-Müllerian hormone (AMH) and inhibin B secretion, whereas the functional activity of Leydig cells is minimal, as evidenced by low testosterone production, and germ cells do not undergo the full spermatogenic process. Klinefelter syndrome is the most frequent cause of hypogonadism in the adult male. In this review, we discuss whether the gonadal failure is already established during infancy and childhood. In Klinefelter syndrome, there is increased germ cells degeneration from mid-foetal life — resulting in a decreased number at birth — which persists during infancy and childhood and becomes dramatic during puberty. Controversial results exist in the literature regarding Leydig cell function in Klinefelter boys: while some authors have found normal to low testosterone levels in infancy and

A   Ontogeny of the pituitary-gonadal hormone levels in the male

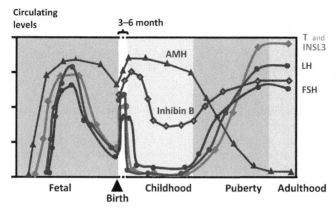

B   Testicular volume changes from birth to adulthood

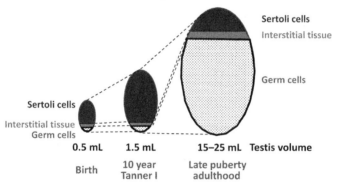

FIGURE 2.—(A) Schematic ontogeny of circulating levels of gonadotrophins (FSH: follicle-stimulating hormone and LH: luteinizing hormone), Leydig cell hormones (T: testosterone and INSL3: insulin-like factor 3) and Sertoli cell hormones (AMH: anti-Müllerian hormone and inhibin B) in the male. (B) Schematic ontogeny of the evolution of testicular volume from birth to adulthood. Seminiferous tubules (Sertoli + germ cells) are always the major component of the testis. From birth and during the whole prepubertal period (Tanner stage I), seminiferous tubule volume depends mainly on Sertoli cells, whereas the significant increase in testicular volume during pubertal development (i.e. between Tanner stages I and V) is mainly because of germ cell proliferation. Reprinted with permission from: (A) Grinspon RP and Rey RA. Anti-mullerian hormone and Sertoli cell function in paediatric male hypogonadism. Horm Res Paediatr 2010; 73: 81—92. Copyright S Karger AG, Basel, 2010, and (B) Rey R. Regulation of spermatogenesis. Endocrine Development 2003; 5:38—55. Söder O (ed): The Developing Testis. Physiology and Pathophysiology. Copyright S Karger AG, Basel, 2003. (Reprinted from Rey RA, Gottlieb S, Pasqualini T, et al. Are Klinefelter boys hypogonadal? *Acta Paediatr.* 2011;100:830-838, with permission from The Author(s)/Acta Pædiatrica.)

childhood, others have reported normal to high values. Sertoli cell products AMH and inhibin B are normal in prepubertal boys and only decline during mid- to late puberty.

Conclusion.—Klinefelter syndrome is a primary hypogonadism affecting all testicular cell populations. Germ cells are affected from foetal life, and a severe depletion occurs at puberty. Leydig cell function may be normal or mildly affected in foetal and early postnatal life. Sertoli cell function is not impaired until mid- to late puberty, as reflected by normal AMH and inhibin B in Klinefelter boys (Fig 2).

▶ Klinefelter's syndrome is defined as an adult with small testes, azoospermia, gynecomastia, and karyotype 47XXY. Rey et al summarize gonadal function in boys with Klinefelter's syndrome at various stages of development.[1] During fetal life, Sertoli cells secrete anti-Müllerian hormone, which suppresses Müllerian ducts. Leydig cells secrete testosterone, resulting in differentiation of the Wolffian ducts. These boys exhibit a neonatal increase in testosterone that then remains quiescent until puberty. During childhood, testes are of normal size, but germ cell numbers decrease, particularly during mid to late puberty when testicular failure develops. Many boys with Klinefelter's syndrome go undiagnosed and present with decreased verbal abilities, decreased motor development, and education problems.[2-7] Many are shy, quiet, immature, and dependent. Despite apparent developmental sexual deficits, they have male gender identity and sexual orientation. After late puberty, germ cell numbers are markedly decreased, and many have low or low normal serum testosterone concentrations. Eunuchoidal features are observed in many associated with hypogonadism.

A. W. Meikle, MD

References

1. Gottlieb S, Rey RA, Malozowski S. Klinefelter syndrome and cryptorchidism. *JAMA.* 2009;301:1436-1437.
2. Bastida MG, Rey RA, Bergadá I, et al. Establishment of testicular endocrine function impairment during childhood and puberty in boys with Klinefelter syndrome. *Clin Endocrinol (Oxf).* 2007;67:863-870.
3. Wikström AM, Dunkel L. Klinefelter syndrome. *Best Pract Res Clin Endocrinol Metab.* 2011;25:239-250.
4. Tartaglia N, Cordeiro L, Howell S, Wilson R, Janusz J. The spectrum of the behavioral phenotype in boys and adolescents 47, XXY (Klinefelter syndrome). *Pediatr Endocrinol Rev.* 2010;8:151-159.
5. Rogol AD, Tartaglia N. Considerations for androgen therapy in children and adolescents with Klinefelter syndrome (47, XXY). *Pediatr Endocrinol Rev.* 2010;8:145-150.
6. Bruining H, Swaab H, Kas M, van Engeland H. Psychiatric characteristics in a self-selected sample of boys with Klinefelter syndrome. *Pediatrics.* 2009;123:e865-e870.
7. Nadworny J, Tarlowski R, Szamborski J. [Klinefelter's syndrome in young boys. pituitary gonadotropic activity and testicular histology]. *Ginekol Pol.* 1965;36:91-93.

Reference Ranges for Testosterone in Men Generated Using Liquid Chromatography Tandem Mass Spectrometry in a Community-Based Sample of Healthy Nonobese Young Men in the Framingham Heart Study and Applied to Three Geographically Distinct Cohorts

Bhasin S, Pencina M, Jasuja GK, et al (Boston Univ School of Medicine, MA; Boston Univ, MA; et al)
J Clin Endocrinol Metab 96:2430-2439, 2011

Context.—Reference ranges are essential for partitioning testosterone levels into low or normal and making the diagnosis of androgen deficiency.

We established reference ranges for total testosterone (TT) and free testosterone (FT) in a community-based sample of men.

Methods.—TT was measured using liquid chromatography tandem mass spectrometry in nonobese healthy men, 19–40 yr old, in the Framingham Heart Study Generation 3; FT was calculated. Values below the 2.5th percentile of reference sample were deemed low. We determined the association of low TT and FT with physical dysfunction, sexual symptoms [European Male Aging Study (EMAS) only], and diabetes mellitus in three cohorts: Framingham Heart Study generations 2 and 3, EMAS, and the Osteoporotic Fractures in Men Study.

Results.—In a reference sample of 456 men, mean (SD), median (quartile), and 2.5th percentile values were 723.8 (221.1), 698.7 (296.5), and 348.3 ng/dl for TT and 141. 8 (45.0), 134.0 (60.0), and 70.0 pg/ml for FT, respectively. In all three samples, men with low TT and FT were more likely to have slow walking speed, difficulty climbing stairs, or frailty and diabetes than those with normal levels. In EMAS, men with low TT and FT were more likely to report sexual symptoms than men with normal levels. Men with low TT and FT were more likely to have at least one of the following: sexual symptoms (EMAS only), physical dysfunction, or diabetes.

Conclusion.—Reference ranges generated in a community-based sample of men provide a rational basis for categorizing testosterone levels as low or normal. Men with low TT or FT by these criteria had higher prevalence of physical dysfunction, sexual dysfunction, and diabetes. These reference limits should be validated prospectively in relation to incident outcomes and in randomized trials.

▶ The diagnosis of androgen deficiency is initiated in men presenting with symptoms of decreased libido, suppressed energy, and mood and erectile dysfunction.[1] Defining testosterone deficiency has been a challenge because serum testosterone concentrations exhibit episodic and circadian variation in section and it is affected strongly by age and other common disorders, such as obesity, the metabolic syndrome, and diabetes. Another variable in establishing reference intervals is the accuracy and specificity of the measurement of serum testosterone. Another issue concerning the reference ranges concerns whether the values should be based on age or based on values for younger healthy men. Another consideration is whether to also base reference values on free testosterone concentrations rather than just total serum testosterone. Bhasin et al included healthy, nonobese men between 19 and 40 years of age.[2] Aging men from 2 other studies were also included in the analysis. Strengths of the study were well characterized healthy men and accurate and specific measurement of testosterone using tandem mass spectrometry.[3,4] A precise cutoff for testosterone concentrations and symptoms of hypogonadism remains to be defined.[5,6]

A. W. Meikle, MD

References

1. Sattler FR, Bhasin S, He J, et al. Durability of the effects of testosterone and growth hormone supplementation in older community dwelling men: the HORMA trial. *Clin Endocrinol (Oxf)*. 2011 Mar 4 [Epub ahead of print].

2. Bhasin S, Basaria S. Diagnosis and treatment of hypogonadism in men. *Best Pract Res Clin Endocrinol Metab.* 2011;25:251-270.
3. Krasnoff JB, Basaria S, Pencina MJ, et al. Free testosterone levels are associated with mobility limitation and physical performance in community-dwelling men: the Framingham Offspring Study. *J Clin Endocrinol Metab.* 2010;95:2790-2799.
4. Kushnir MM, Blamires T, Rockwood AL, et al. Liquid chromatography-tandem mass spectrometry assay for androstenedione, dehydroepiandrosterone, and testosterone with pediatric and adult reference intervals. *Clin Chem.* 2010;56:1138-1147.
5. Kushnir MM, Rockwood AL, Roberts WL, et al. Performance characteristics of a novel tandem mass spectrometry assay for serum testosterone. *Clin Chem.* 2006;52:120-128.
6. Meikle AW, Bishop DT, Stringham JD, Ford MH, West DW. Relationship between body mass index, cigarette smoking, and plasma sex steroids in normal male twins. *Genet Epidemiol.* 1989;6:399-412.

Shorter Androgen Receptor CAG Repeat Lengths Associated with Cryptorchidism Risk among Hispanic White Boys

Davis-Dao C, Koh CJ, Hardy BE, et al (Univ of Southern California, Los Angeles, CA; et al)
J Clin Endocrinol Metab 97:E393-E399, 2012

Context.—Cryptorchidism is the most frequent congenital malformation among males, the major established risk factor for testicular germ cell tumors, and a presumed infertility risk factor. Androgens are essential for testicular descent, and functional genetic polymorphisms in the androgen receptor gene (*AR*) are postulated to influence cryptorchidism risk.

Objective.—The aim of the study was to investigate whether the CAG repeat length polymorphism in exon 1 of the *AR* is associated with cryptorchidism risk.

Design and Setting.—We conducted a family-based genotype-risk association study employing the transmission disequilibrium test for genotypic variants transmitted on the X-chromosome at a university-affiliated regional children's hospital.

Participants.—We studied 127 Hispanic boys with persistent cryptorchidism and comorbidities described in detail and their biological mothers.

Intervention.—Genotypes defined by number of CAG repeats were measured for each member of participating son-mother pairs.

Main Outcome Measure.—Associations between CAG tract length genotype and cryptorchidism risk were estimated using matched-pairs logistic regression.

Results.—Cryptorchidism risk was significantly associated with shorter CAG repeats [CAG ≤ 19 *vs.* CAG ≥ 20, odds ratio (OR) = 0.44; 95% confidence interval (CI), 0.23–0.88]. This association was restricted to cryptorchidism with accompanying comorbidities, which was primarily hernia [CAG ≤ 19 *vs.* CAG ≥ 20, OR = 0.35 (95% CI, 0.16–0.78)], and was strongest for bilateral cryptorchidism [CAG ≤ 19 *vs.* CAG ≥ 20, OR = 0.09 (95% CI, 0.010–0.78)].

TABLE 3.—OR and 95% CI for the Association of CAG Repeat Length with Risk of Cryptorchidism Among All Cases and Stratified by Phenotype, Comparing Case and Control Alleles

	Presence and Type of Accompanying Comorbidity			
	No Comorbidity, Case/Control	Any Comorbidity, Case/Control[a]	Hernia Alone, Case/Control	Any Except Hernia Alone, Case/Control
No. of CAG repeats				
≤19	7/7	24/9	18/8	6/1
≥20	37/37	59/74	46/56	13/18
20−21	13/10	20/22	16/17	
≥22	24/27	39/52	30/39	
OR (95% CI)[b]				
≤19	1.0 (ref)	1.0 (ref)	1.0 (ref)	1.0 (ref)
≥20	1.00 (0.25−3.99)	0.35 (0.16−0.78)	0.41 (0.17−0.99)	0.17 (0.02−1.38)
20−21	1.38 (0.26−7.22)	0.42 (0.16−1.09)	0.49 (0.17−1.43)	
≥22	1.00 (0.25−3.99)	0.31 (0.13−0.74)	0.38 (0.15−0.97)	
	$P_{trend} = 0.67$	$P_{trend} = 0.010$	$P_{trend} = 0.045$	

[a]Comorbidities include: 64 cases with hernia only, three cases with hernia and obesity/morbid obesity, two cases with hernia and hydrocele, and one case with each of the following: hernia and micropenis, penoscrotal transposition, hernia, hypospadias and micropenis, obesity/morbid obesity, cleft palate, Down's syndrome, Miller-Dieker syndrome, phimosis, Kabuki syndrome, mitochondrial disorder, anoxic encephalopathy, renal tubular failure, heart surgery, and congenital syndrome (unspecified).
[b]Conditional logistic regression (comparing transmitted allele to nontransmitted allele).

Conclusions.—Androgen receptor genotypes encoding moderate functional variation may influence cryptorchidism risk, particularly among boys with bilateral nondescent or congenital hernia, and may explain in part the elevated risk of testicular seminoma experienced by ex-cryptorchid boys. Mechanistic research is warranted to examine both classical and nonclassical mechanisms through which androgens may influence risk of cryptorchidism and related conditions (Table 3).

► Cryptorchidism is failure of the descent of the testes into the scrotum with an estimated prevalence of 2% to 8% at birth and 1% to 2% at 1 year of age. It is thus the most common male malformation. The condition has hazards of infertility and testicular germ cell neoplasms. Studies have found that androgen receptor dysfunction might contribute to cryptorchidism.[1-5] This is inferred from animal models, testicular feminization, and the surge of testosterone in boys between 1 and 3 months of age, as testosterone had a function in testicular descent in boys with cryptorchidism at birth. Davis-Dao et al investigated the association between CAG repeat length and cryptorchidism in males undergoing orchiopexy. Shorter CAG repeats with the risk of cryptorchidism was unexpected because shorter repeats have been associated with greater androgen receptor transactivation, and cryptorchidism occurs in men with loss of function and androgen receptor mutations. They suggest that both nongenomic and genomic androgen pathways in testicular descent might unravel this apparent unexpected finding.

A. W. Meikle, MD

References

1. Kaftanovskaya EM, Huang Z, Barbara AM, et al. Cryptorchidism in mice with an androgen receptor ablation in gubernaculum testis. Mol Endocrinol. 2012;26: 598-607.
2. Gabel P, Jensen MS, Andersen HR, et al. The risk of cryptorchidism among sons of women working in horticulture in Denmark: a cohort study. Environ Health. 2011;10:100.
3. Kojima Y, Mizuno K, Kohri K, Hayashi Y. Advances in molecular genetics of cryptorchidism. Urology. 2009;74:571-578.
4. Main KM, Skakkebaek NE, Toppari J. Cryptorchidism as part of the testicular dysgenesis syndrome: the environmental connection. Endocr Dev. 2009;14:167-173.
5. Ferlin A, Zuccarello D, Zuccarello B, Chirico MR, Zanon GF, Foresta C. Genetic alterations associated with cryptorchidism. JAMA. 2008;300:2271-2276.

Osteoporosis in Women

Higher Serum Free Testosterone Concentration in Older Women Is Associated with Greater Bone Mineral Density, Lean Body Mass, and Total Fat Mass: The Cardiovascular Health Study

Rariy CM, Ratcliffe SJ, Weinstein R, et al (Univ of Pennsylvania School of Medicine, Philadelphia; et al)

J Clin Endocrinol Metab 96:989-996, 2011

Context.—The physiological importance of endogenous testosterone (T) in older women is poorly understood.

Objective.—The aim of the study was to determine the association of higher total and free T levels with bone mineral density (BMD), lean body mass, and fat mass in elderly women.

Design.—Total and free T were measured using sensitive assays in 232 community-dwelling women aged 67—94 yr who were enrolled in the Cardiovascular Health Study and had dual-energy x-ray absorptiometry scans. Cross-sectional analyses were performed to examine associations between total and free T and BMD and body composition.

Results.—In adjusted models, total T was directly associated with BMD at the lumbar spine ($P = 0.04$) and hip ($P = 0.001$), but not body composition outcomes, in all women, and after excluding estrogen users and adjusting for estradiol ($P = 0.04$ and 0.01, respectively). Free T was positively related to hip BMD, lean body mass, and body fat (all $P < 0.05$), with more than 10% differences in each outcome between women at the highest and lowest ends of the free T range, with attenuation after excluding estrogen users and adjusting for estradiol.

Conclusions.—In the setting of the low estradiol levels found in older women, circulating T levels were associated with bone density. Women with higher free T levels had greater lean body mass, consistent with the anabolic effect of T, and, in contrast to men, greater fat mass. Mechanistic studies are required to determine whether a causal relationship exists between T, bone, and body composition in this population and the degree to which any T effects are estrogen-independent.

▶ There is limited information concerning the effects of endogenous testosterone on bone mineral density (BMD) in older women.[1-4] While testosterone therapy is known to increase BMD and muscle mass and decrease fat mass in older men with testosterone deficiency, similar results have been observed with testosterone therapy of postmenopausal women. Postmenopausal women with higher endogenous concentrations of testosterone have decreased hip fractures. Rariy et al performed a cross-sectional study in women 65 years or older to determine if endogenous testosterone was associated with BMD and body composition.[1] They observed that older women with high endogenous testosterone concentrations had significantly higher BMD and lean body mass that were independent of body weight and adjusting for endogenous circulating estradiol levels. This study raises a question about the use of testosterone replacement therapy in women to treat or prevent osteoporosis in aging postmenopausal women. Further study is needed to assess the risks and benefits of testosterone therapy in women.

A. W. Meikle, MD

References

1. Rariy CM, Ratcliffe SJ, Weinstein R, et al. Higher serum free testosterone concentration in older women is associated with greater bone mineral density, lean body mass, and total fat mass: the cardiovascular health study. *J Clin Endocrinol Metab*. 2011;96:989-996.
2. Cheung E, Tsang S, Bow C, et al. Bone loss during menopausal transition among southern Chinese women. *Maturitas*. 2011;69:50-56.
3. Ducharme N. Male osteoporosis. *Clin Geriatr Med*. 2010;26:301-309.
4. Kilbourne EJ, Moore WJ, Freedman LP, Nagpal S. Selective androgen receptor modulators for frailty and osteoporosis. *Curr Opin Investig Drugs*. 2007;8: 821-829.

Effects of Risedronate and Low-Dose Transdermal Testosterone on Bone Mineral Density in Women with Anorexia Nervosa: A Randomized, Placebo-Controlled Study

Miller KK, Meenaghan E, Lawson EA, et al (Massachusetts General Hosp, Boston; et al)
J Clin Endocrinol Metab 96:2081-2088, 2011

Context.—Anorexia nervosa is complicated by severe bone loss and clinical fractures. Mechanisms underlying bone loss in adults with anorexia nervosa include increased bone resorption and decreased formation. Estrogen administration has not been shown to prevent bone loss in this population, and to date, there are no approved, effective therapies for this comorbidity.

Objective.—To determine whether antiresorptive therapy with a bisphosphonate alone or in combination with low-dose transdermal testosterone replacement would increase bone mineral density (BMD) in women with anorexia nervosa.

Design and Setting.—We conducted a 12-month, randomized, placebo-controlled study at a clinical research center.

Study Participants.—Participants included 77 ambulatory women with anorexia nervosa.

Intervention.—Subjects were randomized to risedronate 35 mg weekly, low-dose transdermal testosterone replacement therapy, combination therapy or double placebo.

Main Outcome Measures.—BMD at the spine (primary endpoint), hip, and radius and body composition were measured by dual-energy x-ray absorptiometry.

Results.—Risedronate increased posteroanterior spine BMD 3%, lateral spine BMD 4%, and hip BMD 2% in women with anorexia nervosa compared with placebo in a 12-month clinical trial. Testosterone administration did not improve BMD but increased lean body mass. There were few side effects associated with either therapy.

Conclusions.—Risedronate administration for 1 yr increased spinal BMD, the primary site of bone loss in women with anorexia nervosa. Low-dose testosterone did not change BMD but increased lean body mass (Fig 2).

▶ Anorexia nervosa is a primary psychiatric disorder characterized by chronic malnutrition resulting in various complications, including osteoporosis with increased fracture risk.[1-4] The spine is preferentially associated with bone loss. Estrogen therapy has not been shown to benefit these patients, although ovarian dysfunction is common in them. Miller et al conducted a randomized placebo-controlled study to determine the effects of a bisphosphonate alone or with

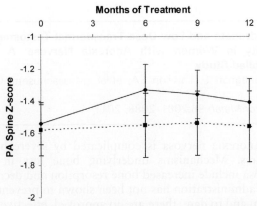

FIGURE 2.—PA spine BMD increased in women receiving risedronate (*solid line*) over a 12-month period compared with those receiving placebo (*dotted line*) (*P* < 0.0001). Z-scores are shown. (Reprinted from Miller KK, Meenaghan E, Lawson EA, et al. Effects of risedronate and low-dose transdermal testosterone on bone mineral density in women with anorexia nervosa: a randomized, placebo-controlled study. *J Clin Endocrinol Metab.* 2011;96:2081-2088, Copyright 2011, with permission from The Endocrine Society.)

testosterone for 1 year on bone mineral density (BMD).[5] While bisphosphonate alone did not benefit BMD, it improved lean body mass, which is interesting since testosterone therapy designed for replacement therapy in women improved lean body mass. Testosterone did not alter a bone formation or bone resorption marker, whereas the bisphosphonate alone or with testosterone did. The study did not include bone microarchitecture or sequential anabolic therapy followed by consolidation antiresorptive therapy. Further study is needed to determine benefit on fracture risk reduction in these patients.

A. W. Meikle, MD

References

1. Mehler PS, Cleary BS, Gaudiani JL. Osteoporosis in anorexia nervosa. *Eat Disord.* 2011;19:194-202.
2. Mehler PS, MacKenzie TD. Treatment of osteopenia and osteoporosis in anorexia nervosa: a systematic review of the literature. *Int J Eat Disord.* 2009;42:195-201.
3. Jayasinghe Y, Grover SR, Zacharin M. Current concepts in bone and reproductive health in adolescents with anorexia nervosa. *BJOG.* 2008;115:304-315.
4. Misra M, Klibanski A. Anorexia nervosa and osteoporosis. *Rev Endocr Metab Disord.* 2006;7:91-99.
5. Miller KK, Grieco KA, Mulder J, et al. Effects of risedronate on bone density in anorexia nervosa. *J Clin Endocrinol Metab.* 2004;89:3903-3906.

Polycystic Ovary Syndrome

Improvement of hyperandrogenism and hyperinsulinemia during pregnancy in women with polycystic ovary syndrome: possible effect in the ovarian follicular mass of their daughters
Crisosto N, Echiburú B, Maliqueo M, et al (Univ of Chile, Santiago)
Fertil Steril 97:218-224, 2012

Objective.—To evaluate the ovarian function during early infancy in daughters of women with polycystic ovary syndrome (PCOS) treated with metformin throughout pregnancy (PCOSd+M), as a means to reduce androgen and insulin levels, compared with daughters of nontreated PCOS women (PCOSd−M) and daughters of women who belong to a healthy comparison group (HCd).
Design.—Descriptive and analytic study.
Setting.—Unit of endocrinology and reproductive medicine.
Patient(s).—Fifteen PCOSd+M, 23 PCOSd−M, and 35 HCd were studied at 2−3 months of age.
Intervention(s).—A GnRH analogue test was performed with determinations of gonadotropins, sex steroids, SHBG, and anti-Müllerian hormone (AMH).
Main Outcome Measure(s).—Differences in AMH levels between PCOSd+M, PCOSd−M and HCd.
Result(s).—AMH and peak E_2 concentrations were significantly higher in PCOSd−M compared with HCd, whereas PCOSd+M exhibited AMH concentrations and peak E_2 levels similar to those observed in HCd.

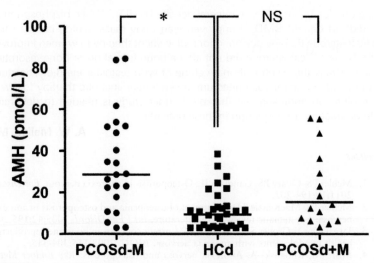

FIGURE 1.—Antimüllerian hormone serum concentrations in daughters of PCOS women treated with metformin (PCOSd+M; *triangles*), of nontreated PCOS women (PCOSd−M; *circles*) and of women who belong to a healthy comparison group (HCd; *squares*). *Adjusted *P* value <.0125 (Bonferroni principle). (Reprinted from Crisosto N, Echiburú B, Maliqueo M, et al, Improvement of hyperandrogenism and hyperinsulinemia during pregnancy in women with polycystic ovary syndrome: possible effect in the ovarian follicular mass of their daughters. *Fertil Steril*. 2012;97:218-224, Copyright 2012, with permission from American Society for Reproductive Medicine.)

Conclusion(s).—The improvement of the altered endocrine-metabolic environment of PCOS mothers reduces AMH levels in their daughters, which might reflect a decrease in their follicular mass (Fig 1).

▶ Polycystic ovary syndrome (PCOS) is common in premenopausal women and is characterized by anovulatory infertility, insulin resistance, excess androgen, and polycystic ovaries.[1] Crisosto et al previously observed that daughters of women with PCOS had higher blood concentrations of anti-Müllerian hormone (AMH),[2] which is a marker of growing ovarian follicles. This resembles observations made in women with PCOS. Crisosto et al intervened with metformin to determine if a reduction in androgens and insulin levels would reduce the occurrence of ovarian follicular mass in their daughters. In daughters of women with PCOS treated with metformin, AMH was reduced, suggesting that improving the hyperinsulinemia and hyperandrogenism in pregnant women with PCOS might reduce ovarian proliferation in their daughters.[3] It was not possible to use a placebo-controlled experimental design. Long-term follow-up is needed to determine if the benefits on the daughters are long-lasting or temporary.[4] The mechanism for the effect of metformin on ovarian function in the daughters requires additional investigation.

A. W. Meikle, MD

References

1. Sir-Petermann T, Codner E, Pérez V, et al. Metabolic and reproductive features before and during puberty in daughters of women with polycystic ovary syndrome. *J Clin Endocrinol Metab.* 2009;94:1923-1930.
2. Crisosto N, Codner E, Maliqueo M, et al. Anti-Müllerian hormone levels in peripubertal daughters of women with polycystic ovary syndrome. *J Clin Endocrinol Metab.* 2007;92:2739-2743.
3. Hickey M, Sloboda DM, Atkinson HC, et al. The relationship between maternal and umbilical cord androgen levels and polycystic ovary syndrome in adolescence: a prospective cohort study. *J Clin Endocrinol Metab.* 2009;94:3714-3720.
4. Franks S, Webber LJ, Goh M, et al. Ovarian morphology is a marker of heritable biochemical traits in sisters with polycystic ovaries. *J Clin Endocrinol Metab.* 2008;93:3396-3402.

Early Metformin Therapy (Age 8–12 Years) in Girls with Precocious Pubarche to Reduce Hirsutism, Androgen Excess, and Oligomenorrhea in Adolescence

Ibáñez L, López-Bermejo A, Díaz M, et al (Univ of Barcelona, Spain; Dr Josep Trueta Hosp and Girona Inst for Biomedical Res, Girona, Spain; et al)
J Clin Endocrinol Metab 96:E1262-E1267, 2011

Context.—Girls with a combined history of low(-normal) birth weight (LBW) and precocious pubarche (PP) are at high risk to develop polycystic ovary syndrome (PCOS).

Objective.—The objective of the study was to compare the capacity of early *vs.* late metformin treatment to prevent adolescent PCOS.

Design.—This was a randomized, open-label study over 7 yr.

Setting.—The study was conducted at a university hospital.

Patients.—Thirty-eight LBW-PP girls were followed up from the mean age 8 until age 15 yr.

Intervention.—Early metformin (study yr 1–4; age 8–12 yr) *vs.* late metformin (yr 6; age 13–14 yr).

Main Outcome Measures.—Measures included height; weight; hirsutism score; menstrual cycle; endocrine-metabolic screening (fasting; follicular phase); C-reactive protein; body composition (absorptiometry); abdominal fat partitioning (magnetic resonance imaging); ovarian morphology (ultrasound); PCOS (National Institutes of Health and Androgen Excess Society definitions) after yr 7 (all girls thus untreated for at least 1 yr).

Results.—None of the girls dropped out of the study. At age 15 yr, early-metformin girls were taller (4 cm), were in a less proinflammatory state, and had less central fat due to reductions in visceral and hepatic fat. Hirsutism, androgen excess, oligomenorrhea, and PCOS were between 2- and 8-fold more prevalent in late- than early-treated girls. Abdominal adiposity was the first variable to diverge (at age 8–10 yr) between girls without *vs.* with PCOS at age 15 yr.

Conclusions.—In LBW-PP girls, early metformin therapy was found to prevent or delay the development of hirsutism, androgen excess, oligomenorrhea, and PCOS more effectively than late metformin. The time

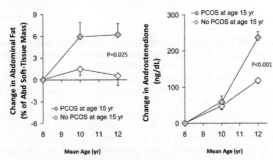

FIGURE 3.—Longitudinal observations in girls with a combined history of low birth weight and precocious pubarche (n = 38), who either were treated with metformin between age 8 and 12 yr (n = 19) or were not (n = 19). Irrespective of such treatment, the girls are subgrouped here by the presence (n = 9) or the absence (n = 29) of PCOS at age 15 yr. Abdominal adiposity diverges between PCOS subgroups by age 10 yr, and circulating androstenedione diverges by age 12 yr. For results at 8 and 15 yr, see Supplemental Table 2 in the original article. Data are shown as mean and SEM. (Reprinted from Ibáñez L, López-Bermejo A, Díaz M, et al. Early metformin therapy (age 8–12 years) in girls with precocious pubarche to reduce hirsutism, androgen excess, and oligomenorrhea in adolescence. *J Clin Endocrinol Metab.* 2011;96:E1262-E1267, Copyright 2011, with permission from The Endocrine Society.)

window of late childhood and early puberty may be more critical for the development, and thus for the prevention, of adolescent PCOS than the first years beyond menarche (Fig 3).

▶ Excess adipose tissue in adolescent girls appears to contribute to androgen excess and polycystic ovary syndrome (PCOS). Precocious pubarche (PP) is associated with low birth weight (LBW) and early PCOS. It is well established that metformin improves the menstrual dysfunction, insulin resistance, and hirsutism in young women.[1-6] The study by Ibanez et al treated girls with PP-LBW at an early age (8–12 years) and later (13–14 years) to determine if metformin would prevent the development of adolescent androgen excess, hirsutism, menstrual dysfunction, and PCOS. They observed that early treatment with metformin was more effective in prevention of these adverse features than late treatment. The mechanism for the benefit is as yet undetermined. The authors proposed that metformin reduced intraabdominal fat, which involved visceral and hepatic fat.[7,8] Further investigation is needed to determine if early metformin treatment can prevent subsequent PCOS later in life. They do provide evidence for consideration of early preventive treatment for PCOS.

A. W. Meikle, MD

References

1. Ibáñez L, Lopez-Bermejo A, Diaz M, Marcos MV, de Zegher F. Early metformin therapy to delay menarche and augment height in girls with precocious pubarche. *Fertil Steril.* 2011;95:727-730.
2. Díaz M, López-Bermejo A, Petry CJ, de Zegher F, Ibáñez L. Efficacy of metformin therapy in adolescent girls with androgen excess: relation to sex hormone-binding globulin and androgen receptor polymorphisms. *Fertil Steril.* 2010;94:2800-2803.
3. Ibáñez L, Lopez-Bermejo A, Diaz M, Marcos MV, de Zegher F. Pubertal metformin therapy to reduce total, visceral, and hepatic adiposity. *J Pediatr.* 2010;156: 98-102.

4. Ibáñez L, Díaz R, López-Bermejo A, Marcos MV. Clinical spectrum of premature pubarche: links to metabolic syndrome and ovarian hyperandrogenism. *Rev Endocr Metab Disord.* 2009;10:63-76.
5. Ibáñez L, López-Bermejo A, Díaz M, Marcos MV, de Zegher F. Metformin treatment for four years to reduce total and visceral fat in low birth weight girls with precocious pubarche. *J Clin Endocrinol Metab.* 2008;93:1841-1845.
6. Ibáñez L, Ong K, Valls C, Marcos MV, Dunger DB, de Zegher F. Metformin treatment to prevent early puberty in girls with precocious pubarche. *J Clin Endocrinol Metab.* 2006;91:2888-2891.
7. Ibáñez L, Valls C, Marcos MV, Ong K, Dunger DB, De Zegher F. Insulin sensitization for girls with precocious pubarche and with risk for polycystic ovary syndrome: effects of prepubertal initiation and postpubertal discontinuation of metformin treatment. *J Clin Endocrinol Metab.* 2004;89:4331-4337.
8. Ibáñez L, Ferrer A, Ong K, Amin R, Dunger D, de Zegher F. Insulin sensitization early after menarche prevents progression from precocious pubarche to polycystic ovary syndrome. *J Pediatr.* 2004;144:23-29.

Effects of Simvastatin and Metformin on Polycystic Ovary Syndrome after Six Months of Treatment

Banaszewska B, Pawelczyk L, Spaczynski RZ, et al (Poznan Univ of Med Sciences, Poland; et al)
J Clin Endocrinol Metab 96:3493-3501, 2011

Context.—A randomized trial on women with polycystic ovary syndrome (PCOS) compared simvastatin, metformin, and a combination of these drugs.

Objective.—The aim of the study was to evaluate long-term effects of simvastatin and metformin on PCOS.

Design.—Women with PCOS (n = 139) were randomized to simvastatin (S), metformin (M), or simvastatin plus metformin (SM) groups. Evaluations were performed at baseline and at 3 and 6 months.

Setting.—The study was conducted at a university medical center.

Primary Outcome.—We measured the change of serum total testosterone.

Results.—Ninety-seven subjects completed the study. Total testosterone decreased significantly and comparably in all groups: by 25.6, 25.6, and 20.1% in the S, M, and SM groups, respectively. Both simvastatin and metformin improved menstrual cyclicity and decreased hirsutism, acne, ovarian volume, body mass index, C-reactive protein, and soluble vascular cell adhesion molecule-1. Dehydroepiandrosterone sulfate declined significantly only in the S group. Total cholesterol and low-density lipoprotein cholesterol significantly declined only in the S and SM groups. Ongoing reduction of ovarian volume, decreased hirsutism, acne and testosterone were observed between 0 and 3 months as well as between 3 and 6 months. Improvement of lipid profile, C-reactive protein, and soluble vascular cell adhesion molecule-1 occurred only during the first 3 months of treatment, with little change thereafter. Treatments were well tolerated, and no significant adverse effects were encountered.

Conclusions.—Long-term treatment with simvastatin was superior to metformin. Improvement of ovarian hyperandrogenism continued throughout the duration of the study.

▶ Polycystic ovary syndrome (PCOS) affects about 10% of women of the reproductive age and is characterized by hyperandrogenism, oligomenorrhea, insulin resistance, the metabolic syndrome, obesity, infertility, and polycystic ovaries. It is associated with a familial risk, but a genetic cause has been elusive. Treatment has been directed at correcting the clinical and laboratory abnormalities, which included agents to improve insulin responsiveness, with agents such as metformin, and suppression of hyperandrogenism, with androgen blockers such as spironolactone.[1-5] Banaszewska et al compared the effectiveness of simvastatin, metformin, and the combination of simvastatin and metformin on various biochemical and clinical aspects of PCOS.[6,7] Hyperandrogenism improved in all treatment groups, but no placebo group was included in the study. Simvastatin improved free and total testosterone.

A. W. Meikle, MD

References

1. Raval AD, Hunter T, Stuckey B, Hart RJ. Statins for women with polycystic ovary syndrome not actively trying to conceive. *Cochrane Database Syst Rev.* 2011;(10). CD008565.
2. Ortega I, Cress AB, Wong DH, et al. Simvastatin reduces steroidogenesis by inhibiting Cyp17a1 gene expression in rat ovarian theca-interstitial cells. *Biol Reprod.* 2012;86:1-9.
3. Economou F, Xyrafis X, Christakou C, Diamanti-Kandarakis E. The pluripotential effects of hypolipidemic treatment for polycystic ovary syndrome (PCOS): dyslipidemia, cardiovascular risk factors and beyond. *Curr Pharm Des.* 2011;17: 908-921.
4. Kaya C, Pabuccu R, Cengiz SD, Dünder I. Comparison of the effects of atorvastatin and simvastatin in women with polycystic ovary syndrome: a prospective, randomized study. *Exp Clin Endocrinol Diabetes.* 2010;118:161-166.
5. Kazerooni T, Shojaei-Baghini A, Dehbashi S, Asadi N, Ghaffarpasand F, Kazerooni Y. Effects of metformin plus simvastatin on polycystic ovary syndrome: a prospective, randomized, double-blind, placebo-controlled study. *Fertil Steril.* 2010;94:2208-2213.
6. Banaszewska B, Pawelczyk L, Spaczynski RZ, Duleba AJ. Comparison of simvastatin and metformin in treatment of polycystic ovary syndrome: prospective randomized trial. *J Clin Endocrinol Metab.* 2009;94:4938-4945.
7. Banaszewska B, Spaczynski RZ, Ozegowska K, Pawelczyk L. The influence of low-dose oral contraceptive pill on clinical and metabolic parameters in young women with polycystic ovary syndrome. *Ginekol Pol.* 2011;82:430-435.

8   Pediatric Endocrinology

Introduction

This year's YEAR BOOK collection is comprised of articles reporting both
negative and positive study results that utilize a variety of methodologies,
including retrospective, cross-sectional, prospective and placebo-controlled
trials. As is customary, the selected papers deal with frequently encountered
conditions as well as rare entities. Some of the topics tackle areas of significant controversy while others touch on spheres in which relative unanimity
within our specialty exists. Within this assortment one finds new insights
pertaining to old clinical quandaries as well as novel discoveries that were
unanticipated decades before. Regardless, each paper contains one or
more important take-home messages that will hopefully aid us in the lifelong
quest of being better thinkers, scientists and clinicians.

The first two selections both deal with human recombinant growth
hormone (GH) and cumulatively provide support for being judicious
with its use. Selection #1 is the report of the high-profile SAGhE study,
the preliminary results of which were widely disseminated by the media
even before the paper underwent thorough peer-review. Even though the
FDA eventually deemed its findings inconclusive, the report of increased
mortality in adults treated with GH during childhood understandably
generated substantial concern. Selection #2 failed to detect a relationship
between quality of life and long term GH therapy in a group of young
women with Turner syndrome (TS), suggesting that height is not the key
factor to success and happiness in these patients. Selection #3 also deals
with TS and is notable for its rigorous study design, a characteristic glar-
ingly lacking in the majority of trials involving children. It represents
a real contribution to clinical care and suggests that oxandrolone still has
a very viable place in the treatment of girls affected with TS. The presentation of primary adrenal insufficiency in children is the focus of selection #4,
which succeeds in providing a fresh look at the baseline clinical and
biochemical features of this condition that challenge some commonly
held assumptions. Selection #5 examines the natural history of mild hypothyroidism in >300 children over 3 years and finds that only ~20% of
subjects required hormone replacement therapy within this timeframe.
Natural history is also a theme of the next selection (#6), as it details the

319

outcome of pediatric patient with presumed idiopathic diabetes insipidus seen at 3 tertiary medical centers. Selection #7 addresses the significance of the mildly elevated TSH values that have become nearly ubiquitous in the setting of exogenous obesity. This paper does a marvelous job of reviewing the existing literature in this area and summarizing the pathophysiology of this phenomenon, which is presumed due to leptin and thought to be driven by an adaptive increase in energy expenditure to compensate for excessive weight gain. Selection #8 pertains to another public health concern — that of a potentially negative impact of endocrine disrupting chemicals on growth and development in children. Although the statistically significant association between higher phthalate concentrations and pubertal gynecomastia is worrisome, further study is clearly needed. Also in the realm of the reproductive system is selection #9, which investigated the obstetric outcome in women with TS. Despite the largely reassuring results from this retrospective study, whether they can truly be generalized to the broader population of TS women is unclear. Selection #10 is devoted to the uncommon but serious diagnosis of differentiated thyroid cancer in children, and found that the sensitivity of fine-needle biopsy in these cases was a sub-optimal 69%. This does not provide ammunition for forgoing routine surgical referral for children found to have a "cold" thyroid nodule, which is the practice currently favored by many pediatric endocrinologists. Finally, the last of this set of YEAR BOOK articles (#11) explores the still unanswered question of whether universal screening of pregnant women for hypothyroidism should be implemented due to concerns regarding neuropsychological development in the offspring should undetected thyroid disease be present. Although the inclusion of nearly 22 000 women is impressive, a closer look at the data gives one pause regarding whether this study's conclusions can be generalized. Thus, the debate surrounding this particular issue will likely continue.

In summary, it is my hope that the selections in this Year Book will provide knowledge, stimulate thought, and perhaps even generate new ideas for research and/or quality improvement initiatives aimed at enhancing the care of children with pediatric endocrine conditions worldwide!

Erica Eugster, MD

Growth/Growth Hormone

Long-Term Mortality after Recombinant Growth Hormone Treatment for Isolated Growth Hormone Deficiency or Childhood Short Stature: Preliminary Report of the French SAGhE Study

Carel J-C, Ecosse E, Landier F, et al (Institut National de la Santé et de la Recherche Mé dicale CIE5, Paris, France; Groupe Hospitalier Cochin-Saint Vincent de Paul and Univ Paris Descartes, France; et al)
J Clin Endocrinol Metab 97:416-425, 2012

Context.—Little is known about the long-term health of subjects treated with GH in childhood, and Safety and Appropriateness of Growth hormone treatments in Europe (SAGhE) is a study addressing this question.

Objective.—The objective of the study was to evaluate the long-term mortality of patients treated with recombinant GH in childhood in France.

Design.—This was a population-based cohort study.

Setting.—The setting of the study was a French population-based register.

Participants.—A total of 6928 children with idiopathic isolated GH deficiency (n = 5162), neurosecretory dysfunction (n = 534), idiopathic short stature (n = 871), or born short for gestational age (n = 335) who started treatment between 1985 and 1996 participated in the study. Follow-up data on vital status were available in September 2009 for 94.7% of the patients.

Main Outcome Measures.—All-cause and cause-specific mortality was measured in the study.

Results.—All-cause mortality was increased in treated subjects [standardized mortality ratio (SMR) 1.33, 95% confidence interval (CI) 1.08–1.64]. In a multivariate analysis adjusted for height, the use of GH doses greater than 50 μg/kg·d was associated with mortality rates using external and internal references (SMR 2.94, 95% CI 1.22–7.07, hazard ratio 2.79, 95% CI 1.14–6.82). All type cancer-related mortality was not increased. Bone tumor-related mortality was increased (SMR 5.00, 95% CI 1.01–14.63). An increase in mortality due to diseases of the circulatory system (SMR 3.07, 95% CI 1.40–5.83) or subarachnoid or intracerebral hemorrhage (SMR 6.66, 95% CI 1.79–17.05) was observed.

Conclusions.—Mortality rates were increased in this population of adults treated as children with recombinant GH, particularly in those who had received the highest doses. Specific effects were detected in terms of death due to bone tumors or cerebral hemorrhage but not for all cancers. These results highlight the need for additional studies of long-term mortality and morbidity after GH treatment in childhood.

▶ The publication of this study has been anxiously awaited ever since news of its findings was leaked to the media well over a year ago. The initial response to those revelations in the pediatric endocrine community ran the gamut from a recommendation to discontinue growth hormone (GH) therapy in all children currently being treated to the decision to carry on as usual until further information emerged. Whether and how to inform patients and families of the potential deleterious effect of GH on long-term health was similarly hotly debated. The Pediatric Endocrine Society itself came under some pressure by a prominent medical bioethicist to divulge to all parents of children receiving GH therapy that their child's increased height was being achieved at no known benefit and at the cost of increased risk of early death.[1] Eventually, the US Food and Drug Administration concluded that the evidence linking human recombinant GH to increased mortality was inconclusive and recommended that no change in prescribing practices for approved indications occur.[2] Now that the complete preliminary results from the Safety and Appropriateness of Growth hormone treatments in Europe (SAGhE) study have seen the light of day, where do they leave us? The study has spawned an impressive number of editorials and commentaries within which internationally renowned pediatric endocrinologists have held forth on a variety of topics including flaws of the SAGhE study, whether the results will change current clinical practice, and how to move forward from here.[3-5] Regardless of whether the safety concerns generated by the SAGhE study are ultimately refuted or confirmed, there is unanimity that rigorous, prospective investigation of the risks and benefits of GH therapy in lifespan cohorts of treated recipients is irrefutably imperative. As in the quote by the famous Jewish scholar Hillel: "If I am not for myself, then who will be for me? And if I am only for myself, then what am I? And if not now, when?"

E. Eugster, MD

References

1. Dreger A. Dying for some standards: broken medical systems as revealed by a new FDA warning. Bioethics Forum 3/21/11.
2. http://www.fda.gov/Safety/MedWatch/SafetyInformation/SafetyAlertsforHuman MedicalProducts/ucm237969.htm. Accessed 4/17/12.
3. Rosenfeld R, Cohen P, Robison LL, et al. Long-term surveillance of growth hormone therapy. *J Clin Endocrinol Metab*. 2012;97:68-72.
4. Sperling MA. Long-term therapy with growth hormone: bringing sagacity to SAGHE. *J Clin Endocrinol Metab*. 2012;97:81-83.
5. Malozowski S. Reports of increased mortality and GH: will this affect current clinical practice? *J Clin Endocrinol Metab*. 2012;97:380-383.

Health-related quality of life of young adults with Turner syndrome following a long-term randomized controlled trial of recombinant human growth hormone
Taback SP, Van Vliet G (Univ of Manitoba, Winnipeg, Canada; Univ of Montreal, Quebec, Canada)
BMC Pediatr 11:49, 2011

Background.—There are limited long-term randomized controlled trials of growth hormone (GH) supplementation to adult height and few published reports of the health-related quality of life (HRQOL) following treatment. The present follow-up study of young adults from a long-term controlled trial of GH treatment in patients with Turner syndrome (TS) yielded data to examine whether GH supplementation resulted in a higher HRQOL (either due to taller stature or from the knowledge that active treatment and not placebo had been received) or alternatively a lower HRQOL (due to medicalization from years of injections).

Methods.—The original trial randomized 154 Canadian girls with TS aged 7-13 years from 13 centres to receive either long-term GH injections at the pharmacologic dose of 0.3 mg/kg/week or to receive no injections; estrogen prescription for induction of puberty was standardized. Patients were eligible for the follow-up study if they were at least 16 years old at the time of follow-up. The instrument used to study HRQOL was the

SF-36, summarized into physical and mental component scales (PCS and MCS); higher scores indicate better HRQOL.

Results.—Thirty-four of the 48 eligible participants (71%) consented to participate; data were missing for one patient. Both groups (GH and no treatment) had normal HRQOL at this post-treatment assessment. The GH group had a (mean ± SD) PCS score of 56 ± 5; the untreated group 58 ± 4; mean score for 16-24 year old females in the general population 53.5 ± 6.9. The GH group had a mean MCS score of 52 ± 6; the untreated group 49 ± 13; mean score for 16-24 year old females in the general population 49.6 ± 9.8. Secondary analyses showed no relationship between HRQOL and height.

Conclusions.—We found no benefit or adverse effect on HRQOL either from receiving or not receiving growth hormone injections in a long-term randomized controlled trial, confirming larger observational studies. We suggest that it remains ethically acceptable as well as necessary to maintain a long-term untreated control group to estimate the effects of pharmacological agents to manipulate adult height. Young adult women with TS have normal HRQOL suggesting that they adjust well to their challenges in life. ClinicalTrials.gov Identifier NCT00191113.

▶ Ever since Turner syndrome (TS) became a Food and Drug Administration—approved indication for growth hormone (GH) therapy, treatment of girls with this condition using recombinant human GH has largely been considered the standard of care. Although the ability of GH to increase stature is undisputed, this study provides a unique opportunity to query whether such treatment actually affects health-related quality of life (HRQOL). Although consisting of a small sample size and not blinded, the prospective-controlled design is a notable strength compared with the vast majority of studies reporting long-term outcomes in this patient population. It is tempting to wonder whether the results would have been different if the GH-treated patients had ended up significantly taller. Because the tallest subset reached a mean adult stature of only 5 feet, the outcome in terms of height can hardly be considered impressive. Only time will tell whether HRQOL might be altered by earlier initiation of GH therapy,[1] which would likely result in a greater gain in adult height standard deviation score. Regardless, this article makes the important point that maintaining an untreated TS control group is ethically acceptable. Although the authors stop short of suggesting this, the implication for parents and providers is that choosing to withhold GH in a girl with TS would be an acceptable option as well.

E. Eugster, MD

Reference

1. Davenport ML, Crowe BJ, Travers SH, et al. Growth hormone treatment of early growth failure in toddlers with Turner syndrome: a randomized, controlled, multicenter trial. *J Clin Endocrinol Metab.* 2007;92:3406-3416. Copyright 2007, with permission from The Endocrine Society.

Effect of oxandrolone and timing of pubertal induction on final height in Turner's syndrome: randomised, double blind, placebo controlled trial
Gault EJ, on behalf of the British Society for Paediatric Endocrinology and Diabetes (Royal Hosp for Sick Children, Glasgow, UK; et al)
BMJ 342:d1980, 2011

Objective.—To examine the effect of oxandrolone and the timing of pubertal induction on final height in girls with Turner's syndrome receiving a standard dose of growth hormone.

Design.—Randomised, double blind, placebo controlled trial.

Setting.—36 paediatric endocrinology departments in UK hospitals.

Participants.—Girls with Turner's syndrome aged 7-13 years at recruitment, receiving recombinant growth hormone therapy (10 mg/m²/week).

Interventions.—Participants were randomised to oxandrolone (0.05 mg/kg/day, maximum 2.5 mg/day) or placebo from 9 years of age. Those with evidence of ovarian failure at 12 years were further randomised to oral ethinylestradiol (year 1, 2 µg daily; year 2, 4 µg daily; year 3, 4 months each of 6, 8, and 10 µg daily) or placebo; participants who received placebo and those recruited after the age of 12.25 years started ethinylestradiol at age 14.

Main Outcome Measure.—Final height.

Results.—106 participants were recruited, of whom 14 withdrew and 82/92 reached final height. Both oxandrolone and late pubertal induction increased final height: by 4.6 (*95%* confidence interval 1.9 to 7.2) cm (*P*=0.001, n=82) for oxandrolone and 3.8 (0.0 to 7.5) cm (*P*=0.05, n=48) for late pubertal induction with ethinylestradiol. In the 48 children who were randomised twice, the effects on final height (compared with placebo and early induction of puberty) of oxandrolone alone, late induction alone, and oxandrolone plus late induction were similar, averaging 7.1 (3.4 to 10.8) cm (*P*<0.001). No cases of virilisation were reported.

Conclusion.—Oxandrolone had a positive effect on final height in girls with Turner's syndrome treated with growth hormone, as did late pubertal induction with ethinylestradiol at age 14 years. However, these effects were not additive, so using both had no advantage. Oxandrolone could, therefore, be offered as an alternative to late pubertal induction for increasing final height in Turner's syndrome.

Trial Registration.—Current Controlled Trials ISRCTN50343149 (Fig 3).

▶ Although randomized placebo-controlled trials are relatively rare in pediatrics, no fewer than 3 rigorously designed prospective studies involving long-term outcomes in girls with Turner syndrome (TS) have been published this year alone. In this particular case, comparisons of the 2 separate randomizations (oxandrolone vs placebo; early vs late pubertal induction) as well as a combinatorial effect yield useful information that can readily be applied to the clinical setting. As seen in Fig 3, both oxandrolone and late pubertal induction were associated with greater gains in height. However, no additional benefit was observed from pursuing both. Several other aspects of the study are worth noting. One is the

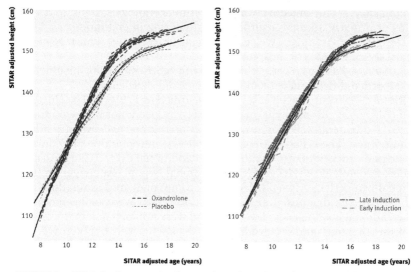

FIGURE 3.—SITAR fitted summary height curves by trial arm for randomisation 1 (left) and randomisation 2 (right). (Reprinted from Gault EJ, on behalf of the British Society for Paediatric Endocrinology and Diabetes. Effect of oxandrolone and timing of pubertal induction on final height in Turner's syndrome: randomised, double blind, placebo controlled trial. *BMJ*. 2011;342:d1980.)

use of a low and slow protocol for estrogen replacement, which is supported by several other studies demonstrating better height outcomes in girls with TS when this approach is followed. Another point is that even the "early pubertal induction" group in whom E2 was initiated at age 12 was in fact "late" compared with the average age of pubertal onset in the general population. Because later pubertal induction has been associated with lower quality of life in young adults with TS, consideration should be given to starting estrogen therapy at an even younger age. Lastly, many clinicians who prescribe oxandrolone to girls with TS typically discontinue it once sex steroid replacement is underway. This study suggests that continuing oxandrolone throughout pubertal induction may in fact optimize height without undo side effects. On balance, this elegantly conducted multicenter study represents a significant contribution to the care of girls with TS.

E. Eugster, MD

Miscellaneous

Presentation of Primary Adrenal Insufficiency in Childhood
Hsieh S, White PC (Univ of Texas Southwestern Med Ctr, Dallas)
J Clin Endocrinol Metab 96:E1-E4, 2011

Context.—Primary adrenal insufficiency is usually diagnosed in infancy or adulthood, and cases presenting in childhood have not been systematically reviewed.

Objective.—Our objective was to determine etiologies, signs, and symptoms of primary adrenal insufficiency presenting in childhood.

Design and Setting.—We conducted a retrospective chart review at a tertiary-care pediatric hospital.

Patients.—Patients were children with corticoadrenal insufficiency, glucocorticoid deficiency, or mineralocorticoid deficiency.

Results.—Seventy-seven cases were identified in 1999—2010. Thirty-five had congenital adrenal hyperplasia (CAH) and were not reviewed further. Forty-two patients (20 diagnosed at our institution) had primary adrenal insufficiency. These had etiologies as follows: autoimmune (18), autoimmune polyendocrinopathy syndrome (an additional five), ACTH resistance (four), adrenoleukodystrophy (three), adrenal hypoplasia congenita (two), adrenal hemorrhage (two), IMAGe syndrome (one), and idiopathic (two). Of 20 patients diagnosed at our institution, two were being monitored when adrenal insufficiency developed and were not included in the analysis of presenting signs and symptoms: 13 of 18 patients were hypotensive; 12 of 18 had documented hyperpigmentation. Hyponatremia (<135 mEq/liter) occurred in 16 of 18. However, hyperkalemia (>5.0 mEq/liter) was noted in only nine. Hypoglycemia and ketosis were documented in four of 15 and four of six patients in whom it was sought, respectively. Fifteen patients underwent cosyntropin stimulation testing with median baseline and stimulated cortisol of 1.1 and 1.2 μg/dl, respectively. ACTH and renin were markedly elevated in all patients.

Conclusions.—Hyperkalemia is not a consistent presenting sign of primary adrenal insufficiency in childhood, and its absence cannot rule out this condition. A combination of chronic or subacute clinical symptoms, hypotension, and hyponatremia should raise suspicion of adrenal insufficiency.

▶ This retrospective study represents a careful, systematic characterization of the clinical features of children presenting to a tertiary care children's hospital with primary adrenal insufficiency not due to congenital adrenal hyperplasia (CAH). Although the findings are hardly earth shattering, they highlight the variability and nonspecific nature of the presenting signs and symptoms of this potentially lethal condition and serve as a useful reminder that presumed classic features may in fact not be present. This was particularly true of hyperkalemia, which was found in only half of this cohort, despite the old adage that an elevation in potassium is the first electrolyte abnormality seen in an impending adrenal crisis. The study also emphasizes the high incidence of gastrointestinal complaints, including nausea, vomiting and weight loss, as well as the potential for spurious diagnoses such as anorexia nervosa, before the true inciting etiology comes to light. On balance, it underlines the need for all pediatric health care providers to maintain a high index of suspicion for primary adrenal insufficiency to ensure expeditious diagnosis and treatment.

E. Eugster, MD

The natural history of the normal/mild elevated TSH serum levels in children and adolescents with Hashimoto's thyroiditis and isolated hyperthyrotropinaemia: a 3-year follow-up

Radetti G, Maselli M, Buzi F, et al (Regional Hosp of Bolzano, Italy; Regional Hosp of Brescia, Italy; et al)

Clin Endocrinol 76:394-398, 2012

Objective.—The natural history of Hashimoto's thyroiditis (HT) and isolated hyperthyrotropinaemia (IH) is not well defined. We therefore studied the natural course of patients with HT and IH and looked for possible prognostic factors.

Design.—This is retrospective cross-sectional study.

Patients.—Three hundred and twenty-three patients with HT (88 boys and 235 girls) and 59 with IH (30 boys and 29 girls), mean age $9 \cdot 9 \pm 3 \cdot 8$ years were included in the study. When first examined, 236 of the children with HT had a normal TSH (G0) and in 87, it was elevated but <100% of the upper limit (G1). All IH subjects had elevated TSH. Potential risk factors for thyroid failure were evaluated after 3 years and included the presence or familiarity for endocrine/autoimmune diseases, premature birth, signs and symptoms of hypothyroidism, TSH levels, antithyroid antibodies and thyroid volume.

Results.—HT: Of those with HT, 170 G0 patients remained stable, 31 moved to G1 and 35 to G2 (hypothyroidism). Thirty-six G1 children moved to G0, 17 remained stable and 34 moved to G2. Of patients with IH: 23 normalized, 28 remained stable and eight became overtly hypothyroid. In patients with HT, the presence of coeliac disease, elevated TSH and thyroid peroxidase antibodies (TPOAb) increased the risk of developing hypothyroidism by $4 \cdot 0$-, $3 \cdot 4$- and $3 \cdot 5$-fold, respectively. The increase in TSH levels during follow-up was strongly predictive of the development of hypothyroidism. In patients with IH, no predictive factor could be identified.

Conclusions.—Coeliac disease, elevated TSH and TPOAb at presentation and a progressive increase in TSH are predictive factors for thyroid failure in HT patients.

▶ The appropriate management of patients with mild compensated hypothyroidism has long been a subject of debate among pediatric endocrinologists. Specifically, whether subtle biochemical abnormalities in thyrotropin (TSH) are clinically significant, and at what point treatment with levothyroxine should be initiated, is unclear. Therefore, additional information regarding the natural history of such abnormalities in pediatric patients is particularly welcome. Although retrospective, this 3-year study is strengthened by its sample size, the exclusion of overweight children, and the considerable number of evaluations performed in the subjects at annual intervals, which included thyroid ultrasounds, antithyroid antibodies, and thyroid function tests. Thus, the authors were able to separate their subjects into those with Hashimoto thyroiditis (HT) and those with isolated hyperthyrotropinemia (IH). It is striking that after

3 years of follow-up approximately 80% did not require thyroid hormone replacement. While certain factors were noted to increase the risk of progression in HT, no such prognostic variables were identified in the IH group. Although the lack of any change in height and body mass index standard deviation score during the 3 years of follow-up was reassuring, this particular study did not include any assessment of cognitive function. However, it does lend support for an interval of watchful waiting in children and adolescents with mild compensated hypothyroidism, even in the presence of positive antithyroid antibodies.

E. Eugster, MD

Natural History of Idiopathic Diabetes Insipidus
Richards GE, Thomsett MJ, Boston BA, et al (Seattle Children's Hosp and Univ of Washington; Mater Children's and Royal Children's Hosps, Brisbane, Queensland, Australia; Doernbecher Children's Hosp and Oregon Health and Science Univ, Portland; et al)
J Pediatr 159:566-570, 2011

Objective.—To determine what percentage of diabetes insipidus (DI) in childhood is idiopathic and to assess the natural history of idiopathic DI.

Study Design.—We conducted a retrospective chart review of 105 patients with DI who were born or had DI diagnosed between 1980-1989 at 3 medical centers. A second cohort of 30 patients from 6 medical centers in whom idiopathic DI was diagnosed after 1990 was evaluated retrospectively for subsequent etiologic diagnoses and additional hypothalamic/pituitary deficiencies and prospectively for quality of life.

Results.—In the first cohort, 11% of patients had idiopathic DI. In the second cohort, additional hypothalamic/pituitary hormone deficiencies developed in 33%, and 37% received an etiologic diagnosis for DI. Health-related quality of life for all the patients with idiopathic DI was comparable with the healthy reference population.

Conclusions.—Only a small percentage of patients with DI will remain idiopathic after first examination. Other hormone deficiencies will develop later in one-third of those patients, and slightly more than one-third of those patients will have an etiology for the DI diagnosed. Long-term surveillance is important because tumors have been diagnosed as long as 21 years after the onset of DI. Quality of life for these patients is as good as the reference population.

▶ The topic of this retrospective review is not new, and the authors' findings are in line with previous reports. However, this article does offer a concise summary of the literature and adds reassuring data regarding quality of life to the existing knowledge about children and adolescents with central diabetes insipidus (DI). Thus, it provides helpful prognostic information for pediatric endocrinologists and for parents of children in whom a diagnosis of apparent "idiopathic" DI has been made. A few specific aspects of the article are noteworthy. One is the implication of a subsequent diagnosis of growth hormone deficiency, which clearly portends a greater chance of identifying an underlying pathologic process. Although this point is well taken, readers could legitimately have issues with some of the ways in which the data are presented. As the authors' themselves suggest, labeling children who have a positive family history of DI as "idiopathic" hardly seems appropriate. Along the same lines is that a subsequent etiology and additional hormonal deficiencies were identified as soon as 1 month after the initial diagnosis of DI, again raising into question the validity of the "idiopathic" designation. The paper would have been strengthened by a more precise temporal definition of initial evaluation, and, because most lesions become apparent within the first 3 to 5 years, by the inclusion of suggested guidelines for the frequency of central nervous system imaging and hormonal surveillance.

E. Eugster, MD

Thyroid function in the nutritionally obese child and adolescent

Reinehr T (Univ of Witten/Herdecke, Datteln, Germany)
Curr Opin Pediatr 23:415-420, 2011

Purpose of Review.—In recent years, there has been an increasing focus on thyroid function in obese children. There is controversy concerning whether the changes in the levels of thyroid hormones and thyroid-stimulating hormone (thyrotropin − TSH) in obesity are causes or consequences of weight status and whether these subtle differences merit treatment with thyroxine. This review aimed to study the prevalence of disturbed thyroid hormone and TSH values in childhood obesity and the underlying pathophysiologic mechanisms linking obesity to thyroid function.

Recent Findings.—In the past 18 months, four studies demonstrated moderate elevation of TSH concentrations in 10−23% of obese children, which was associated with normal or slightly elevated thyroxine and triiodothyronine values. Two studies reported ultrasonographic hypoechogenicity of the thyroid in obese children with hyperthyrotropinemia, which was not caused by autoimmune thyroiditis; therefore, the authors hypothesized a link to chronic inflammation in obesity. Weight loss led to a normalization of elevated TSH levels in two studies. The adipokine leptin is the most promising link between obesity and hyperthyrotropinemia since leptin stimulates the hypothalamic−pituitary−thyroid.

Summary.—The elevated TSH levels in obesity seem a consequence rather than a cause of obesity. Therefore, treatment of hyperthyrotropinemia with thyroxine seems unnecessary in obese children (Fig 1).

▶ Pediatric endocrine clinics are inundated with referrals for abnormal thyroid function tests in obese children. These typically consist of a minimally-elevated thyrotropin (TSH) with a normal total or free thyroxine. More often than not, the family has been given the message that this biochemical abnormality is the cause of the child's difficulty with weight control and that consequently the endocrinologist holds the key to fixing it. Sadly, much of our time is spent in correcting this misconception and in educating parents about the interplay between energy

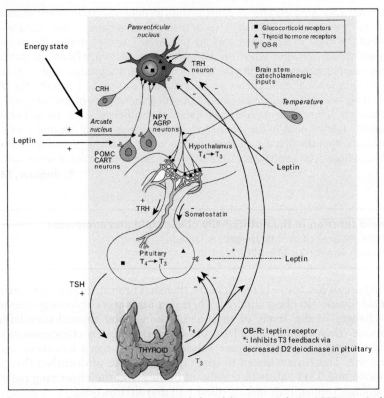

FIGURE 1.—Relationship between leptin and thyroid hormone synthesis. AGRP, agouti-related peptide; CART, cocaine and amphetamine-regulated transcript; CRH, corticotropin-releasing hormone; NPY, neuropeptide γ; TRH, thyrotropin-releasing hormone; TSH, thyroid-stimulating hormone. Adapted from [27]. *Editor's Note*: Please refer to original journal article for full references. (Reprinted from Reinehr T. Thyroid function in the nutritionally obese child and adolescent. *Curr Opin Pediatr.* 2011;23: 415-420, with permission from Lippincott Williams & Wilkins.)

intake and energy utilization. Despite long-standing recognition of the childhood obesity epidemic, the increased incidence of an elevated TSH in this setting has only recently been established. This article is a concise and informative review of recent literature in this area that addresses prevalence, radiographic and laboratory features, pathophysiology, and clinical implications. As shown in Fig 1, the putative mechanism for an elevated TSH in obesity involves leptin, which is known to stimulate the hypothalamic-pituitary-thyroid axis, and the postulated etiology is an adaptive increase in energy expenditure to avoid additional weight gain. In fact, as the author points out, the decrease in TSH that accompanies initial weight loss may in part explain the notorious difficulty in maintaining weight control and progressively shedding pounds that is encountered by many individuals. Regardless, ample evidence now exists to support a policy of lifestyle counseling rather than levothyroxine therapy in obese children with a mildly-elevated TSH and no evidence of thyroid autoimmunity.

E. Eugster, MD

Plasma Phthalate Levels in Pubertal Gynecomastia

Durmaz E, Özmert EN, Erkekoğlu P, et al (Hacettepe Univ, Ankara, Turkey)
Pediatrics 125:e122-e129, 2010

Objective.—Several untoward health effects of phthalates, which are a group of industrial chemicals with many commercial uses including personal-care products and plastic materials, have been defined. The most commonly used, di-(2-ethylhexyl)-phthalate (DEHP), is known to have anti-androgenic or estrogenic effects or both. Mono-(2-ethylhexyl)-phthalate (MEHP) is the main metabolite of DEHP. In this study, we aimed to determine the plasma DEHP and MEHP levels in pubertal gynecomastia cases.

Patients and Methods.—The study group comprised 40 newly diagnosed pubertal gynecomastia cases who were admitted to Hacettepe University Ihsan Doğramacı Children's Hospital. The control group comprised 21 age-matched children without gynecomastia or other endocrinologic disorder. Plasma DEHP and MEHP levels were measured by using high-performance liquid chromatography. Serum hormone levels were determined in some pubertal gynecomastia cases according to the physician's evaluation.

Results.—Plasma DEHP and MEHP levels were found to be statistically significantly higher in the pubertal gynecomastia group compared with the control group $(P < .001)$ (DEHP, 4.66 ± 1.58 and 3.09 ± 0.90 $\mu g/mL$, respectively [odds ratio: 2.77 (95% confidence interval: $1.48-5.21$)]; MEHP, 3.19 ± 1.41 and 1.37 ± 0.36 $\mu g/mL$ [odds ratio: 24.76 (95% confidence interval: $3.5-172.6$)]). There was a statistically significant correlation between plasma DEHP and MEHP levels $(r: 0.58; P < .001)$. In the pubertal gynecomastia group, no correlation could be determined between plasma DEHP and MEHP levels and any of the hormone levels.

Conclusions.—DEHP, which has antiandrogenic or estrogenic effects, may be an etiologic factor in pubertal gynecomastia. These results may pioneer larger-scale studies on the etiologic role of DEHP in pubertal gynecomastia.

▶ Although some degree of pubertal gynecomastia occurs in the majority of adolescent boys, it is usually mild and self-limited. However, a subset developed marked and persistent breast enlargement, which may result in significant psychological distress. Because the endocrinologic evaluation is almost always normal, the precise etiology of this phenomenon in otherwise healthy boys is unclear. This study offers an intriguing explanation in the form of a link between elevated plasma phthalate levels and gynecomastia in 40 pubertal boys compared with controls. A few aspects of the study are particularly noteworthy. Although the inclusion of an age-matched control group was obviously a strength, the sample size was only half that of the affected individuals. It is also striking that 45% of those in the study group had been hospitalized for gynecomastia, of whom, 9 reportedly had severe pain, suggesting that the entity described here is substantially different from the garden variety pubertal gynecomastia often encountered in the outpatient setting. Still, the finding of statistically higher di-(2-ethylhexyl)-phthalate and mono-(2-ethylhexyl)-phthalate levels in those with the more symptomatic cases of gynecomastia is intriguing. Although it would not prove causality, a documented increase in the incidence of pubertal gynecomastia coinciding with the exponential increase in environmental phthalate exposure that has occurred during recent decades would certainly lend support to the author's hypothesis.

E. Eugster, MD

Obstetric Outcomes in Women with Turner Karyotype
Hagman A, Källén K, Barrenäs M-L, et al (Sahlgrenska Academy at Univ of Gothenburg, Sweden; et al)
J Clin Endocrinol Metab 96:3475-3482, 2011

Context.—Women with Turner syndrome (TS) have high risk of cardiovascular complications and hypertensive disorders. Few studies have analyzed obstetric outcome in women with TS.

Objective.—This study compared obstetric outcome in women with TS karyotype with women in the general population.

Design.—The Swedish Genetic Turner Register was cross-linked with the Swedish Medical Birth Register between 1973 and 2007. Obstetric outcome in singletons was compared with a reference group of 56,000 women from the general population. Obstetric outcome in twins was described separately.

Results.—A total of 202 singletons and three sets of twins were born to 115 women with a TS karyotype that was unknown in 52% at time of pregnancy. At first delivery, TS women of singletons were older than controls (median 30 vs. 26 yr, P < 0.0001). Preeclampsia occurred in 6.3 vs. 3.0% (P = 0.07). Aortic dissection occurred in one woman. Compared with the general population, the gestational age was shorter in children born by TS women (−6.4 d, P = 0.0067), and median birth weight was lower (−208 g, P = 0.0012), but SD scores for weight and length at birth were similar. The cesarean section rate was 35.6% in TS women and 11.8% in controls (P < 0.0001). There was no difference in birth defects in children of TS women as compared with controls.

Conclusions.—Obstetric outcomes in women with a TS karyotype were mostly favorable. Singletons of TS women had shorter gestational age, but similar size at birth, adjusted for gestational age and sex. Birth defects did not differ between TS and controls.

▶ Although the subjects of this retrospective study are obviously not children, the topic of reproductive potential is one that is frequently raised during discussions with girls with Turner syndrome (TS) and their parents. As the authors indicate, the main strength of this report is the sample size and the impressive 34-year interval of time available for analysis. Utilization of the Swedish Genetic Turner Register, which collects from all Swedish cytogenetic laboratories and was cross-referenced with the enviable Swedish Medical Birth Register, allows us to feel confident that all births to women with TS that occurred within the prescribed data collection years were included. On balance, the findings are reassuring, although several important questions do remain. On the positive side was the lack of any increased incidence of birth defects, stillbirths, or intrauterine growth restriction in the offspring of mothers with TS compared with the reference population. Notably, however, no information regarding rates of spontaneous abortions is provided. The implication that the majority of the pregnancies in this cohort were spontaneous and the fact that more than 50% of the women with TS were undiagnosed at the time of first delivery indicate that this population was not representative of the majority of girls with TS who we care for in the pediatric endocrine clinic. This is further supported by the very small number of women with a monosomy X karyotype, who comprised less than 10% of the study population. Thus, additional investigations of fetal and maternal complications in women with TS with classic phenotypes who are recipients of donor oocytes are badly needed.

E. Eugster, MD

Sensitivity of Fine-Needle Biopsy in Detecting Pediatric Differentiated Thyroid Carcinoma

Redlich A, Boxberger N, Schmid KW, et al (Otto-von-Guericke-Univ Magdeburg, Germany; Univ Duisburg-Essen, Germany; et al)
Pediatr Blood Cancer 2011 [Epub ahead of print]

Background.—Differentiated thyroid carcinomas (DTC) are uncommon in children. Since the frequency of malignancy is assumed to be high in pediatric symptomatic thyroid nodules, carcinomas should be ruled out reliably. The objective of this study was to assess the sensitivity of fine-needle biopsy (FNB) in diagnosing children with DTC.

Procedure.—We retrospectively analyzed 15 years of data from the GPOH-MET registry, a database by the German Society for Pediatric Oncology and Hematology (GPOH) with a focus on malignant endocrine tumors (MET). We reviewed data on pediatric patients with DTC who had undergone FNB. FNB results were classified according to well-established guidelines.

Results.—During the study period, 206 children with a histological diagnosis of DTC were entered into the GPOH-MET database. Fifty of those patients aged 3.6–17.3 years (mean, 12.3 years) had undergone FNB preoperatively. Forty-one were diagnosed with papillary thyroid carcinoma (PTC), seven with follicular thyroid carcinoma (FTC), and two had DTC not otherwise specified. Of the first FNB performed on each patient, the cytological specimens were diagnosed as benign in 13 cases, malignant in 14, suspicious in 9, follicular neoplasms in 6, and unsatisfactory in 8. The sensitivity of FNB in detecting DTC was 69.0%.

Conclusions.—Our results reflect the current practice of pediatric thyroid FNB in Germany. In order to improve its usefulness, FNB should always be performed by experienced physicians. Furthermore, a central review of all specimens is necessary to ascertain the validity of the cytological diagnosis

TABLE 5.—FNB in Children and Adolescents

	Patients	Age at Diagnosis, Years (Range)	Histology (%)	DTC	Follow-up, Years (Range)	Sensitivity (%)	Unsatisfactory (%)
Bargren et al. [43]	110	14.6 (5−19)	100	31	n. a.	88.1	9.0
Willgerodt et al. [44]	169	14.9 (5.1−17.8)	69.8	13	n. a.	63.6	13.8
Hosler et al. [45]	82	14.6 (8−18)	54.9	20	n. a.	80.0	13
Amrikachi et al. [15]	185	17 (10−21)	17.3	14	1−17	100	28
Corrias et al. [14]	42	13.1 (8.6−17.9)	100	20	0	95.0	0
Khurana et al. [12]	57	16.5 (9−20)	42.1	14	1.5 (1−4)	92.9	0
Belfiore et al. [22]	109	16.3 (4−20)	20.2	11	n. a.	100	2.8
Raab et al. [9]	57	13.1 (1−18)	22.8	10	1-5	90.0	4.5
Chang et al. [46]	51	17 (2−21)	33.3	9	n. a.	100	7
Degnan et al. [11]	18	14.2 (8−18)	88.8	5	n. a.	40.0	5.8
Giard and Hermans [23]	507	51.1 (7−93)	100	507	n. a.	54.8−68.3	13.9
GPOH-MET	50	12.3 (3.6−17.3)	100	50	5.1 (0.1−12.1)	69.0−71.7	16.0

n.a., not available.
Editor's Note: Please refer to original journal article for full references.

and to introduce immunocytological and molecular methods. Pediatr Blood Cancer (Table 5).

▶ The role of fine needle aspiration (FNA) in the evaluation of pediatric thyroid nodules is controversial. At many children's hospitals, patients are referred for surgery on the basis of imaging studies alone. This is based on the relatively high incidence of papillary thyroid cancer in cold thyroid nodules in children, as well as a general lack of comfort among pediatric endocrinologists regarding the accuracy of FNA in this setting. Unfortunately, this particular study is unlikely to alter that perception. Strengths of this analysis include the sample size as well as the fact that all subjects had histologically confirmed differentiated thyroid carcinoma (DTC). As the authors point out, this makes it difficult to compare their findings with those of other studies in which a negative FNA result was assumed to be true and surgery was not performed. As is illustrated in Table 5, published estimates of the sensitivity of FNA vary considerably. The authors also emphasize the importance of the experience of the clinician and pathologist performing the procedure in terms of the accuracy of FNA. Regrettably, no information regarding the correlation between the observed sensitivities and the 6 types of specialists who performed the FNAs in the present study is provided. Until additional information comes to light, this article will likely simply reinforce, rather than change, current practice regarding management of pediatric thyroid nodules in Germany and elsewhere.

E. Eugster, MD

Antenatal Thyroid Screening and Childhood Cognitive Function

Lazarus JH, Bestwick JP, Channon S, et al (Cardiff School of Medicine, Wales, UK; Queen Mary Univ of London, UK; St David's Hosp, Cardiff, UK; et al)
N Engl J Med 366:493-501, 2012

Background.—Children born to women with low thyroid hormone levels have been reported to have decreased cognitive function.

Methods.—We conducted a randomized trial in which pregnant women at a gestation of 15 weeks 6 days or less provided blood samples for measurement of thyrotropin and free thyroxine (T_4). Women were assigned to a screening group (in which measurements were obtained immediately) or a control group (in which serum was stored and measurements were obtained shortly after delivery). Thyrotropin levels above the 97.5th percentile, free T_4 levels below the 2.5th percentile, or both were considered a positive screening result. Women with positive findings in the screening group were assigned to 150 μg of levothyroxine per day. The primary outcome was IQ at 3 years of age in children of women with positive results, as measured by psychologists who were unaware of the group assignments.

Results.—Of 21,846 women who provided blood samples (at a median gestational age of 12 weeks 3 days), 390 women in the screening group and 404 in the control group tested positive. The median gestational age at the start of levothyroxine treatment was 13 weeks 3 days; treatment was adjusted as needed to achieve a target thyrotropin level of 0.1 to 1.0 mIU per liter. Among the children of women with positive results, the mean IQ scores were 99.2 and 100.0 in the screening and control groups, respectively (difference, 0.8; 95% confidence interval [CI], -1.1 to 2.6; $P = 0.40$ by intention-to-treat analysis); the proportions of children with an IQ of less than 85 were 12.1% in the screening group and 14.1% in the control group (difference, 2.1 percentage points; 95% CI, -2.6 to 6.7; $P = 0.39$). An on-treatment analysis showed similar results.

Conclusions.—Antenatal screening (at a median gestational age of 12 weeks 3 days) and maternal treatment for hypothyroidism did not result in improved cognitive function in children at 3 years of age. (Funded by the Wellcome Trust UK and Compagnia di San Paulo, Turin; Current Controlled Trials number, ISRCTN46178175.)

▶ Whether or not to implement universal screening of pregnant women for hypothyroidism has been highly controversial. This debate was fueled largely by the landmark 1999 *NEJM* article by Haddow et al,[1] which demonstrated a decrement in neurocognitive functioning in 7- to 9-year old offspring of women with hypothyroidism during pregnancy compared with controls. However, that study had its share of critics, who argued among other things that the differences in intelligence quotient (IQ) were not significant and that the authors had failed to investigate the prevalence of maternal hypothyroxinemia, which has been linked to poorer postnatal neuropsychological outcome in previous studies. Thus, this important issue has remained unresolved awaiting additional data. At first blush, the present study appears to represent the definitive answer that obstetricians and pediatricians alike have been waiting for. The authors are to be commended for their rigorous study design, the successful recruitment of nearly 22 000 women from 11 centers in 2 different countries, and their very respectable retention rate. The lack of a difference in IQ at age 3 years between children in the screening group and those in the control group appears highly reassuring. Unfortunately, scrutiny of the data makes one less confident that the results reported here can reasonably be compared with those of Haddow et al. At issue are the median thyrotropin (TSH) values in the treated versus control groups, which are well within the normal range and only significantly different in the group from the United Kingdom. How these women compare to the maternal hypothyroidism group in the 1999 study, who had an average TSH level of 13 mU/L, is unclear. Similarly, the number of women in the treated group who actually had thyroid function test results outside of the normal reference ranges is not provided. Therefore, while this is a noteworthy trial that certainly contributes to the ongoing debate, it does not provide sufficient evidence to be the final word on this weighty topic.

E. Eugster, MD

Reference

1. Haddow JE, Palomaki GE, Allan WC, et al. Maternal thyroid deficiency during pregnancy and subsequent neuropsychological development of the child. *N Eng J Med.* 1999;341:549-555.

Article Index

Chapter 1: Diabetes

Chapter 2: Lipoproteins and Atherosclerosis

Chapter 3: Obesity

Chapter 4: Thyroid

Chapter 5: Calcium and Bone Metabolism

Chapter 6: Adrenal Cortex

Chapter 7: Reproductive Endocrinology

Chapter 8: Pediatric Endocrinology

Author Index